Melanoma

Editors

BRIAN R. GASTMAN
MICHAEL W. NEUMEISTER

CLINICS IN
PLASTIC SURGERY

www.plasticsurgery.theclinics.com

October 2021 • Volume 48 • Number 4

ELSEVIER

1600 John F. Kennedy Boulevard • Suite 1800 • Philadelphia, Pennsylvania, 19103-2899

http://www.theclinics.com

CLINICS IN PLASTIC SURGERY Volume 48, Number 4
October 2021 ISSN 0094-1298, ISBN-13: 978-0-323-81321-1

Editor: Stacy Eastman
Developmental Editor: Jessica Nicole B. Cañaberal

Clinics in Plastic Surgery (ISSN 0094-1298) is published quarterly by Elsevier Inc., 360 Park Avenue South, New York, NY 10010-1710. Months of issue are January, April, July, and October. Business and Editorial Offices: 1600 John F. Kennedy Blvd., Suite 1800, Philadelphia, PA 19103-2899. Periodicals postage paid at New York, NY and additional mailing offices. Subscription prices are $543.00 per year for US individuals, $1210.00 per year for US institutions, $100.00 per year for US students and residents, $607.00 per year for Canadian individuals, $1252.00 per year for Canadian institutions, $675.00 per year for international individuals, $1252.00 per year for international institutions, $100.00 per year for Canadian and $305.00 per year for international students/residents. To receive student/resident rate, orders must be accompanied by name of affiliated institution, date of term, and the *signature* of program/residency coordinator on institution letterhead. Orders will be billed at individual rate until proof of status is received. Foreign air speed delivery is included in all *Clinics* subscription prices. All prices are subject to change without notice. **POSTMASTER:** Send address changes to *Clinics in Plastic Surgery*, Elsevier Health Sciences Division, Subscription Customer Service, 3251 Riverport Lane, Maryland Heights, MO 63043. **Customer Service: 1-800-654-2452 (US and Canada). From outside of the United States and Canada, call 314-447-8871. Fax: 314-447-8029. E-mail: JournalsCustomerService-usa@elsevier.com (for print support); JournalsOnlineSupport-usa@elsevier.com (for online support).**

Reprints. For copies of 100 or more of articles in this publication, please contact the Commercial Reprints Department, Elsevier Inc., 360 Park Avenue South, New York, New York 10010-1710. Tel.: +1-212-633-3874; Fax: +1-212-633-3820; E-mail: reprints@elsevier.com.

Clinics in Plastic Surgery is covered in *Current Contents, EMBASE/Excerpta Medica, Science Citation Index, MEDLINE/PubMed (Index Medicus), ASCA, and ISI/BIOMED.*

Contributors

EDITORS

BRIAN R. GASTMAN, MD, FACS
Surgical and Co-director of the CCF Melanoma and High Risk Skin Cancer Program, Professor of Surgery, Cleveland Clinic Lerner College of Medicine, Staff, CCF, Dermatology and Plastic Surgery Institute, Department of Plastic Surgery, Taussig Cancer Center, Lerner Research Institute, Department of Immunology, Head and Neck Institute, Cleveland Clinic, Cleveland, Ohio

MICHAEL W. NEUMEISTER, MD, FRCSC, FACS
Professor and Chair, Department of Surgery, Elvin G. Zook Endowed Chair, Institute for Plastic Surgery, Southern Illinois University School of Medicine, Springfield, Illinois

AUTHORS

GHAITH ALRAHAWAN, MS
University of Missouri School of Medicine, Columbia, Missouri

JOSHUA ARBESMAN, MD
Department of Dermatology, Cleveland Clinic, Cleveland Clinic Lerner Research Institute, Cleveland, Ohio

PAOLA BARRIERA-SILVESTRINI, MD
Department of Dermatology, MetroHealth System, Cleveland, Ohio

C. MATTHEW BRADBURY, MD, PhD
Springfield Clinic Cancer Center and Southern Illinois University School of Medicine, Springfield, Illinois

AMANDA BROWN, BS
The Institute for Plastic Surgery, Southern Illinois University School of Medicine, Springfield, Illinois

WILLIAM J. BRUCE, MD
Institute for Plastic Surgery, Southern Illinois University School of Medicine, Springfield, Illinois

PARINAZ J. DABESTANI, BS
Creighton University School of Medicine, Omaha, Nebraska

AMANDA J. DAWSON, MD
Department of Surgery, Plastic and Reconstructive Surgery Division, Creighton University School of Medicine, Omaha, Nebraska

C. MARCELA DIAZ-MONTERO, PhD, LRI/CCF
Scientific Director, Cleveland Clinic, Lerner Research Institute, Center for Immunotherapy and ImmunoOncology, Cleveland, Ohio

WILLIAM W. DZWIERZYNSKI, MD
Professor and Program Director, Department of Plastic Surgery, Medical College of Wisconsin, Milwaukee, Wisconsin

JACOB D. FRANKE, BS
Southern Illinois University School of Medicine, Springfield, Illinois

BRIAN R. GASTMAN, MD, FACS
Surgical and Co-director of the CCF Melanoma and High Risk Skin Cancer Program, Professor

of Surgery, Cleveland Clinic Lerner College of Medicine, Staff, CCF, Dermatology and Plastic Surgery Institute, Department of Plastic Surgery, Taussig Cancer Center, Lerner Research Institute, Department of Immunology, Head and Neck Institute, Cleveland Clinic, Cleveland, Ohio

ALADDIN H. HASSANEIN, MD, MMSc, FACS
Assistant Professor, Division of Plastic Surgery, Indiana University School of Medicine, Indianapolis, Indiana

JULIE IACULLO, MD
Department of Dermatology, MetroHealth System, Cleveland, Ohio

AZIZ U. KHAN, MD
Division of Hematology/Oncology, Department of Internal Medicine, Southern Illinois University School of Medicine, Springfield, Illinois

REBECCA KNACKSTEDT, MD, PhD
Department of Plastic Surgery, Cleveland Clinic, Cleveland, Ohio

THOMAS J. KNACKSTEDT, MD
Department of Dermatology, MetroHealth System, Case Western Reserve University, School of Medicine, Cleveland, Ohio

JESSIE L. KOLJONEN, MD
Institute for Plastic Surgery, Southern Illinois University School of Medicine, Springfield, Illinois

JEFFREY H. KOZLOW, MD, MS
Section of Plastic and Reconstructive Surgery, University of Michigan School of Medicine, Ann Arbor, Michigan

BRIAN A. MAILEY, MD, FACS
Associate Professor of Surgery, Vice-Chair of Research, Hand Fellowship Program Director, Director, Brachial Plexus and Tetraplegia Clinic, Director, Congenital Head and Neck Anomalies Clinic, Institute for Plastic Surgery, Southern Illinois University School of Medicine Springfield, Illinois

ALAA MANSOUR, MS3
Medical Student, Southern Illinois University School of Medicine, Springfield, Illinois

SAMEER MASSAND, MD
Division of Plastic Surgery, Penn State University, Hershey, Pennsylvania

MICHAEL W. NEUMEISTER, MD, FRCSC, FACS
Professor and Chair, Department of Surgery, Elvin G. Zook Endowed Chair, Institute for Plastic Surgery, Southern Illinois University School of Medicine, Springfield, Illinois

ROGERIO I. NEVES, MD, PhD, FACS, FSSO
Reconstructive Oncology Program Leader, Senior Member, Department of Cutaneous Oncology, H. Lee Moffitt Cancer Center and Research Institute, Professor of Oncologic Sciences, University of South Florida, Tampa, Florida

DANIELLE OLLA, MD
Resident Physician, Institute for Plastic Surgery, Southern Illinois University, Springfield, Illinois

YEE PENG PHOON, PhD, LRI/CCF
Post Doctoral, Cleveland Clinic, Lerner Research Institute, Department of Inflammation and Immunity, Cleveland, Ohio

MICHAEL R. ROMANELLI, MD, MA
Resident Physician, Institute for Plastic Surgery, Southern Illinois University School of Medicine, Springfield, Illinois.

ALEXIS M. RUFFOLO, MD
Division of Plastic Surgery, Southern Illinois University School of Medicine, Springfield, Illinois

ASHWATH J. SAMPATH, MD
Department of Internal Medicine, St. Louis University School of Medicine, St Louis, Missouri

JUSTIN D. SAWYER, MD
The Institute for Plastic Surgery, Southern Illinois University School of Medicine, Springfield, Illinois

LILLIAN SUN, MD
Cleveland Clinic, Lerner College of Medicine at Case Western Reserve University, Cleveland, Ohio

TIMOTHY SMILE, MD
Department of Radiation Oncology,
Cleveland Clinic, Taussig Cancer Center,
Cleveland, Ohio

CHARLES TANNENBAUM, PhD, LRI/CCF
Project Scientist, Cleveland Clinic, Lerner
Research Institute, Department of
Inflammation and Immunity, Cleveland, Ohio

ALLYNE TOPAZ, MD
Fellow Physician, Institute for Plastic Surgery,
Southern Illinois University, Springfield, Illinois

ANTHONY P. TUFARO, DDS, MD, FACS
Professor of Surgery, Surgical Oncology and
Plastic Surgery, Case Western Reserve
University School of Medicine, University
Hospitals Cleveland Medical Center,
Cleveland, Ohio

KAVITA T. VAKHARIA, MD, MS
Department of Plastic Surgery, Cleveland
Clinic, Cleveland, Ohio

MORGAN L. WILSON, MD
Associate Professor of Dermatology, Division
of Dermatology, Southern Illinois University
School of Medicine, Springfield, Illinois

KATLYN M. WOOLFORD, BS
Southern Illinois University School of Medicine,
Springfield, Illinois

MAKI YAMAMOTO, MD, FACS
Health Sciences Associate Professor of
Surgery, Division of Surgical Oncology,
Department of Surgery, University of California,
Irvine, Orange, California

JENNIFER YU, MD, PhD
Department of Radiation Oncology, Cleveland
Clinic, Taussig Cancer Center, Cleveland, Ohio

Contents

Melanoma Risk Factors and Prevention   543

William W. Dzwierzynski

> In the Western population, 1 out of every 50 individuals will develop melanoma. The incidence of melanoma is increasing faster than any other malignancy. The development of melanoma is multifactorial arising from an interaction between genetic susceptibility and environmental exposures. Sixty to seventy percent of melanomas are thought to be caused by ultraviolet radiation. Most cutaneous melanomas are of increased risk. Prevention strategies involve mitigating the environmental risk factors and identifying individuals with phenotypic risk factors for increased surveillance.

Canonical Signaling Pathways in Melanoma   551

Lillian Sun and Joshua Arbesman

> Melanoma is the most lethal type of skin cancer, originating from the uncontrolled proliferation of melanocytes. The transformation of normal melanocytes into malignant tumor cells has been a focus of research seeking to better understand melanoma's pathogenesis and develop new therapeutic targets. Over the past few decades, a conglomeration of studies has pinpointed several driver mutations and their associated signaling pathways. In this review, we summarize the key signaling pathways and the driver mutations involved in melanoma tumorigenesis and also discuss the potential underlying mechanisms.

Immunobiology of Melanoma   561

Yee Peng Phoon, Charles Tannenbaum, and C. Marcela Diaz-Montero

> Despite the ability of immune-based interventions to dramatically increase the survival of patients with melanoma, a significant subset fail to benefit from this treatment, underscoring the need for accurate means to identify the patient population likely to respond to immunotherapy. Understanding how melanoma evades natural or manipulated immune responses could provide the information needed to identify such resistant individuals. Efforts to address this challenge are hampered by the vast immune diversity characterizing tumor microenvironments that remain largely understudied. It is thus important to more clearly elucidate the complex interactions that take place between the tumor microenvironment and host immune system.

Clinical Diagnosis and Classification: Including Biopsy Techniques and Noninvasive Imaging   577

Kavita T. Vakharia

> Early detection of melanoma is important in improving patient survival. The treatment of melanoma is multidisciplinary and begins by obtaining an accurate diagnosis. The mainstays of melanoma diagnosis include examination of the lesion and surrounding areas and an excisional biopsy so that a pathologic diagnosis

can be obtained. The pathology results will help guide treatment recommendations, and some information can be used for prognosis. Further workup of the patient may include laboratory studies and imaging for staging and surveillance.

Conventional histopathology is the primary means of melanoma diagnosis. Both architectural and cytologic features aid in discrimination of melanocytic nevi from melanoma. Communication between the clinician and pathologist regarding the history, examination, differential diagnosis, prior biopsy findings, method of sampling, and specimen orientation is critical to an accurate diagnosis. A melanoma pathology report includes multiple prognostic indicators to guide surgical and medical management. In challenging cases, immunohistochemistry and molecular diagnostics may be of benefit.

The eighth edition of the American Joint Committee on Cancer melanoma staging system relies on assessments of the primary tumor (T), regional lymph nodes (N), and distant metastatic sites (M). Its notable updates include tumor thickness measurements to the nearest 0.1 mm, revision of T1a and T1b definitions, re-evaluation of N category descriptors, increased number of stage III subgroupings, and incorporation of a new M1d designation, among others. These changes were based on analyses of a large contemporary international melanoma database. Ultimately, these revisions were made to improve staging and prognostication, risk stratification, and selection of patients for clinical trials.

Melanoma tumor thickness and ulceration are the strongest predictors of nodal spread. The recommendations for sentinel lymph node biopsy (SLNB) have been updated in recent American Joint Committee on Cancer and National Comprehensive Cancer Network guidelines to include tumor thickness $\geq$0.8 mm or any ulcerated melanoma. Mitotic rate is no longer considered an indicator for determining T category. Improvements in disease-specific survival conferred from SLNB were demonstrated through level I data in the Multicenter Selective Lymphadenectomy Trial (MSLT) I. The role for completion lymph node dissection has evolved to less surgery in lieu of recent domestic (MSLT II) and international (Dermatologic Cooperative Oncology Group Selective Lymphadenectomy Trial [DeCOG-SLT]) level I data having similar melanoma-specific survival. Treatment options for the prevention of treatment of lymphedema have progressed to include immediate lymphatic reconstruction, lymphovenous anastomosis, and vascularized lymph node transfer.

As our knowledge and understanding of melanoma evolve, melanoma surveillance guidelines will reflect these findings. Currently, there is no consensus across international guidelines for melanoma follow-up. However, it is accepted that more aggressive surveillance is recommended for more advanced disease. When examining high-risk individuals, a systematic approach should be followed. Future considerations include the use of noninvasive imaging techniques, 'liquid biopsies,' and artificial intelligence to enhance detection of melanomas.

Malignant melanoma is the 5th most common cancer and stage IV melanoma accounts for approximately 4% of new melanoma diagnoses in the United States. The prognosis for regionally advanced disease is poor, but there have been numerous recent advances in the medical management of melanoma in-transit metastases. The goal of this paper is to review currently accepted treatment options for in-transit metastases and introduce emerging therapies. Therapies to be discussed include limb perfusion and infusion, immunotherapy, checkpoint inhibitors, and radiation therapy.

While primary treatment for melanoma consists of surgical resection and chemotherapeutics, radiation can be used as either definitive or adjuvant therapy in certain clinical scenarios. This chapter aims to explore the indications for primary definitive radiotherapy as well as adjuvant treatment following resection. Delivery, dose, fractionation, and toxicity of radiation treatment will be discussed. As our understanding of melanoma tumor biology increases, the role of radiotherapy may expand for more effective treatment of oligometastatic disease.

Adjuvant therapy plays an integral role in the treatment algorithm for stage III and stage IV cutaneous melanoma. Current ongoing clinical trials are exploring the effects of neoadjuvant therapeutics, specifically for the presurgical treatment of high-risk, borderline resectable disease. In both the adjuvant and neoadjuvant settings, the early chemotherapeutic and biochemical antitumor agents are making way to newer immune therapies, mutation-specific targeted therapies, and oncolytic vaccines that are transforming the treatment of malignant melanoma. The use of these systemic therapies in addition to surgical resection has been shown to increase both overall and progression-free survival.

Contents

surgical excision and reconstruction. The goal for the surgeon is to maintain the function and anatomy of the hand or foot.

CLINICS IN PLASTIC SURGERY

ISSUE OF RELATED INTEREST

Facial Plastic Surgery Clinics
https://www.facialplastic.theclinics.com/
Otolaryngologic Clinics
https://www.oto.theclinics.com/

THE CLINICS ARE AVAILABLE ONLINE!
Access your subscription at:
www.theclinics.com

Preface
A Melanoma Update

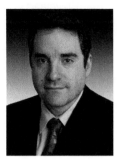

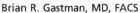

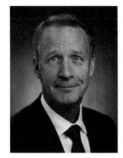

Brian R. Gastman, MD, FACS   Michael W. Neumeister, MD, FRCSC, FACS

Editors

Malignant melanoma, a potentially lethal cutaneous cancer, represents around 5% of all cancers in patients. Melanoma was the third most common cancer in patients between the ages of 20 and 39 and the fifth most common cancer overall in men and women.

Our knowledge of melanoma has grown significantly over the years. Indeed, the first reported case of melanoma was recorded by Hippocrates in the fifth century BC. In the Pre-Colombian found in the Peruvian archeological digs have demonstrated many pathologic conditions, including conditions such as metastatic melanoma. Once termed "fatal black tumors" or "cancerous fungous excrescence," the tumor was described as "melanoses" in 1806 by Rene Theophile Hyancinthe Laennec, who is also known for his invention of the stethoscope. It was not until 1838 that Sir Robert Carswell, a pathologist, coined the term "melanoma." It was clear long ago that surgery was warranted for the management of melanoma. While not the first to perform surgery for melanoma, William Handley, a research fellow in Middlesex Hospital, London, England, suggested that a 5-cm margin was appropriate for the surgical management of melanoma based on one anecdotal case of lymphatic spread of melanoma in a young woman's leg in 1905. The management of melanoma has improved vastly over the years, incorporating contributions from Wallace Clark and Alexander Breslow in the mid to late twentieth century.

It is estimated there will be more than 200,000 new cases of melanoma reported in 2021. About half of these cases will be invasive malignant melanoma, and the other half will be melanoma in situ. The incidence of melanoma has doubled over the last 30 years. In fact, in the last 10 years, newly diagnosed cases of melanoma has increased more than 40%. UV light is the leading known

Clin Plastic Surg 48 (2021) xiii–xiv
https://doi.org/10.1016/j.cps.2021.07.001

cause of melanoma. The sunbelts of California and Florida represent the highest rates of new melanomas reported each year in the United States. But there is good news on the horizon, as the death rate from melanoma has recently decreased by at least 5% per year due to new treatment modalities. These changes indicate major improvements in the detection of early melanoma, when it's most likely to be cured. In addition, immunotherapies and target molecules against the mutation in the BRAF molecule (found in 45% of cutaneous melanomas) have driven 5-year survival for unresectable, stage IV disease to 50% or higher. With dozens of potential new therapies and novel therapeutic combinations on the horizon, the major changes seen in the last 5 years will likely be overshadowed by those in the upcoming 5 years.

The intent of this issue of *Clinics in Plastic Surgery* was to provide an updated knowledge of various aspects of melanoma to surgeons and treating health care providers. A multidisciplinary approach is paramount in the care of stricken patients as we continue to find new ways to decrease progression and fatality of melanoma. Although melanoma as a subject will evolve quickly, this up-to-date expert compilation of where the field stands now will give those treating the disease the tools they need to make the most informed decision to do so.

Brian R. Gastman, MD, FACS
Cleveland Clinic
Lerner College of Medicine
Dermatology and Plastic Surgery Institute
Department of Plastic Surgery
Taussig Cancer Center
Lerner Research Institute
Department of Immunology, Head and Neck
Institute
Cleveland Clinic
9500 Euclid Avenue
Desk A60
Cleveland, OH 44195, USA

Michael W. Neumeister, MD, FRCSC, FACS
Department of Surgery
Institute for Plastic Surgery
Southern Illinois University
School of Medicine
3rd Floor Baylis, Suite 357
747 North Rutledge
Springfield, IL 62702, USA

E-mail addresses:
gastmab@ccf.org (B.R. Gastman)
mneumeister@siumed.edi (M.W. Neumeister)

Melanoma Risk Factors and Prevention

William W. Dzwierzynski, MD

KEYWORDS

• Melanoma • Risk factors • Prevention • UV radiation

KEY POINTS

- The development of melanoma is multifactorial arising from an interaction between genetic suscep-tibility and environmental exposure.
- 60 to 70% of melanomas are thought to be caused by ultraviolet (UV) radiation. Most cutaneous melanomas are caused by the indirect DNA damage initiated by UVA radiation.
- The phenotypic characteristics of decreased melanin production: light complexion, blue or green eyes and freckling are markers for greater susceptibility to melanoma.
- Melanoma prevention strategies involve mitigating the environmental risk factors and identifying in-dividuals with phenotypic risk factors for increased surveillance.

INTRODUCTION

The incidence of new skin cancer diagnosed each year is greater than all other forms of cancers com-bined.[1] Of these cancers, cutaneous melanoma, the deadliest, is increasing faster than any other malignancy. A century ago, cutaneous melanoma was rare; in 1935, a person's lifetime risk of devel-oping melanoma was one in 500.[2] Now, in the Western population, one in 50 individuals will develop melanoma.[3] Over the past 2 decades, the incidence rates have doubled each decade. Mortality rate have also increased, but fortunately at only 5%/year.[4] In the 1960s, 60% of patients diagnosed with melanoma died of the disease, now the mortality rate is 11%, albeit the signifi-cantly increased incidence.[5]

Most cases of melanoma are in the elderly, but it is the third most common cancer in adolescence and young adults aged 15 to 39 years. The most significant increased incidence has been in mela-nomas in the lower legs in middle-aged women and in the head and neck regions in older men.[4] Causes of the extreme rise in melanoma incidence are only partially elucidated. One cause is certainly increased awareness of the disease and early detection; however, this does not account for the entire precipitous rise in cases.

Risk Factors

The development of melanoma is multifactorial, arising from an interaction between genetic sus-ceptibility and environmental exposure.[3] Genetic studies of melanoma suggest that there may be two or more populations prone to the disease. The first population is in individuals with inherently low propensity for melanocyte proliferation and who require chronic sun exposure which drives clonal expansion. The second pathway is in pa-tients with a high propensity for melanocyte prolif-eration (eg, genetic or phenotypic predisposition or high nevi count) and less sun exposure early in the process. Individual risk is determined by inherited mutations, melanoma susceptibility, and genes or polymorphism in secondary risk modifier genes and how much acute or chronic sun exposure modifies risk.[6]

Ultraviolet Exposure

Sixty to seventy percent of melanomas are thought to be caused by ultraviolet (UV) radiation.[7] The sun emits UVA (320–400 nm), UVB (280–315 nm), and UVC (200–280 nm). Our ozone layer and oxygen generally absorb all the UVC before it reaches the surface. Both UVA and UVB are thought to play a role in melanoma development.

Department of Plastic Surgery, Medical College of Wisconsin, 1155 N. Mayfair Road, Milwaukee, WI 53226, USA
E-mail address: billd@mcw.edu

Clin Plastic Surg 48 (2021) 543–550
https://doi.org/10.1016/j.cps.2021.05.001
0094-1298/21/Published by Elsevier Inc.

plasticsurgery.theclinics.com

Of the UV radiation that reaches the earth's surface, 98.7% is UVA.[2]

UVB causes direct damage by the formation of cyclobutene pyrimidine dimers and 6 to 4 photoproducts which can cause direct DNA damage and cell apoptosis.[8] While it was earlier believed that cancers were mostly caused by UVB, it is now known that most cutaneous melanomas are caused by the indirect DNA damage initiated by UVA radiation. UVA penetrates fivefold deeper into skin. The deeper penetration of the UVA photons allows transfer of energy to the oxygen molecules, and these molecules become highly reactive. These molecules include singlet oxygen hydroxy radicals and hydrogen peroxide. These reactive chemical species reach the DNA by diffusion and cause damage to the DNA.[2]

Human skin has evolved to form a very efficient process to minimize the damage caused by exposure to UV radiation. This is believed to have evolved over four billion years ago. UV protection is achieved by internal conversion of molecules which absorbs the energy of the UV photons. The internal conversion converts the energy into small amounts of heat. The conversion is ultrafast with the DNA being in the excited state for only femtoseconds (10^{-15}s). However, the energy of the UV photon which is not converted into heat can generate harmful reactive chemical species including hydroxyl radicals and free oxygen. The absorption spectrum of DNA has a strong absorption for UVB radiation but a much lower absorption of UVA radiation.[2]

A second significant mechanism for photoprotection is provided by melanin. Melanin is thought to have developed much later in human evolutionary development. There are two types of melanin, eumelanin and pheomelanin. Eumelanin is a brown black pigment found in brown and black hair, brown eyes, and all healthy skin. Pheomelanin is a reddish pigment found only in red hair. It is hypothesized that higher levels of eumelanin and deeply pigmented skin developed as a protective mechanism for people living under high continuous UVB radiation.[2] Eumelanin protects against nutrient photolysis, especially that of folate. Increased eumelanin prevents both direct and indirect DNA damage. Eumelanin can convert 99.9% of the absorbed UV radiation to heat.

Sunburn is the result of direct DNA damage as it absorbs UVB photons. UVB radiation causes a covalent linkage between thymine and cystine bases in the DNA forming dimers. During DNA replication, an incorrect base is incorporated causing a mutation. These mutations can subsequently lead to the development of skin cancers. It is estimated that each cell in the skin experiences between 15 and 100 reactions during every second of sunlight exposure. Most of these genetic alterations are corrected by nucleotide excision repair before replication. Chronic lifelong UV exposure with high cumulative UV hours is significant to development of skin cancers, most notably squamous cell carcinoma. In contrast, melanoma is related to more acute intermittent intense exposure in nonacclimated (fair skin) patients.[9] The predominate sites of melanoma are those in exposed intermittent intense sunlight, and these include the backs of men and the legs in women.[4] Early age intermittent high-intensity sun exposure appears to be the major risk factor for development of melanoma, especially associated with sunburns in childhood.[10] Lifetime sunburns history is not as significant predictor of risk as childhood sunburns.

Individuals who had 2 to 5 severe sunburns had a 2.40 relative risk compared with patients who had only one sunburn. In individuals with 6 and more sunburns, the risk was increased to 3.30.

Sun exposure during vacations has conferred an increased risk for melanoma. The number of sunny location vacations, childhood sunny vacations, and sun days during childhood summers increased the risk of melanoma development.[7] This may also be the reason that melanoma is seen more frequently in individuals of higher social economic status. These individuals may have the luxury of being able to take vacations to sunny locations.

Tanning Beds and UV Lights

In the United States, tanning beds are classified in the same cancer risk category as cigarettes. Tanning beds can have UVA doses 12 times greater than those of the sun.[8] Clear relationships between UV exposure from tanning beds and skin cancer has been demonstrated in laboratory studies as well as epidemiologic studies. Individuals who have used a tanning bed before the age of 25 years have a 6-fold increase in melanoma risk. One to 14 lifetime tanning sessions increased melanoma risk by 19%; individuals with 15 to 30 sessions had a 31% increased risk, and 40 hours of indoor intentional tanning can result in a 55% increased melanoma risk.[2]

In a large multinational study of individuals with biopsy-proven cutaneous melanoma, over 70% of respondents reported some degree of intentional tanning in the past year. Individuals younger than 25 years are less likely to perceive the risk of intentional tanning. Surprisingly even individuals with previous melanomas reported frequent intentional tanning.[11]

Tanning bed use is associated with a younger age of melanoma diagnosis. The more frequent use of tanning in young women than in men is postulated to be the reason that there is increased incidence of melanoma in younger women.[12]

Indoor Light Exposure

Paradoxically, several epidemiologic studies comparing indoor workers to outdoor workers have found a lower risk of cutaneous melanoma in individuals working outdoors. This may be due to blockage of UVB by windows while allowing the full transmission of UVA.[2] Paradoxically while UVB can cause direct skin damage, it is also responsible for making vitamin D, which may be protective for cancers. It is postulated that the increase ratio of UVA/UVB exposure may decrease vitamin D levels and increase the tendency for malignancy. A Canadian case-control study showed an elevated risk of melanoma associated with fluorescent light exposure in men (but not in women). Relationship of indoor light exposure to melanoma is uncertain currently.[13]

Skin Type and Tanning

Pale skin and blue eyes may have offered an evolutionary benefit to the ancient humans who migrated from areas of intense sun and abundant fish to more temperate climates. The evolutionary protection of melanin may have become a liability. Vitamin B folate is destroyed by UV radiation, where vitamin D is synthesized by UV radiation. In the tropics where sunlight is plentiful, abundant melanin production and darker complexion protects folate stores and allows enough UV penetration to synthesize vitamin D. The evolutionary protection that allowed light-skinned individuals to synthesize vitamin D now can lead to increased skin cancer risk, especially that of melanoma. Dark- and light-skin individuals generally both have the same relative number of melanocytes; however, in light-skinned individuals, the melanocytes generally do not produce melanin. Caucasians account for 70% of melanoma cases. Black population may have a different biology and unfortunately an increased mortality.[6]

The phenotypic characteristics of decreased melanin production—light complexion, blue or green eyes, and freckling—all serve to be markers for greater susceptibility to melanoma. Blue eyes have a relative risk of 1.6 to 3.00 compared with dark eyes for the development of melanoma Green eyes has a relative risk of 1.06 to 2.45 compared with dark eyes.[1] Blonde hair is associated with a relative risk of 1.6 to 9.7 compared with dark hair. Red hair has a relative risk in the range of 2.3 to 5.59.[7] Freckles are also an important marker in identifying patients prone to melanoma. Freckles do not appear until an individual is exposed to sunlight. Patients with xeroderma pigmentosa (XP) have a significant increased rate of freckling and risk of melanoma. Twenty percent of XP individuals will develop melanoma.

Tanning inability is almost certainly an increased risk for melanoma. The inability to tan has an increased relative risk of 1.4 to 4.5. The ability to tan may be considered as a protection against sunburn and melanoma. Tanning ability is characterized by the Fitzgerald scale (**Table 1**).

Sex and Age

Males are 1.5 times more likely develop melanoma than females.[1] Melanoma is the fifth most common cancer in men. By the age of 75 years, the incidence of cutaneous melanoma is almost 3 times higher in men than in women.[9] Males, especially those of older age, have a more unfavorable prognosis than females.[14] It is not clear why males have a higher risk, but it is thought that this may be behaviorally related to sun protection strategies and less frequent use of sun protection as well as skin type.[3]

Melanoma in the sixth most common cancer in women. The incidence of melanomas in women is higher than that in men until they reached the age of 40 years. The increase in melanomas in younger women is postulated to be caused by the increased use of indoor tanning.

During pregnancy, melanocytic activity normally increases. Hyperpigmentation is frequently seen during this time. Several studies have examined melanoma risk in pregnancy. Controlled studies do not support any increased melanoma risk, thicker tumors, increase in risk of metastasis, or worse prognosis in pregnant women.[2]

Middle-aged patients, regardless of sex, often have a history of excessive intermittent sun exposure and a history of sunburns. Melanomas in middle-aged patients are likely to be thinner and associated with dysplastic nevus. Young patients are more likely to have a family history of melanoma.[14]

Melanocytic Nevi

In almost all studies, the presence of acquired melanocytic nevus is a risk factor for the development of melanoma. While some nevus may be congenital, many are acquired with sun exposure. Genetic factors, immune function, and sun exposure are all thought to be determinants of nevi proliferation. Generally, individuals do not develop nevi after the age of 50 years. It is controversial whether

Table 1
Fitzpatrick skin classification

Skin Type	Skin Color	Hair Color	Eye Color	Tanning Ability	Sunburns
I	Pale	Red, blonde	Blue, gray, green	Never tans	Always burns
II	Light	Red, blonde, light brown	Blue, gray, green, hazel	Tans poorly	Burns easily
III	Medium	Blonde, brown	Blue, green, brown	Tans gradually	Mild burns
IV	Olive	Brown	Hazel, brown	Tans very easily	Burns minimally
V	Brown	Dark brown	Brown	Tans very easily	Rarely burns
VI	Black	Black	Brown	Tans very easily	Never burns

nevi represent a true precursor lesion to melanoma or more of a marker for further melanoma risk. Twenty-five percent of melanomas are thought to occur within pre-existing nevi.[3] Retrospectively, almost 80% of patients with melanoma report a change in a pre-existing mole.[4] An individual's total number of nevi confers the greatest risk to the development of melanoma. In general, the greater the number of atypical nevi, the greater the melanoma risk. Patients with greater than 100 nevi with or without atypia or 50 nevi with one or several atypical nevi are considered to be at increased risk. Patients with greater than 100 nevi have almost a seven-fold relative risk of melanoma. The presence of clinically atypical moles, despite the total number of moles, is a strong predictor of future melanoma.[10]

The presence a giant congenital nevus greater than 20 cm also has an increased risk. The malignant transformation of giant congenital nevus has been hotly debated with estimates between 4% and 40% chances of malignant transformation. It is generally believed that the risk is less than 8%.

Family and Genetic Factors

Family history is one of the most significant risk factors for melanoma. Approximately, 5% to 10% of melanomas occur in families with a hereditary predisposition. Melanoma has one of the highest rates of mutation of any cancer. The BRAF mutation is found in 60% of melanomas. NRAS mutations are found in 15% to 20% of melanomas.[8] BRAF mutation alone probably does not cause melanoma, but when associated with environmental factors, it increases melanoma risk. BRAF mutations are found mostly in melanoma arising in skin intermittently exposed to sun and less often in chronic sun-exposed sites.[5] Germ line mutations in the CDKN2A or CDK4 genes, involved in controlling cell division, are relatively rare but are associated with a significant melanoma risk.[8] B–K mole syndrome and familial atypical mole/melanoma (FAMM) syndrome are associated with an increased number of dysplastic nevi and an increased risk of melanomas. These syndromes are both autosomal dominant traits with incomplete penetrance and may be related to an abnormality on chromosome 1P.[4] The incidence of melanoma in FAMM patients is as high as 85% by middle age.[15] Parents with a melanoma risk increases relatively the risk by 2.4. A sibling with melanoma increases relative risk to 2.98.[1]

Dietary factors

Citrus consumption is associated with an increased risk of melanoma. This is somewhat paradoxic because vitamin C had been shown to have an in vitro toxicity for melanoma cells. Consuming greater than 1.6 servings of citrus fruits daily increases melanoma risk. The postulated mechanism is due to the presence of psoralens and furocoumarins in these fruits, which interacts with UV light to stimulate melanoma cell proliferation.[11]

Increased alcohol intake has been shown to have an association with elevated cutaneous melanoma risk. This risk is associated more with sunlight-spared sites, such as the trunk, as opposed to the head, neck, and extremities. Alcohol intake can increase the severity of sunburns. Alcohol acts as a photosensitizer in combination with UV light generating reactive oxygen species.[11]

Personal History of Melanoma

One of the greatest risk factors for developing a melanoma is a previous history of melanoma. Whatever be the etiology of the primary melanoma, whether it is a genetic aberration, deficiency in skin repair mechanism, or previous excess UV radiation, these factors do not disappear at the first melanoma. The site of a melanoma does not necessarily correlate with area of previous sunburn or tanning. Greatest attention should be given to surveillance of individuals with a previous history of melanoma. A previous melanoma has a 3% to 8% chance of developing another melanoma. Patients with a history of non-melanoma skin cancer have a relative risk of between two and seven times.[1]

Immunosuppression

Individuals with HIV have an increased incidence of melanoma.[4] Patients receiving long-term immunosuppression have an increased risk of skin cancers including melanoma. Kidney transplant recipients have a relative risk of 3.6 for developing a melanoma.[6]

Prevention

Prevention of melanoma should theoretically be straightforward because the lesions are in a superficial location and risk factors are well known. Cancer-prevention strategies are either primary or secondary. The purpose of primary preventions is to mediate risk factors and to identify precursor lesions. Secondary prevention serves to identify established premalignant lesions and early cancers to decrease morbidity and mortality. Since melanoma involves both phenotypic and environmental risk factors, prevention strategies involve mitigating the environmental risk factors and identifying individuals with phenotypic risk factors for increased surveillance.

Primary Prevention

The greatest environmental risk factor for melanoma is UV radiation; primary prevention involves limiting the amount of UV radiation, especially the high-intensity intermittent UV radiation which causes sunburns. Peak UVB radiation occurs between the hours of 10 AM and 4 PM. Minimalized sun exposure during this time can avoid sunburns.[15] If exposure cannot be avoided, the use of protective clothing, wide-brimmed hats, sunglasses, and sunscreen is recommended.[16]

Sunscreens prevent sunburns; however, there is little conclusive evidence currently available that sunscreens prevent melanomas.[2] In fact, one study found that males who use sunscreens have a 1.7x increased risk for the development of melanoma.[7] Sunscreen may be either organic (chemical absorbers) or inorganic (physical absorbers). The organic compounds include a variety of compounds, the most common being para-aminobenzoic acid. The organic sunscreens absorb high-intensity UV rays, releasing energy by a photochemical process in the epidermis. Organic agents may however penetrate the epidermis and can come in contact with living cells. There, they can generate reactive oxygen species causing DNA damage.[2] The vehicle of the sunscreen has a significant effect on its absorption into the skin. Alcohol-based formulations can increase absorption. Inorganic agents physically block the skin by reflecting the UV radiation; most of these contain titanium dioxide or zinc oxide. These physical blockers are quite efficient at blocking both UVA and UVB. The American Academy of Dermatology (AAD) and American Cancer Society (ACS) recommend application of a waterproof UVA/UVB sunscreen with an SPF of at least 30; reapplication every 2 to 4 hours.[15] Newer broad-spectrum sunscreens are 4 times as effective as older sunscreens. Ultimately protective clothing, hats, sunglasses, and sun avoidance provides the best protection.[17]

The ACS and AAD have initiated national and local programs to alert the public on sun dangers. Outcome measurements for successful prevention includes improved knowledge and attitudes about sun protection, decreased rates of deliberate sunbathing, increased rates of use of sunscreen and protective clothing, decreased use of tanning salons, and changing societal norms about sun safety. Prevention targets are most importantly directed at limiting exposure in children, adolescences, and college students. Although education begins in childhood, it is important to be continued throughout adulthood because individuals receive 75% of their total UV radiation after the age of 18 years.[16]

The first country to initiate a public health campaign was Australia. In Victoria, almost two-third of its residents developed skin cancer by the age of 70 years. The Sun Smart program, otherwise known as Slip! Slot! Slap! Seek! Slide! advocated slipping on clothing, slopping on sunscreen, slapping on a hat, seeking shade, and sliding on sunglasses. It was broadly successful with an estimate of prevention of 50,000 cancers and 1400 lives.[18] Also in Australia, over a 2-year period, three episodes featuring melanoma and sun safety and an Australian equivalent of "60 Minutes" were aired. After airing these programs, melanoma diagnoses increased 167% in the subsequent 3 months.[13] Sun safe programs in the United States include the Ray program, Sunbeatibles, and the MD Anderson Safety Curriculum.

Chemoprevention is the use of natural or synthetic agents to prevent premalignant lesions from progressing into invasive cancers. While there are limited data supporting their widespread use, several agents show promise in laboratory studies.[10] Coffee is the only agent that has well-documented epidemiologic efficacy. This effect may be due to caffeine's ability to inhibit UV-induced sunburns. The Norwegian Woman and Cancer Study found that melanoma risk among high-caffeine drinkers was significantly lower than that among those with a lower caffeine intake. The NIH-AARP Diet and Health Study detected moderate decrease in melanoma risk among patients drinking more than 4 cups of coffee a day.[19]

A product in green tea, epigallocatechin gallate, is associated with antitumor activities, having an antimetastatic effect on melanoma cells. Genistein is a flavonoid present in soybeans and other legumes that has been shown experimentally to reduce tumor size, impair extracellular signaling, and prevent cancer cells from establishing metastasis by suppression of adhesion proteins.[10] Resveratrol, found in grapes, berries, and peanuts, and lupeol, found in mango pulp, roots of cucumbers, and soybeans, have anticancer properties. They can inhibit growth of metastatic melanoma through induction of an apoptosis.[10] Curcumin can inhibit cell migration and tumor growth. Fisetin, found in strawberries and apples, experimentally prevents oxidative stress and has been shown to induce apoptosis in cancer cells. Silymarin extracted from milk thistle is protective against photo carcinogenesis. Long-chain omega-3 fatty acids, which are abundant in fish and seafood, have an antineoplastic effect that may decrease UV-related immunosuppression in the skin. This role of omega-3s has been postulated by the relatively low rates of melanoma in the Eskimo population which has a large fish-based diet.[19]

Vitamins have many potential antitumor properties. Niacin (vitamin B3) can reduce UV damage by reducing UV-induced immunosuppression and facilitating DNA repair.[19] Folic acid (vitamin B9) has a controversial role in cancer reduction. High folate intake may suppress lesion development in normal tissue but may facilitate the growth of premalignant lesions. Folic acid is also associated with phototoxicity.[19] Vitamin D's role in melanoma is also controversial. UV exposure by sunlight is a major source of vitamin D, while UV exposure is a risk factor in development of melanoma. Vitamin D may paradoxically reduce the risk of melanoma and autoimmune diseases. Higher levels of vitamin D from food intake are associated with lower melanoma risk. Patients with lower serum vitamin D levels have a greater tumor thickness, more advanced tumor stage, and worse survival outcome than patients with a higher vitamin D level. It is uncertain if these finding are independent or only an association with excess sun exposure.[19]

Secondary Prevention

Secondary prevention seeks to identify at-risk individuals to detect melanomas at an early stage and prevent deaths. Their rationale of screening for melanomas has been debated, mostly regarding the societal cost of screening.[20–22] Large-scale screening is clearly labor-intensive and may be cost-prohibitive for many medical systems. Self-examination is the simplest, most convenient, and most cost-effective method of screening. In 1985, the "ABCD" criterion was developed. ABCD stands for asymmetry, border irregularity, color variation, and diameter greater than 6 mm. Later an E was added for evolving lesions. Adapting the ABCDE criterion to skin self-examination can increase detection of suspicious lesions from 57% to 90%.[3] In Australia, melanoma mortality was reduced by 63% by early melanoma diagnosis through skin self-examination.[1]

In 1985, the AAD sponsored population-based screening starting with screening of family members of melanoma patients.[13] In Queensland, Australia, patients had a 14% lower risk of thick melanomas if they received a clinical skin examination within 3 years. There was 26% fewer melanoma deaths once routine screening was established.[1] Risk stratification rules can improve the efficiency and cost-effectiveness of early detection.[23] Currently, in the United States, screening is recommended only for individuals at high risk for melanoma, which include those with a personal or family history, dysplastic nevus syndrome, and frequent sunburns as a child or phenotypic factors (light hair color, increased burning tenderness, limited tanning ability). Sunburns are one of the best markers of high-intensity intermittent sun exposure. A history of sunburn in children is associated with a high risk of melanoma development.[3] A population at increasing risk is older white males, and this may be due to a variety of factors, including more sunny vacations, poor-quality sunscreen available when they were children, and poorer attitude of males about applying sunscreen. Almost half of melanoma-specific deaths currently occur in white males older than 50 years. The AAD screening program suggest the highest yield of screening is from this population. Currently this represents only 25% of individuals screened.[6]

Optimal screening would best be provided by trained skin specialist, yet limitations in numbers currently prevent this. Screening by primary care physicians during routine yearly examinations is currently recommended for individuals at lower risk. The utility of this is somewhat controversial. One study showed that only 12% of nondermatologists could correctly identify five of six melanomas compared with 69% of dermatologists.[16] Patient self-reported data suggest that primary care skin examinations are currently quite low. Only 46% of patients with a high school degree or less reported having a physician perform a skin examination. Among patients with a college degree, 65% reported having a skin examination.[16] Close surveillance every 3 to 4 months is warranted for high-risk individuals. Biopsy should be performed on lesions that are clinically suspicious of melanoma. Typically, new moles do not arise after the age of 50 years. All new moles should be assessed and biopsied in middle-aged patients.[15] Even a trained dermatologist can increase their diagnostic accuracy. The use of dermoscopy can increase diagnostic accuracy 27% when used by a trained dermatologist. Total body photography can be used to detect evolving lesions. Artificial intelligence (AI) is a potential emerging technology to identify high-risk lesions. Photographs or smartphone images of lesions can be uploaded into deep learning image analysis algorithms; initial data suggest AI can outperform even skilled dermatologists.[1] Further research is needed to validate this innovative technology.

SUMMARY

The estimated direct medical expenditure for skin cancer care is over $8 billion annually; over $3.3 billion for melanoma care alone. Additional indirect costs related to workday loss are estimated at $106.2 million annually.[1] Just the use of tanning beds in the United States is estimated to lead to an economic loss of $127.3 billion over the lifetime of individuals.[12] Identifying risk factors and prevention strategies for melanoma will not only result in cost-savings but ultimately save lives.

CLINICS CARE POINTS

- The most significant risk factor to the development of melanoma is acute intermittent intense UV exposure in non-acclimated fair skinned patients.

- Individuals who have used a tanning bed before the age of 25 have a 6-fold increase in melanoma risk.

- Patients with greater than 100 nevi with or without atypia or 50 nevi with one or several atypical nevi have almost a seven-fold relative risk of melanoma.

- Sunscreens prevent sunburns, however there is little conclusive evidence currently available that sunscreen use prevents melanomas.

DISCLOSURE

The author has no significant financial disclosures.

REFERENCES

1. O'Neill CH, Scoggins CR. Melanoma. J Surg Oncol 2019;120(5):873–81.
2. Volkovova K, Bilanicova D, Bartonova A, et al. Associations between environmental factors and incidence of cutaneous melanoma. Rev Environ Health 2012;11(Suppl 1):S12.
3. Rastrelli M, Tropea S, Rossi CR, et al. Melanoma: epidemiology, risk factors, pathogenesis, diagnosis and classification. In Vivo 2014;28(6):1005–11.
4. Williams ML, Sagebiel RW. Melanoma risk factors and atypical moles. West J Med 1994;160(4):343–50.
5. Lipsker D. Growth rate, early detection, and prevention of melanoma: melanoma epidemiology revisited and future challenges. Arch Dermatol 2006;142(12):1638–40.
6. Demierre MF. Epidemiology and prevention of cutaneous melanoma. Curr Treat Options Oncol 2006;7(3):181–6.
7. Evans RD, Kopf AW, Lew RA, et al. Risk factors for the development of malignant melanoma–I: Review of case-control studies. J Dermatol Surg Oncol 1988;14(4):393–408.
8. Sample A, He YY. Mechanisms and prevention of UV-induced melanoma. Photodermatol Photoimmunol Photomed 2018;34(1):13–24.
9. MacKie RM. Incidence, risk factors and prevention of melanoma. Eur J Cancer 1998;34(Suppl 3):S3–6.
10. Syed DN, Mukhtar H. Botanicals for the prevention and treatment of cutaneous melanoma. Pigment Cell Melanoma Res 2011;24(4):688–702.
11. Bränström R, Chang YM, Kasparian N, et al. Melanoma risk factors, perceived threat and intentional tanning: an international online survey. Eur J Cancer Prev 2010;19(3):216–26.
12. Suppa M, Gandini S. Sunbeds and melanoma risk: time to close the debate. Curr Opin Oncol 2019;31(2):65–71.
13. Goldstein AM, Tucker MA. Etiology, epidemiology, risk factors, and public health issues of melanoma. Curr Opin Oncol 1993;5(2):358–63.
14. Palve JS, Korhonen NJ, Luukkaala TH, et al. Differences in risk factors for melanoma in young and middle-aged higher-risk patients. In Vivo 2020;34(2):703–8.

15. Calianno C. Influencing melanoma prevention. Nurse Pract 2011;36(3):6–10.

16. Koh HK, Geller AC, Miller DR, et al. Prevention and early detection strategies for melanoma and skin cancer. Current status. Arch Dermatol 1996;132(4): 436–43.

17. Wang J, Li X, Zhang D. Coffee consumption and the risk of cutaneous melanoma: a meta-analysis. Eur J Nutr 2016;55(4):1317–29.

18. Trager MH, Queen D, Samie FH, et al. Advances in prevention and surveillance of cutaneous Malignancies. Am J Med 2020;133(4):417–23.

19. Yang K, Fung TT, Nan H. An epidemiological Review of diet and cutaneous malignant melanoma. Cancer Epidemiol Biomarkers Prev 2018;27(10): 1115–22.

20. Quéreux G, N'guyen JM, Cary M, et al. Validation of the self-Assessment of melanoma risk Score for a melanoma-targeted screening. Eur J Cancer Prev 2012;21(6):588–95.

21. Curiel-Lewandrowski C, Chen SC, Swetter SM. Melanoma Prevention Working Group-Pigmented Skin Lesion Sub-Committee. Screening and prevention measures for melanoma: is there a survival advantage? Curr Oncol Rep 2012;14(5):458–67.

22. Olsen CM, Pandeya N, Thompson BS, et al. Risk stratification for melanoma: Models Derived and Validated in a purpose-Designed Prospective Cohort. J Natl Cancer Inst 2018;110(10):1075–83.

23. Watts CG, Madronio C, Morton RL, et al. Clinical Features Associated With Individuals at Higher Risk of Melanoma: A Population-Based Study. JAMA Dermatol 2017;153(1):23–9.

Canonical Signaling Pathways in Melanoma

Lillian Sun, MD[a], Joshua Arbesman, MD[b],*

KEYWORDS

• Melanoma • Signaling pathways • Mutations • Tumorigenesis • Drug targets

KEY POINTS

• Understanding critical mutations in melanoma tumorigenesis and their impact on the signaling pathways can hopefully further advances in prevention, screening, and treatment.
• Hot-spot mutations in melanoma often occur in genes encoding key regulators for cell growth and differentiation, leading to aberrant activation of downstream signaling pathways.
• Based upon the causative role of these mutations and dysregulated pathways in melanoma, therapies targeting these mutations and pathways have been developed with promising efficacy.

INTRODUCTION

Melanoma is the most lethal type of skin cancer, originating from the uncontrolled proliferation of melanocytes. Although it has been historically considered a rare cancer, its incidence has steadily risen in the last 50 years.[1] The transformation of normal melanocytes into malignant tumor cells has been a focus of research seeking to better understand melanoma's pathogenesis and develop new therapeutic targets. Over the past few decades, a conglomeration of studies have pinpointed several driver mutations (**Table 1**) and their associated signaling pathways (**Fig. 1**). Understanding these critical mutations and their impact on the signaling pathways has already led to new advances in treatment and will hopefully further advances in prevention, screening, and therapy. In this review, we summarize the key signaling pathways and the driver mutations involved in melanoma tumorigenesis and also discuss the potential underlying mechanisms.

Mitogen-Activated Protein Kinase

The mitogen-activated protein kinase (MAPK) signal cascades regulate physiologic cell growth, survival, and migration. However, in the tumor environment, the signal cascades promote cancer cell proliferation, survival, dissemination, and even drug resistance.[2] Overall, the MAPK signaling pathways are composed of 4 independent signaling families: the MAPK/ERK (extracellular signal-regulated kinase) family, the big MAP kinase-1, c-Jun N-terminal kinase (JNK), and p38 signaling family.[3]

In the canonical MAPK/ERK pathway, there are three types of MAPK kinase-kinase (MAPKKK): A-RAF, B-RAF, and C-RAF kinases, among which, BRAF is highly mutated in melanoma. Downstream of MAPKKK are two MAPK kinases MEK1 and MEK2, while the final effectors of this signaling pathway are ERK1/2.[4]

Many oncogenic driver mutations that have recently been mapped activate the MAPK pathway during tumorigenesis. These mutations include v-Ki-ras Kirsten rat sarcoma viral oncogene

[a] Cleveland Clinic, Lerner College of Medicine at Case Western Reserve University, 9501 Euclid Avenue, Cleveland, OH 44106, USA; [b] Department of Dermatology, Cleveland Clinic, Cleveland Clinic Lerner Research Institute, 9500 Euclid Avenue, Cleveland, OH 44195, USA
* Corresponding author:
E-mail address: ARBESMJ@ccf.org

Clin Plastic Surg 48 (2021) 551–560
https://doi.org/10.1016/j.cps.2021.05.002

Table 1
Genetic mutations in melanoma

Gene	Mutation	Function	Frequency in Melanoma	Reference
BRAF	V600E	MAPK kinase-kinase	Somatic; 50%–70%	5,7,8
NRAS	Q61	GTPase, NRAS activation	Somatic; 15%–20%	5
	G12/13	GTPase, NRAS activation	Somatic; 7%/5%	5
RAC1	P29S	GTPase, PAK signaling	Somatic; 9.2% in sun-exposed melanoma	14
CDKN2A p16[INK4a]	Missense, nonsense, frame shift splice site mutation	Cyclin-dependent kinase inhibitor 2A	Germline mutation, 20%–40% in familial melanomas	52,53
CDKN2A p16[INK4a]	Deletion, nonsense, missense, splice site mutation	Cyclin-dependent kinase inhibitor 2A	Up to 50% in sporadic melanomas	52,54
CDKN2A p14[ARF]	Deletion and insertion	P53 destabilization	Germline mutation; rare	53
CDK4	R24C, R24H	Cyclin-dependent kinase	Germline mutation; found in familial melanoma families	8,64
MITF	E318K	Transcription regulation	Germline variant; 1.4%	49
DDX3X	LOF mutation	RNA helicase	Somatic; around 5.8% in cancer	69–71
TERT	c.-146C > T;c.-124C > T	Telomerase reverse transcriptase	Somatic mutation with frequency 33% in Melanoma	76
TERT	c.-57 T>G	Telomerase reverse transcriptase	Germline mutation; rare	76
POT1	LOF mutation	Protection of telomere 1 gene	Germline mutation; in almost 4% of familial melanoma	81,82
ACD	Q320X, N249S	Shelterin complex encoding gene	Germline; 6 out of 510 melanoma families	83
TERF2IP	R364X	Shelterin complex encoding gene	Germline; 4 out of 510 melanoma families	83
MC1R	D84E	Melanocortin 1 receptor	Germline; ~10% in melanoma	94,95

Abbreviations: ACD, adrenocortical dysplasia protein homolog; TERF2IP, telomeric repeat-binding factor 2-interacting protein.

homolog (KRAS) and the valine to glutamic acid (V600E) *BRAF* mutation.[5–7] *BRAF* mutations have been found in 50% to 70% of malignant melanomas, while the V600E mutation is the most frequent mutation among all the *BRAF* mutations (up to 80%).[6,8,9] The V600E *BRAF* is a gain-of-function mutant that has a 10-fold greater kinase activity than the wild-type *BRAF*.[6] The overactivated BRAF eventually activates ERK, triggering downstream effects including cancer cell proliferation, increased survival, reduced apoptosis, and increased capability of invasion and metastasis, thus leading to tumor formation and progression.[10]

It is noteworthy that *BRAF*[V600E] alone might not be sufficient to drive tumorigenesis as normal nevi also harbor a high frequency of V600E mutation akin to melanoma (~85%).[8] However, only 23% of the common nevi with *BRAF* mutations have activated MAPK.[11] In contrast, approximately 93% of melanomas harboring *BRAF* mutations have MAPK activation,[11] suggesting the essential role of MAPK activation in melanoma development

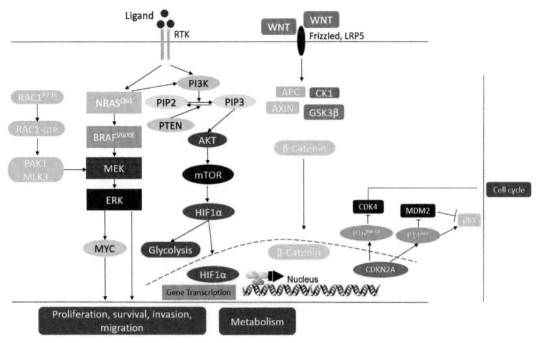

Fig. 1. Key signaling pathways in melanoma.

and the decoupling of BRAF from its downstream MAPK effectors in normal nevi.

Ras-related C3 Botulinum Toxin Substrate 1

Ras-related C3 botulinum toxin substrate 1 (Rac 1) is a GTPase that belongs to the rat sarcoma (RAS) superfamily.[12] As a small GTPase, Rac1 switches between the guanosine triphosphate (GTP)-bound state and guanosine diphosphate–bound state, alternating between the active and inactive forms. Once in its active form, Rac1 can interact with various effector proteins that mediate different biological functions, including nicotinamide adenine dinucleotide phosphate oxidase activation (for the production of reactive oxygen species [ROS]), formation of membrane ruffles (a meshwork of actin filaments close to the cell membrane for cell motility), and lamellipodia (protrusion of the leading edge of the cells to facilitate cell movement). One important outcome of Rac1's impact on actin polymerization/assembly is epithelial-mesenchymal transition, a hallmark of cancer progression.

Notably, Rac1 has been implicated in cancer progression and metastasis because of its ability to promote cell proliferation and cell migration.[13] A recent exciting discovery is the identification of a Rac1 hotspot mutation (Rac1^P29S), with a frequency of 9.2% in primary melanoma.[14] Rac1^P29S is the third most common driver mutation in sun-induced melanoma,

following BRAF and NRAS. Unlike the BRAF and NRAS hotspot mutations, the Rac1^P29S mutation carries a distinctive signature for ultraviolet B–induced DNA damage (CCT>TCT), which in turn corroborates the critical role of Rac1^P29S in sun-induced melanoma. Moreover, Rac1^P29S is absent from normal nevi and more prevalent in BRAF and NRAS wild-type carrying melanomas. When Rac1^P29S is introduced into normal melanocytes, it increases the ability of Rac1 to promote cell proliferation and migration, accompanied by enhanced ERK activation and cell membrane ruffling, the process of forming actin-rich membrane protrusions, which is essential for cell motility and a signature of Rac1 activation.[14] Mechanistically, it was shown that Rac1^P29S has substantially enhanced ability in binding with PAK1 and MLK3 compared with the wild-type Rac1. Structurally, the switch I region of Rac1 is crucial for nucleotide binding and effector protein interaction. Simultaneously, the alteration of Pro29Ser releases the conformational restraint, allowing for GTP binding in the switch I loop and enhancing the effector activation. In addition, one recent study pointed out that Rac1^P29S in melanoma activated an serum response factor/myocardin-related transcription factor transcriptional program that drives melanocytes into a mesenchymal state, while these melanocytes and melanoma cells driven by Rac1^P29S are dependent on AKT and MRTF for survival.[15] Moreover, Rac1^P29S can also confer resistance to BRAF inhibition in melanoma cells.[16]

Wnt Signaling Pathway

Wnt signaling pathway is crucial in cell polarity, proliferation, and migration.[17] In skin, Wnt signaling is important in the development of melanocytes and their migration to the epidermis or hair follicles.[18] Mutations of β-catenin have been described in both melanoma cell lines and primary melanoma. The Wnt signaling can be relayed through three different paths by different mediators: the canonical Wnt pathway mediated by β-catenin, the noncanonical pathway mediated by protein kinase c/Ca^{2+}, and the planar cell polarity pathway mediated by JNK.[19] Nuclear β-catenin was detected in melanoma tissues suggesting the activation of the Wnt signaling pathway. The constitutively activated Wnt signaling acts in concordance with MAPK in melanoma formation and development.

Canonical Wnt signaling was found to delay the oncogene-induced senescence in either $BRAF^{V600E}$- or $NRAS^{Q61K}$-carrying melanocytes, indicating its importance to tumor development.[20,21] The noncanonical signaling pathway mediated by Wnt5a increased cell motility and pseudo-senescence and conferred an invasive phenotype in melanoma.[22–24] In addition, the Wnt5a ligand can also bind to some coreceptors to activate the canonical Wnt signaling,[25,26] suggesting that the two divergent pathways converge somewhere along the way during melanoma tumorigenesis.

PI3K Signaling Pathway

PI3K is also important for cell growth, proliferation, and metabolism.[27] Its downstream effector is AKT. Upon PI3K activation by extracellular stimuli, Akt is phosphorylated and activated, resulting in the phosphorylation of an array of substrates, including GSK3β.[28] The phosphorylation of GSK3β frees β-catenin, which in turn translocates to the nucleus to induce the expression of oncogenes, such as myelocytomatosis and cyclin D1.[29] As a result, phosphorylated AKT inhibits apoptosis and promotes cell proliferation, resulting in cancer progression.

Another critical molecule involved in this signaling pathway is phosphatase and tensin homolog (PTEN). The PTEN functions as a phosphatase that can dephosphorylate PIP3 into PIP2, dampen AKT phosphorylation, and thus inhibit PI3K signaling.[30] In melanoma cell lines, it was observed that around 30% to 50% of these cell lines had a loss of PTEN expression, while in primary melanoma, this percentage was around 5%-20%.[31]

Interestingly, concurrent *BRAF* and *PTEN* mutations have been detected in melanoma patients. In a mouse model, the $BRAF^{V600E}$ expression only led to benign melanocytic hyperplasia, but not the development of melanoma. However, when $BRAF^{V600E}$ expression was combined with PTEN silencing, melanoma developed with complete penetrance, and metastases were observed in lymph nodes and lungs. This result might be mediated by β-catenin signaling.[32]

Metabolism Reprogramming in Melanoma

While cancer cells have upregulated glycolysis and increased lactate production from pyruvate, normal cells use oxygen and glucose to produce adenosine triphosphate (ATP) for energy supply.[33–35] This phenomenon was first noted as the Warburg effect by the Nobel laureate Otto Heinrich Warburg in 1924. Metabolic reprogramming is a hallmark of all malignant tumors. Compared with normal melanocytes, melanoma cells presented a higher sensitivity to glycolysis inhibition and a higher rate of glutaminolysis.[36]

As noted before, $BRAF^{V600E}$ is one of the most highly mutated genes in melanoma. It has been reported that genetic or chemical inhibition of $BRAF^{V600E}$ expression leads to the downregulation of glycolytic enzymes and glucose transporters.[37,38] Consequently, the downstream ERK activation and expression of transcription factors, including MYC, are suppressed.[38,39] MYC can upregulate several glucose metabolism genes, including lactate dehydrogenase A, glucose transporter 1, and hexokinase 2, all of which concomitantly increase glucose uptake and glycolytic activity.[39] Thus, these findings suggest that $BRAF^{V600E}$ increases glycolysis partially through the action of MYC.

The other genes that are crucial in the $BRAF^{V600E}$-mediated metabolism reprogramming include *HIF-1α* and *PGC1α*.[40,41] HIF-1α allows cells to become accustomed to hypoxia by upregulating an array of glycolytic enzymes and glucose transporters. In contrast, the normal expression of PGC1α increases the capacity of ATP production and protects against oxidative stress.[37,42] These two genes form a balance and are dynamically regulated by metabolic demands. Melanoma cells always have a skewed balance with activated HIF-1α and suppressed PGC1α, creating an environment beneficial to aerobic glycolysis.[37] The constitutively activated BRAF upregulates HIF-1α[41,43,44] and inhibits PGC1α signaling.[40,45]

The transcription level of PGC1α is activated by a microphthalmia-associated transcription factor

(MITF).[40] MITF functions as a regulator of melanocyte development, survival, and differentiation through MITF's impact on the expression of various differentiation and cell-cycle genes.[46,47] Functional experiments also demonstrated that MITF is a dominant oncogene and that disruption of MITF sensitizes melanoma to conventional chemotherapeutic drugs.[48] While *MITF* gene amplification was found to affect around 15% to 20% of melanomas, gain-of-function mutations were found in familial and sporadic melanoma patients.[49] It was reported that the germline mutation *MITF* E318 K was reported in familial melanoma patients with a five-fold increased risk for melanoma.[49] This site is located in a small-ubiquitin-like modifier (SUMO) consensus site, and the mutation interferes with the SUMOylation of MITF. In addition, *MITF* E318K has a higher transcriptional activity than the wild-type *MITF*, promoting melanocyte clonogenicity, migration, and invasion, consistent with its role in tumorigenesis and metastasis.

Another characteristic of melanoma cells is to have suppressed energy-stress-mediated activation of LKB1 and AMPK signaling pathway. The melanoma $BRAF^{V600E}$ mutation functions to dismantle the LKB1 and AMPK complex by compromising LKB1 phosphorylation and reducing the binding and activation of AMPK, which is a key signaling pathway in regulating $BRAF^{V600E}$-mediated metabolism.[50,51]

Other melanoma-related susceptibility genes and pathways

CDKN2A and CDK4
CDKN2A is a tumor suppressor gene located on chromosome 9p21. It is frequently mutated in melanoma patients, accounting for up to 50% in sporadic melanomas,[52] and has high penetrance in familial melanoma.[53–55] *CDKN2A* encodes two proteins p16^{INK4A} and p14^{ARF}, both of which function as tumor suppressor proteins. P16^{INK4A} can bind to cyclin-dependent kinase 4 (CDK4), dismantling the cyclin D-CDK4 complex and the subsequent phosphorylation of retinoblastoma (Rb) family protein. The hypophosphorylated state of Rb protein facilitates its interaction with transcription factor E2F1,[56] leading to cell cycle arrest in G1 phase.[57,58] Mice lacking p16^{INK4A} have increased tumor formation, suggesting the critical role of p16^{INK4A} in restricting aberrant cell proliferation.[59] p14^{ARF}, another tumor suppressor, is encoded by exon 1β and exon 2 of *CDKN2A*. Interestingly, ARF is overexpressed in p53-deficient cells, suggesting an interplay between ARF and p53.[60] For instance, ARF was reported to inhibit

cell transformation induced by murine double minute 2 (MDM2), but this activity was abolished in p53-deficient cells.[61] Furthermore, biochemical studies demonstrated that ARF interacted with MDM2, inhibiting the degradation of p53.[62] Interestingly, mice with ARF deficiency develop lymphoma and carcinoma,[60] attesting to the tumor suppressor role of p14^{ARF}.

CDK4 is one member of the cyclin-dependent kinase family, which is responsible for cell-cycle progression and controls the transcriptional process. CDK4 is known as an oncogene, and germline mutations in CDK4 have been detected in a handful of familial melanoma patients. It has been shown that CDK4 is able to cooperate with active *BRAF* or *NRAS* mutants[63,64] to promote cancer progression. As mentioned previously, CDK4 interacts with p16^{INK4A}, which specifically hampers the assembly of cyclin D-CDK4 complex. Therefore, in melanoma, the loss of p16^{INK4A} unleashes the cyclin D-CDK4 complex, driving cell cycle progression and leading to aberrant proliferation. In addition, the germline mutation Arg24Cys of *CDK4* (R24C) was identified in two melanoma-prone families. *CDK4* (R24C) can function as a tumor-specific antigen in sporadic melanoma.[65] Mechanistically, R24C is located in the *CDK4* binding domain to prevent p16^{INK4A}-CDK4 complex formation.[66] Mice harboring the *CDK4* R24C mutation phenocopied the p16^{INK4A}-deficient mice, displaying increased carcinogen-induced melanoma formation.[67,68] These findings indicate that although the loss of p16^{INK4A} or activation of CDK4 alone is not sufficient to induce melanoma, it does predispose mice to tumorigenesis.

DDX3X

In a recent study conducted by Alkallas and colleagues, they found a previously unrecognizable RNA helicase, DDX3X, to be highly associated with cutaneous melanoma.[69] *DDX3X* is a tumor suppressor gene that escapes X chromosome inactivation.[70] Alkallas and colleagues found that this gene is more frequently mutated in males, with its loss of function (LOF) mutations found exclusively in males with reduced protein expression levels as a consequence of the mutations.[69] Through gene set enrichment analysis, patients with DDX3X LOF mutations had upregulated genes involved in tumor metastasis, including *RAS*, *PI3K*, and β-Catenin signaling pathways, and had downregulated genes involved in the cell cycle and RNA metabolism. These results suggest that the *DDX3X* LOF mutation plays an important role in melanoma tumorigenesis.[69,71]

Telomeres

Telomeres are repetitive DNA sequences located at the end of chromosomes. The existence of telomeres helps to protect the end of chromosomes from random DNA breaks and avoid inappropriate end-to-end fusion among different chromosomes.[72] The telomeres represent the fragile sites in chromosomes, which are protected by "capping," a combination of high-order DNA structure and telomere-binding proteins, which helps reduce the DNA damage response and unwanted DNA repair. It has been well documented that cell proliferation is invariably accompanied by telomere shortening,[73] implying that the gradual overall decrease in telomere length over time is due to aging.

One mechanism that counteracts the shortening of telomere is telomerase. Telomerase is a ribonucleoprotein enzyme that synthesizes new telomeric DNA to compensate for the telomere attrition during replication.[74] Telomerase is a protein-RNA complex consisting of telomerase reverse transcriptase (TERT), telomerase RNA, and dyskerin. Compared with normal cells, cancer cells have a higher level of telomerase, due to increased TERT expression or enhanced TERT activity.[74,75] TERT promoter mutations are common in melanoma patients.[76,77] These mutations correlated with disease severity and poor prognosis.[78] Through linkage analysis and high-throughput sequencing in the melanoma-prone families not carrying germline mutations in CDKN2A or CDK4, a new germline mutation (c.-57 T>G) in TERT promoter was identified.[76] In addition, somatic mutations in TERT promoter including c. −124 C>T (C228T) and c. −146 C>T (C250T) were also found in melanoma samples.[77] All these mutations enhanced the expression of TERT[79,80] and telomerase activity, thereby preventing the shortening of telomeres.

In addition, exome and whole-genome sequencing revealed that protection of telomeres 1 gene (POT1) variants are a new predisposition factor to familial melanoma.[81,82] POT1, a component of the shelterin complex (a hexameric nucleoprotein complex), is known to have critical functions in maintaining telomere integrity, by binding directly to single-stranded telomeric DNA. Missense variants in POT1 disrupt the interaction of POT1 with telomeres and are associated with increased telomere length,[82] thus increasing the risk of melanoma. Another study reported the role of the other shelterin complex members besides POT1 in cutaneous malignant melanoma.[83] It concluded that mutations in adrenocortical dysplasia protein homolog and telomeric repeat-binding factor 2-interacting protein are associated with melanoma occurrence,[83] further suggesting that telomere dysregulation is important for melanoma development.

DNA Repair

DNA repair process protects the human genome from damage caused by DNA lesions, mutations, and DNA strand breaks.[84] The fulfillment of the DNA repair process includes several parallel pathways, such as excision repair, mismatch repair, and recombination repair.[85] Although DNA repair can help clear damaged DNA, the residual lesions can accumulate and drive the cell to carcinogenic transformation.[86] When mutation numbers reach up to 10^5 per cell, this is regarded as a driving force for tumorigenesis.[85,87] In terms of response to drug therapy, low activity of DNA repair genes renders tumor cells more sensitive to drugs, while high activity of DNA repair genes might confer tumor cell drug resistance.[88]

Xeroderma pigmentosum (XP) is an autosomal recessive disorder, which is caused by a disruption in DNA repair. Clinically, the symptoms include photosensitivity, actinic skin damage, and UV radiation–induced skin cancer, including melanoma.[89] In vitro cultured cells from XP patients manifested hypersensitivity to UV radiation and its mimetic chemical compounds.[90] UV exposure is thought to cause DNA breaks, which are typically mended by the nucleotide excision repair pathway. However, in XP cells, DNA breaks cannot be properly repaired. Thus, these XP cells become precancerous and carry the characteristic sign of UV mutagenesis, a C-to-T mutation.[90]

Melanocortin Receptor Mutations

Human melanin pigmentation protects the skin from damage caused by ultraviolet radiation.[91] It comprises two different types: the red phaeomelanin and the black eumelanin. The black eumelanin is photoprotective, while the red phaeomelanin might promote UV-induced skin damage because of its ROS production.[91] However, one recent study indicates phaeomelanin can generate ROS without UV exposure,[92] suggesting a completely UV-independent pathway leading to carcinogenesis.

The relative amount of these two melanins is regulated by melanocyte-stimulating hormone, which acts on its receptor melanocortin 1 receptor (MC1R) to increase the synthesis of eumelanin.[91] It was first reported that more than 80% of the people who had red hair or fair skin that tanned poorly had MC1R variations, but this percentage dropped sharply in people with brown or black hair (~20%) or people who had good tanning response (<4%).[93] In the wake of this study, accumulating studies showed that MC1R Asp84Glu variation is highly associated with an increased risk of melanoma.[94,95] Other variations such as Arg151Cys, Arg160Trp, and Asp294His are also reported to be melanoma risk factors.[94]

As mentioned previously, the tumorigenesis of melanoma can be independent of UV exposure, but the underlying mechanism is not fully understood. One recent case-control study recruited melanoma patients with and without sunburns and control participants in an attempt to dissect out MC1R variants as a potential risk factor for melanoma while controlling for previous UV exposure. They found that individuals carrying MC1R variants had a higher risk of melanoma than the wild-type carriers, irrespective of UV exposure history, implicating MC1R as a UV-independent intrinsic risk factor.[96]

Overall, MC1R mutations conferred individuals with a higher intrinsic risk of melanoma, which can work in conjunction with UV exposure to contribute to melanoma formation. The presented evidence also highlights the need to take both MC1R risk variants and UV-induced ROS into consideration regarding precaution against melanoma.

SUMMARY

Our review summarizes the most recent, emerging pathways critical in melanoma development and discusses how genetic and environmental factors contribute to melanoma formation and progression. The hot-spot mutations found in melanoma often occur in genes that encode key regulators for cell growth and differentiation (see **Table 1**), invariably leading to aberrant activation of downstream signaling pathways (see **Fig. 1**). This dysregulation, either inherited from germline mutation or caused by somatic mutation, confers a higher risk of tumorigenesis to mutation carriers and/or increases the aggressiveness of melanomas that develop. In light of the causative role of these mutations and dysregulated pathways in melanoma formation and progression, targeted therapies against these mutations and pathways have been developed with promising efficacy. Future studies are required to continue the discovery of genetic mutations and their impact on signaling pathways and cellular behavior to facilitate the development of new strategies for melanoma prevention, screening, and treatment.

DISCLOSURE

The authors have no disclosures or conflicts of interest.

REFERENCES

1. Matthews NH, Li WQ, Qureshi AA, et al. Epidemiology of melanoma. In: Ward WH, Farma JM, editors. Cutaneous melanoma: etiology and therapy. 2017.
2. Fecher LA, Amaravadi RK, Flaherty KT. The MAPK pathway in melanoma. Curr Opin Oncol 2008; 20(2):183–9.
3. Cossa G, Gatti L, Cassinelli G, et al. Modulation of sensitivity to antitumor agents by targeting the MAPK survival pathway. Curr Pharm Des 2013; 19(5):883–94.
4. Burotto M, Chiou VL, Lee JM, et al. The MAPK pathway across different malignancies: a new perspective. Cancer 2014;120(22):3446–56.
5. Colombino M, Capone M, Lissia A, et al. BRAF/NRAS mutation frequencies among primary tumors and metastases in patients with melanoma. J Clin Oncol 2012;30(20):2522–9.
6. Davies H, Bignell GR, Cox C, et al. Mutations of the BRAF gene in human cancer. Nature 2002; 417(6892):949–54.
7. Nikolaev SI, Rimoldi D, Iseli C, et al. Exome sequencing identifies recurrent somatic MAP2K1 and MAP2K2 mutations in melanoma. Nat Genet 2011;44(2):133–9.
8. Pollock PM, Harper UL, Hansen KS, et al. High frequency of BRAF mutations in nevi. Nat Genet 2003;33(1):19–20.
9. Curtin JA, Fridlyand J, Kageshita T, et al. Distinct sets of genetic alterations in melanoma. N Engl J Med 2005;353(20):2135–47.
10. Cohen JV, Sullivan RJ. Developments in the space of new MAPK pathway inhibitors for BRAF-mutant melanoma. Clin Cancer Res 2019;25(19):5735–42.
11. Uribe P, Andrade L, Gonzalez S. Lack of association between BRAF mutation and MAPK ERK activation in melanocytic nevi. J Invest Dermatol 2006;126(1): 161–6.
12. Halaban R. RAC1 and melanoma. Clin Ther 2015; 37(3):682–5.
13. Bauer NN, Chen YW, Samant RS, et al. Rac1 activity regulates proliferation of aggressive metastatic melanoma. Exp Cell Res 2007;313(18):3832–9.
14. Krauthammer M, Kong Y, Ha BH, et al. Exome sequencing identifies recurrent somatic RAC1 mutations in melanoma. Nat Genet 2012;44(9):1006–14.
15. Lionarons DA, Hancock DC, Rana S, et al. RAC1(P29S) induces a mesenchymal phenotypic switch via serum response factor to promote melanoma development and therapy resistance. Cancer cell 2019;36(1):68–83.e9.
16. Watson IR, Li L, Cabeceiras PK, et al. The RAC1 P29S hotspot mutation in melanoma confers resistance to pharmacological inhibition of RAF. Cancer Res 2014;74(17):4845–52.

17. Zhan T, Rindtorff N, Boutros M. Wnt signaling in cancer. Oncogene 2017;36(11):1461–73.

18. Chien AJ, Moore EC, Lonsdorf AS, et al. Activated Wnt/beta-catenin signaling in melanoma is associated with decreased proliferation in patient tumors and a murine melanoma model. Proc Natl Acad Sci U S A 2009;106(4):1193–8.

19. Mosimann C, Hausmann G, Basler K. Beta-catenin hits chromatin: regulation of Wnt target gene activation. Nat Rev Mol Cell Biol 2009;10(4):276–86.

20. Delmas V, Beermann F, Martinozzi S, et al. Beta-catenin induces immortalization of melanocytes by suppressing p16INK4a expression and cooperates with N-Ras in melanoma development. Genes Dev 2007;21(22):2923–35.

21. Pawlikowski JS, McBryan T, van Tuyn J, et al. Wnt signaling potentiates nevogenesis. Proc Natl Acad Sci U S A 2013;110(40):16009–14.

22. O'Connell MP, Fiori JL, Baugher KM, et al. Wnt5A activates the calpain-mediated cleavage of filamin A. J Invest Dermatol 2009;129(7):1782–9.

23. Webster MR, Xu M, Kinzler KA, et al. Wnt5A promotes an adaptive, senescent-like stress response, while continuing to drive invasion in melanoma cells. Pigment Cell Melanoma Res 2015;28(2):184–95.

24. Anastas JN, Kulikauskas RM, Tamir T, et al. WNT5A enhances resistance of melanoma cells to targeted BRAF inhibitors. J Clin Invest 2014;124(7):2877–90.

25. Grossmann AH, Yoo JH, Clancy J, et al. The small GTPase ARF6 stimulates beta-catenin transcriptional activity during WNT5A-mediated melanoma invasion and metastasis. Sci Signal 2013; 6(265):ra14. https://doi.org/10.1126/scisignal.2003398.

26. Mikels AJ, Nusse R. Purified Wnt5a protein activates or inhibits beta-catenin-TCF signaling depending on receptor context. PLoS Biol 2006;4(4):e115.

27. Davies MA. The role of the PI3K-AKT pathway in melanoma. Cancer J 2012;18(2):142–7.

28. Mancinelli R, Carpino G, Petrungaro S, et al. Multifaceted roles of GSK-3 in cancer and autophagy-related diseases. Oxid Med Cell Longev 2017;2017: 4629495.

29. Gajos-Michniewicz A, Czyz M. WNT signaling in melanoma. Int J Mol Sci 2020;21(14). https://doi.org/10.3390/ijms21144852.

30. Lee YR, Chen M, Pandolfi PP. The functions and regulation of the PTEN tumour suppressor: new modes and prospects. Nat Rev Mol Cell Biol 2018; 19(9):547–62.

31. Wu H, Goel V, Haluska FG. PTEN signaling pathways in melanoma. Oncogene 2003;22(20): 3113–22.

32. Damsky WE, Curley DP, Santhanakrishnan M, et al. beta-catenin signaling controls metastasis in Braf-activated Pten-deficient melanomas. Cancer Cell 2011;20(6):741–54.

33. Deberardinis RJ, Sayed N, Ditsworth D, et al. Brick by brick: metabolism and tumor cell growth. Curr Opin Genet Dev 2008;18(1):54–61.

34. Lunt SY, Vander Heiden MG. Aerobic glycolysis: meeting the metabolic requirements of cell proliferation. Annu Rev Cell Dev Biol 2011;27:441–64.

35. Ratnikov BI, Scott DA, Osterman AL, et al. Metabolic rewiring in melanoma. Oncogene 2017;36(2): 147–57.

36. Scott DA, Richardson AD, Filipp FV, et al. Comparative metabolic flux profiling of melanoma cell lines: beyond the Warburg effect. J Biol Chem 2011; 286(49):42626–34.

37. Abildgaard C, Guldberg P. Molecular drivers of cellular metabolic reprogramming in melanoma. Trends Mol Med 2015;21(3):164–71.

38. Parmenter TJ, Kleinschmidt M, Kinross KM, et al. Response of BRAF-mutant melanoma to BRAF inhibition is mediated by a network of transcriptional regulators of glycolysis. Cancer Discov 2014;4(4): 423–33.

39. Zeller KI, Jegga AG, Aronow BJ, et al. An integrated database of genes responsive to the Myc oncogenic transcription factor: identification of direct genomic targets. Genome Biol 2003;4(10):R69. https://doi.org/10.1186/gb-2003-4-10-r69.

40. Haq R, Shoag J, Andreu-Perez P, et al. Oncogenic BRAF regulates oxidative metabolism via PGC1alpha and MITF. Cancer cell 2013;23(3):302–15.

41. Kumar SM, Yu H, Edwards R, et al. Mutant V600E BRAF increases hypoxia inducible factor-1alpha expression in melanoma. Cancer Res 2007;67(7):3177–84.

42. Chau MD, Gao J, Yang Q, et al. Fibroblast growth factor 21 regulates energy metabolism by activating the AMPK-SIRT1-PGC-1alpha pathway. Proc Natl Acad Sci U S A 2010;107(28):12553–8.

43. Damsky W, Micevic G, Meeth K, et al. mTORC1 activation blocks BrafV600E-induced growth arrest but is insufficient for melanoma formation. Cancer cell 2015;27(1):41–56.

44. Haq R, Fisher DE, Widlund HR. Molecular pathways: BRAF induces bioenergetic adaptation by attenuating oxidative phosphorylation. Clin Cancer Res 2014;20(9):2257–63.

45. Vredeveld LC, Possik PA, Smit MA, et al. Abrogation of BRAFV600E-induced senescence by PI3K pathway activation contributes to melanomagenesis. Genes Dev 2012;26(10):1055–69.

46. Levy C, Khaled M, Fisher DE. MITF: master regulator of melanocyte development and melanoma oncogene. Trends Mol Med 2006;12(9):406–14.

47. Widlund HR, Fisher DE. Microphthalamia-associated transcription factor: a critical regulator of pigment cell development and survival. Oncogene 2003;22(20):3035–41.

48. Garraway LA, Widlund HR, Rubin MA, et al. Integrative genomic analyses identify MITF as a lineage

survival oncogene amplified in malignant melanoma. Nature 2005;436(7047):117–22.

49. Bertolotto C, Lesueur F, Giuliano S, et al. A SUMOylation-defective MITF germline mutation predisposes to melanoma and renal carcinoma. Nature 2011;480(7375):94–8.

50. Zheng B, Jeong JH, Asara JM, et al. Oncogenic B-RAF negatively regulates the tumor suppressor LKB1 to promote melanoma cell proliferation. Mol Cell 2009;33(2):237–47.

51. Esteve-Puig R, Canals F, Colome N, et al. Uncoupling of the LKB1-AMPKalpha energy sensor pathway by growth factors and oncogenic BRAF. PLoS One 2009;4(3):e4771.

52. Zhao R, Choi BY, Lee MH, et al. Implications of genetic and epigenetic alterations of CDKN2A (p16(INK4a)) in cancer. EBioMedicine 2016;8:30–9.

53. Paluncic J, Kovacevic Z, Jansson PJ, et al. Roads to melanoma: key pathways and emerging players in melanoma progression and oncogenic signaling. Biochim Biophys Acta 2016;1863(4):770–84.

54. Hussussian CJ, Struewing JP, Goldstein AM, et al. Germline p16 mutations in familial melanoma. Nat Genet 1994;8(1):15–21.

55. ul Alam MN. Computational assessment of somatic and germline mutations of p16INK4a: Structural insights and implications in disease. Inform Med Unlocked 2019;17:100208.

56. Serrano M. The tumor suppressor protein p16INK4a. Exp Cell Res 1997;237(1):7–13.

57. Serrano M, Hannon GJ, Beach D. A new regulatory motif in cell-cycle control causing specific inhibition of cyclin D/CDK4. Nature 1993;366(6456):704–7.

58. Goldstein AM, Struewing JP, Chidambaram A, et al. Genotype-phenotype relationships in U.S. melanoma-prone families with CDKN2A and CDK4 mutations. J Natl Cancer Inst 2000;92(12):1006–10.

59. Krimpenfort P, Quon KC, Mooi WJ, et al. Loss of p16Ink4a confers susceptibility to metastatic melanoma in mice. Nature 2001;413(6851):83–6.

60. Kamijo T, Zindy F, Roussel MF, et al. Tumor suppression at the mouse INK4a locus mediated by the alternative reading frame product p19ARF. Cell 1997;91(5):649–59.

61. Pomerantz J, Schreiber-Agus N, Liegeois NJ, et al. The Ink4a tumor suppressor gene product, p19Arf, interacts with MDM2 and neutralizes MDM2's inhibition of p53. Cell 1998;92(6):713–23.

62. Kamijo T, Weber JD, Zambetti G, et al. Functional and physical interactions of the ARF tumor suppressor with p53 and Mdm2. Proc Natl Acad Sci U S A 1998;95(14):8292–7.

63. Chudnovsky Y, Adams AE, Robbins PB, et al. Use of human tissue to assess the oncogenic activity of melanoma-associated mutations. Nat Genet 2005;37(7):745–9.

64. Sheppard KE, McArthur GA. The cell-cycle regulator CDK4: an emerging therapeutic target in melanoma. Clin Cancer Res 2013;19(19):5320–8.

65. Zuo L, Weger J, Yang Q, et al. Germline mutations in the p16INK4a binding domain of CDK4 in familial melanoma. Nat Genet 1996;12(1):97–9.

66. Coleman KG, Wautlet BS, Morrissey D, et al. Identification of CDK4 sequences involved in cyclin D1 and p16 binding. J Biol Chem 1997;272(30):18869–74.

67. Rane SG, Cosenza SC, Mettus RV, et al. Germ line transmission of the Cdk4(R24C) mutation facilitates tumorigenesis and escape from cellular senescence. Mol Cell Biol 2002;22(2):644–56.

68. Sotillo R, Dubus P, Martin J, et al. Wide spectrum of tumors in knock-in mice carrying a Cdk4 protein insensitive to INK4 inhibitors. EMBO J 2001;20(23):6637–47.

69. Alkallas R, Lajoie M, Moldoveanu D, et al. Multi-omic analysis reveals significantly mutated genes and DDX3X as a sex-specific tumor suppressor in cutaneous melanoma. Nat Cancer 2020;1(6):635–52.

70. Dunford A, Weinstock DM, Savova V, et al. Tumor-suppressor genes that escape from X-inactivation contribute to cancer sex bias. Nat Genet 2017;49(1):10–6.

71. Phung B, Ciesla M, Sanna A, et al. The X-Linked DDX3X RNA helicase dictates translation reprogramming and metastasis in melanoma. Cell Rep 2019;27(12):3573–3586 e7.

72. Wong JMY, Collins K. Telomere maintenance and disease. Lancet 2003;362(9388):983–8.

73. Harley CB, Futcher AB, Greider CW. Telomeres shorten during ageing of human fibroblasts. Nature 1990;345(6274):458–60.

74. Reddel RR. Telomere maintenance mechanisms in cancer: clinical implications. Curr Pharm Des 2014;20(41):6361–74.

75. Wu KJ, Grandori C, Amacker M, et al. Direct activation of TERT transcription by c-MYC. Nat Genet 1999;21(2):220–4.

76. Horn S, Figl A, Rachakonda PS, et al. TERT promoter mutations in familial and sporadic melanoma. Science 2013;339(6122):959–61.

77. Huang FW, Hodis E, Xu MJ, et al. Highly recurrent TERT promoter mutations in human melanoma. Science 2013;339(6122):957–9.

78. Populo H, Boaventura P, Vinagre J, et al. TERT promoter mutations in skin cancer: the effects of sun exposure and X-irradiation. J Invest Dermatol 2014;134(8):2251–7.

79. Heidenreich B, Nagore E, Rachakonda PS, et al. Telomerase reverse transcriptase promoter mutations in primary cutaneous melanoma. Nat Commun 2014;5:3401.

80. Heidenreich B, Kumar R. TERT promoter mutations in telomere biology. Mutat Res 2017;771:15–31.

81. Shi J, Yang XR, Ballew B, et al. Rare missense variants in POT1 predispose to familial cutaneous malignant melanoma. Nat Genet 2014;46(5):482–6.

82. Robles-Espinoza CD, Harland M, Ramsay AJ, et al. POT1 loss-of-function variants predispose to familial melanoma. Nat Genet 2014;46(5):478–81.

83. Aoude LG, Pritchard AL, Robles-Espinoza CD, et al. Nonsense mutations in the shelterin complex genes ACD and TERF2IP in familial melanoma. J Natl Cancer Inst 2015;107(2). https://doi.org/10.1093/jnci/dju408.

84. Chatterjee N, Walker GC. Mechanisms of DNA damage, repair, and mutagenesis. Environ Mol Mutagen 2017;58(5):235–63.

85. Kiwerska K, Szyfter K. DNA repair in cancer initiation, progression, and therapy-a double-edged sword. J Appl Genet 2019;60(3–4):329–34.

86. Jackson SP, Bartek J. The DNA-damage response in human biology and disease. Nature 2009; 461(7267):1071–8.

87. Broustas CG, Lieberman HB. DNA damage response genes and the development of cancer metastasis. Radiat Res 2014;181(2):111–30.

88. Housman G, Byler S, Heerboth S, et al. Drug resistance in cancer: an overview. Cancers (Basel) 2014;6(3):1769–92.

89. Kraemer KH, Lee MM, Andrews AD, et al. The role of sunlight and DNA repair in melanoma and nonmelanoma skin cancer. The xeroderma pigmentosum paradigm. Arch Dermatol 1994;130(8):1018–21.

90. DiGiovanna JJ, Kraemer KH. Shining a light on xeroderma pigmentosum. J Invest Dermatol 2012;132(3 Pt 2):785–96.

91. Brenner M, Hearing VJ. The protective role of melanin against UV damage in human skin. Photochem Photobiol 2008;84(3):539–49.

92. Mitra D, Luo X, Morgan A, et al. An ultraviolet-radiation-independent pathway to melanoma carcinogenesis in the red hair/fair skin background. Nature 2012;491(7424):449–53.

93. Valverde P, Healy E, Jackson I, et al. Variants of the melanocyte-stimulating hormone receptor gene are associated with red hair and fair skin in humans. Nat Genet 1995;11(3):328–30.

94. Kennedy C, ter Huurne J, Berkhout M, et al. Melanocortin 1 receptor (MC1R) gene variants are associated with an increased risk for cutaneous melanoma which is largely independent of skin type and hair color. J Invest Dermatol 2001;117(2): 294–300.

95. Valverde P, Healy E, Sikkink S, et al. The Asp84Glu variant of the melanocortin 1 receptor (MC1R) is associated with melanoma. Hum Mol Genet 1996;5(10): 1663–6.

96. Wendt J, Rauscher S, Burgstaller-Muehlbacher S, et al. Human determinants and the role of melanocortin-1 receptor variants in melanoma risk independent of UV radiation exposure. JAMA Dermatol 2016;152(7): 776–82.

Immunobiology of Melanoma

Yee Peng Phoon, PhD, LRI/CCF[a], Charles Tannenbaum, PhD, LRI/CCF[a], C. Marcela Diaz-Montero, PhD, LRI/CCF[b],*

KEYWORDS

- Immunoediting • Immunosurveillance • Immunosuppression • Melanoma

KEY POINTS

- Interaction between the host immune system and the tumor microenvironment is explored.
- Regulation and modulation of host immune networks are highly dependent on host–tumor interaction.
- Suppression of immunity in the tumor microenvironment is reviewed.

INTRODUCTION

Skin cancer is one of the most common cancers. Although melanoma accounts for only a very small percentage of skin cancers, it is one of the most aggressive forms of skin cancer in the United States.[1] For the past 5 decades, the incidence of melanoma has increased significantly as compared with other cancers.[2] A 47% increase year over year in new invasive melanoma cases from 2010 to 2020[3,4] has been observed, with approximately 100,000 new cases and nearly 7000 deaths in the United States[5] in 2020 alone.

In addition to acting as a protective, physical barrier, the skin also functions as an immunologic barrier capable of responding to environmental risk factors such as the sun's UV rays, chemical carcinogens, and pathogens including oncogenic viruses.[2,6] An immune monitoring system termed "immunosurveillance" protects the tissues by eliminating both damaged cells, and foreign pathogens and restoring homeostasis by the synergistic interaction of leukocytes and lymphocytes that are recruited to sites of infection.

Failing to achieve equilibrium or the restoration of homeostasis often leads to chronic local inflammation, which in addition to genetic instability can lead to cancer progression. Aberrant cells that successfully escape immunosurveillance will continue to thrive, proliferate and eventually develop into melanoma.[7–10] **Fig. 1** illustrates the key role that immunosurveillance plays in preventing disease progression.

Melanoma is one of the most immunogenic forms of human cancer, rendering it particularly susceptible to immunotherapy. Indeed, it was for metastatic melanoma[11] that the US Food and Drug Administration (FDA) first approved immune checkpoint inhibition (ICI) as an antitumor, immunopotentiating intervention. Despite recent advances in ICI, only 50% of treated patients show favorable outcomes, with the remaining nonresponders failing to achieve any sustained therapeutic benefits.[12] What distinguishes those who respond to ICI from those who do not remains unclear, although it is thought that the heterogeneity and complexity of patient tumor microenvironment (TMEs) likely play a role. Therefore, despite the decades-long advancements we have achieved in understanding the mechanisms by which various molecular mediators of ICI enhance antitumor immune responses (**Fig. 2**), the immunobiology of melanoma remains understudied.[6,13,14] It is imperative that continued effort is exerted to understand the immune biology of melanoma. This article provides an overview of the immunobiology of melanoma in the context of immunoediting, immune evasion and escape, highlighting too the key

[a] Cleveland Clinic, Lerner Research Institute, Department of Inflammation and Immunity, 9500 Euclid Avenue, Cleveland, Ohio 44195, USA; [b] Cleveland Clinic, Lerner Research Institute, Center for Immunotherapy and ImmunoOncology, 9500 Euclid Avenue, Cleveland, Ohio 44195, USA
* Corresponding author.
E-mail address: diazc2@ccf.org

Clin Plastic Surg 48 (2021) 561–576
https://doi.org/10.1016/j.cps.2021.06.005
0094-1298/21/© 2021 Elsevier Inc. All rights reserved.

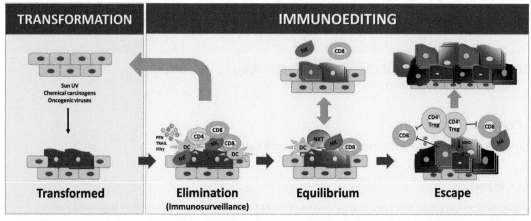

Fig. 1. Cancer immunoediting process.

immune mediators of the antitumor immune response, and the contribution that the extensive heterogeneity of melanoma plays in evading those interventions.

CANCER IMMUNOEDITING AND IMMUNOSURVEILLANCE

Immunology is now center stage owing to current coronavirus pandemic. However, immunologic concepts have been appreciated as early as 2000 BC, when the very first disease and pestilence was documented in the Babylonian Epic of Gilgamesh[6,13,14] (see **Fig. 2**). In fact, the word "immunity" was derived from the Latin word "immunitas" (meaning exemption from liability or taxes), describing protection and resistance to

diseases or infections.[13] The field of immunology has progressed tremendously since then, not only in the context of infection diseases, but also for cancer treatment. The earliest evidence that immune responses might be effective against cancer was reported in 1893 by a surgeon in New York, William Coley.[13–15]

The concept that immune surveillance plays a role in preventing tumor development was introduced more than one century ago. In the early twentieth century (1909), it was Paul Ehrlich who first proposed that the immune system prevented and repressed tumor progression.[8,16] It was not until 50 years later that F. Macfarlane Burnet and Lewis Thomas reintroduced the concept of immune surveillance and natural defense against cancer, hypothesizing that malignant cells are

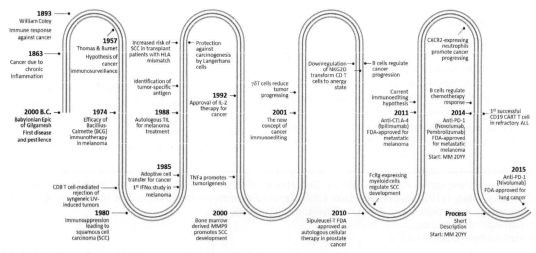

Fig. 2. Timeline of the development of immunobiology and immunotherapy.

eliminated by the recognition of tumor specific neoantigens on cancer cells. Then, in 1953, using in vivo mouse models[7,8,16,17] Gross and then Foley independently demonstrated that immune response could be stimulated against sarcoma and methycholantrene-induced tumors, respectively. Building on these classic hypotheses, the concept of immunosurveillance was introduced and validated in the 1990s.[7-9,18] More recent work demonstrated that the interaction between host immune systems TME are not 1 dimensional but a dynamic process, which is now known as immunoediting.[7-9,19] Immunosurveillance and immunoediting of cancer are now understood to be integral to both tumor eradication and tumor evasion, respectively. In fact, both processed involve a continuous dynamic interplay between the innate immune response, the adaptive immune milieus, and the TME throughout the entire cycle of tumorigenesis.[7-9,20] The process of immunoediting comprises of 3 main phases: elimination (also known as immunosurveillance), equilibrium, and escape (see **Fig. 1**)

Elimination, classically known as immunosurveillance, represents the first phase of immunoediting and involves the recruitment of innate and adaptive immune cells to identify and eradicate tumor cells, thus protecting the host from developing cancer. If tumors are not destroyed during the elimination phase, they enter the equilibrium phase, an immune-mediated tumor dormancy stage in which tumor variants with acquired resistance to immune system evolve. Finally, these tumor variants may eventually enter the escape phase by evading the immune system and successfully proliferating unimpeded.[7-9,21]

The notion that immunosurveillance normally plays a role in preventing human cancer was revisited when researchers started to ask whether immunodeficient or immunosuppressed patients are more prone to develop malignant neoplasms.[7-9,22] As a result of those studies, it is now established that immunologic deficiencies are key promoters of tumorigenesis, and that immunosurveillance is an extrinsic tumor suppressor, safeguarding immunocompetent hosts from cancer development.[7-9,20,22,23]

In this regard, it is not surprising that melanoma, known for being a highly immunogenic tumor, undergoes dynamic immunomodulation and immunoediting. Throughout the elimination phase of immunosurveillance, a series of immunologic events leading to antimelanoma cytotoxicity occurs within the TME involving both the innate and adaptive immune response,[7-9,16,24] and the recruitment of various immune effectors including T cells, B cells, natural killer (NK) cells, and

dendritic cells (DCs). Indeed, to effectively eradicate melanoma, a sequence of immune responses need to transpire, including T-cell activation, homing of activated T cells to the TME or peripheral tissues, and the identification and targeting of melanoma cells by activated T cells, leading to the apoptosis and death of tumor cells[24] (**Fig. 3**).

Despite vigorous immune surveillance and an initial elimination of neoplastic cells, some resilient tumor variants arise through mutations that are capable of eluding the immunosurveillance armory and enter into equilibrium phase. These surviving tumor cells achieve dynamic equilibrium and initially coexist with host immune cells, creating an extended period of latency. This tumor dormancy phase triggers a selection process that favors tumor cells that can escape the host immune system and subsequently proliferate to cause clinical disease. Unlike the elimination stage, the major player in the equilibrium phase is adaptive immunity, which is comprised of cytokines (eg, IFN-γ, IL-12 and IL-23), CD4$^+$ regulatory T cells, CD8$^+$ T cells, and NK T cells; innate immunity plays only a minimal role in this phase.[7-9,20,23] The tumor variants that eventually emerge from the equilibrium phase are those that were initially conditioned in the TME to escape during the immunoediting process.

The edited tumor cells that successfully enter the escape phase can now progress unimpeded because the host immune cells is lees effective at constraining their growth. Depending on the immune components that sculpted the tumor cells in the latency period, each tumor cell that escapes may possess a unique mechanistic signature that allowed it to survive; thus, different means of escape are due to different immunologic mechanisms.[8,20,21,25] Some tumor cells elude adaptive immune detection by altering the antigen presentation pathway. Numerous studies have shown that many tumor cells exhibit decreased expression of immunogenic tumor antigens and either fewer major histocompatibility complex class 1 (MHC) molecules or a complete loss of HLA class I proteins.[8,26,27] Another possible escape mechanism involves upregulation of antiapoptotic pathways and oncogenes, which inhibits immune-mediated cytotoxicity.[8,20] Recently, additional evidence demonstrates that tumors also circumvent host immune defenses by activating immunosuppressive mechanisms. Tumors actively elicit the generation of immunosuppressive T-cell subpopulations such as CD4$^+$CD25$^+$FOXP3$^+$ regulatory T cells, IL-13–producing NKT cells, and myeloid-derived suppressor cells (MDSC).[8,20,23,28,29] In addition to immunosuppressive T cells, tumors also generate and activate immunosuppressive cytokines

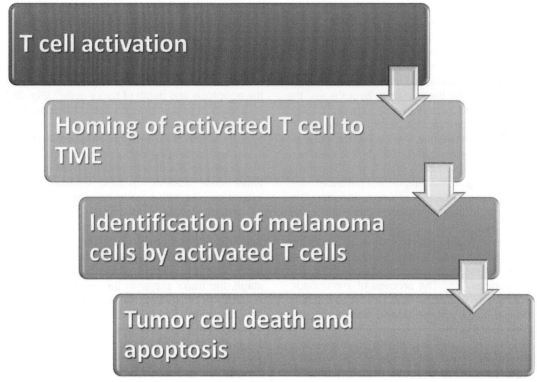

Fig. 3. Immune mechanisms during tumor cells eradication.

including transforming growth factor beta (TGF-β), IL-10, and vascular endothelial growth factor (VEGF).[8,30] Moreover, tumor cells possess the ability to acquire immune resistance by overexpressing immune checkpoint ligands (eg, programmed death ligand 1 [PD-L1]), which have the capacity to turn off tumor-specific T cells that enter the TME.

Decades of study have led to the development of immunotherapies that revolutionized the treatment of cancers, particularly advanced melanoma.[12,31,32] Nevertheless, nearly one-half of the patients with advanced melanoma receiving immunotherapy still fail to benefit from an attempt to reinvigorate the antitumor immune response.[12] Therefore, further studies are needed to more definitively elucidate how key immunologic players do effectively mediate each phase of tumor cell immunoediting. Only with such in depth understanding will we discover novel targets against refractory cancers.

Immune Response to Melanoma

The optimal goal of immunotherapy is to orchestrate a sustained immune response against tumors with minimal deleterious effects on normal tissues. To achieve an effective antitumor immune response, the host immune system must initiate the series of immune reactions described by Chen and Mellman.[33] Their "cancer immunity cycle" describes the 7-step process by which the host immune system interacts with the TME to eliminate cancer cells, including: (1) the release of tumor antigen, (2) tumor antigen presentation, (3) T-cell priming and activation, (4) T-cell trafficking, (5) T-cell infiltration into tumors, (6) T-cell recognition of tumor cells, and (7) T-cell killing of tumor cells (**Fig. 4**). Despite the existence of this protective response, there are inhibitory and negative regulatory mechanisms capable of interfering with each of the steps, any one of which could minimize the effectiveness of the cancer immunity cycle.[20,33]

The first evidence that an immune response to melanoma existed was the recognition that a spontaneous regression of primary tumors occurred mainly when lymphocytes were found to infiltrate the TME. In fact, the existence of melanoma-specific cytotoxic lymphocytes (CTL) was discovered in the early 1980s.[34–40] To date, numerous unique melanoma tumor antigens that promote melanoma-associated CTL activity have been identified and reported including melanoma antigen family A1 (MAGE-A1), and a tyrosinase family melan-A and gp100. These melanoma-specific antigens have been shown to be

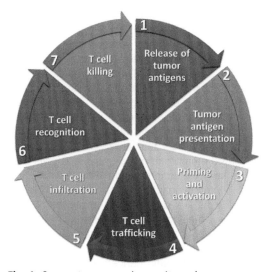

Fig. 4. Seven-step cancer immunity cycle.

recognized by autologous CD8[+] CTL in an MHC-1 restricted manner. Recently, apart from CD8[+] CTL responses, CD4[+] T cells and NK cells were also found to be involved in antitumor response in melanoma.[34,41] However, melanoma tumors seem to have only low expression levels of MHC molecules, minimizing antigen presentation and eventually facilitating immune escape.[34,42] Importantly, melanoma cells also seem to possess the ability to induce T-cell anergy by downregulating costimulatory molecules like B7-1 and B7-2. Decreased signaling by these costimulatory molecules impaired immune responses.[34,43,44]

To achieve sustained antitumor responses, the elements of the immune system need to work synergistically to fight tumors. Hence, the primary focus of this section is to provide a basic introduction to the major immune players that interact in a melanoma TME, including tumor-infiltrating lymphocytes (TILs), DC and NK cells. In addition, the role of tumor antigens and cytokines in eradicating melanoma will also be covered in this section.

Tumor Antigens

In 1991, MAGE-A1[20,45] was identified as the first human gene known to encode a human tumor antigen. MAGE-A1 was also found to be expressed by numerous other malignant tissues, including lung and breast cancers.[20,46] Although primary melanomas express MAGE-A1 in only 16% to 20% of their tumor cells, metastatic melanomas express the antigen at levels that are more than 2-fold higher (48%–50%).[46] Interestingly, MAGE-A1 is not found in normal tissues.[20,47] Since the first discovery of human tumor antigens,

significant effort has been devoted to grouping them into 3 main categories based on their expression patterns and origins: (1) antigens stemming from mutations, translocations, and other genetic modifications, or that are virally encoded genes, collectively known as tumor-specific antigens or neoantigens (eg, the BCR/ABL fusion protein in leukemia), (2) overexpression of proto-oncogenes, as compared with their levels in normal tissues (eg, human epidermal growth factor 2 [HER2 or ERBB2] in breast cancer), and (3) nonmutated genes expressed at elevated levels in tumor cells and germline cells, known as cancer–testis antigens (eg, MAGE). Other cancer–testis antigens include G antigen, B-M antigen-1, New York esophageal squamous cell carcinoma-1 (NY-ESO-1), and preferentially expressed antigen of melanoma (PRAME) families that are mostly melanoma associated.[20,48–50]

Tumor antigens have been used for multiple purposes, such as cancer vaccines, biomarkers of disease for diagnostic purposes, targeted adoptive T-cell therapy, and complementary target in combination immunotherapy.[20,48,49,51,52] Despite being used as targets for immunotherapy, most tumor antigens only elicit weak antitumor responses. Hence, it is not surprising that tumor antigen-targeted therapies have not resulted in sustained regressions of melanoma lesions.[20,53,54] Among the tumor antigens that have been targeted for melanoma immunotherapy to date are MAGE, NY-ESO-1 and melanoma-associated tyrosinase family protein (eg, tyrosinase, tyrosinase-related proteins 1 and 2), tyrosinase family melan-A-1, and gp100 (pmel17), all of which are mainly restricted to having their peptides presented on HLA-A2.[20,48,55,56]

Immunotherapy targeting the MAGE family proteins initially showed encouraging results in phase I and II studies. After these apparent successes, a vaccine targeting MAGE-A3 protein was developed and assessed in the DERMA phase III clinical trial in combination with an immune stimulant in patients with melanoma after surgery.[20,57] Disappointingly, this trial was ended in 2016 without demonstrating antitumor efficacy (NCT 00796445). The NY-ESO-1 antigen also continues to be used in immunotherapy trials either as a tumor vaccine or for adoptive transfer therapy.[20,58,59] The adoptive transfer trial using transgenic T cells with NY-ESO-1–specific T-cell receptors showed promising results, with 55% of treated patients with melanoma exhibiting positive responses.[20,58,59] Immunotherapies targeting NY-ESO-1 continue to be assessed for their efficacy in numerous clinical trials.[60] The PRAME tumor antigen family is another group of tumor antigens that is being assessed for safety, immunogenicity and clinical activity. A dose escalation phase I and II study of PRAME-directed immunotherapy that combined recombinant PRAME protein (recPRAME) and the AS15 immuno-stimulant to treat advanced patients with melanoma reported an acceptable safety profile and displayed similar humoral and cellular immune responses in all cohorts (NCT01149343).[61] These studies led to the realization that other factors need to be taken into consideration when attempting to develop effective tumor antigen-based immunotherapies, including the delivery vector, the immunogen (RNA, DNA, or protein), and suitable adjuvants, and not just the specific type of tumor antigen.

Tumor-Infiltrating Lymphocytes

As noted elsewhere in this article, multiple elements of the immune system need to work in concert for immunotherapy to work effectively and safely. Unfortunately, the TME is typically in an immunosuppressive state, particularly in advanced cancers, which is a key stumbling block to effective immunotherapy that renders a patient susceptible to unabated tumor progression.[62] Tumor-mediated immunosuppression can result from activation of regulatory T cells or impaired tumor infiltration of T cells. Additionally, T cells that manage to infiltrate the TME are frequently in an exhausted or dysfunctional state.[20,63] Exhausted T cells are hyporesponsive to antigen, resulting in minimal cytokine release and diminished cytotoxic activity, often termed a state of anergy.[63,64] Nonetheless, many studies have demonstrated that there is a direct correlation of TIL, especially CTLs, with a better disease prognosis.[20,65,66] In contrast, the infiltration of tumors by regulatory T cells such as $CD4^+CD25^+FOXP3^+$ lymphocytes (Treg) correlates with negative disease outcomes for many forms of cancer.[20,67,68]

Cells infiltrating the TME are highly heterogeneous and consist of a large array of immune cells including lymphocytes (eg, $CD4^+$ and $CD8^+$ T cells), B cells, NK cells, macrophages, and DCs.[20,66,69] The specific cells infiltrating a TME can be prognostic for patient outcome.[20,70–73] $CD3^+CD8^+$ TILs are often considered a critical prognostic marker in disease stage classification and for predicting clinical responses. The importance of $CD3^+$ and $CD8^+$ TILs, in combination with cells bearing the CD45RO T-cell memory marker, is exemplified by their use in an "immunoscore," a novel classification system for cancer. In fact, this immunoscore classification system surpasses the conventional American Joint Commission on Cancer TNM system for prognosis of early stage colorectal cancer. Although it is currently being evaluated in melanoma, it has yet to be tested in large patient cohorts.[20,71] Tertiary lymphoid structures (TLS) in cancers have also been gaining more interest lately. These structures consist of immune cell aggregates within complex immune structures, and seem to have favorable predictive and prognostic value.[73–75] The TLS are rich in mature DCs that express DC–lysosomal associated membrane protein, and in B cells that play a key role in producing essential chemokines.[20] Interestingly, the discovery of a 12-chemokine signature identified the existence of TLS in late stage melanoma, and importantly their presence positively correlated with better overall survival.[20,76] The presence of TLS in colorectal, breast, and pancreatic cancers was also shown to have a good prognostic value.[73] These findings strongly suggest an important role of TLS in protective immunity against cancer.

It is now understood that tumors synthesize molecules such as PD-L1, PD-L2, VEGF, and $TGF\beta$[20,77] that can either suppress effector T cell responses or even render tumor infiltrating T cells anergic and incapable of mediating protective activities. Tumors also chemoattract immunosuppressive cell types such as MDSCs. MDSCs are a highly heterogenous cell population. Based on their similarities to either monocytes or neutrophiles they are grouped as monocytic MDSC or polymorphonucleated-MDSC, respectively. MDSCs are known to promote tumor progression by suppressing antitumor immune responses and by inducing angiogenesis, which synthesize a panel of immunoinhibitory molecules such as indoleamine-2,3-dioxygenase (IDO), which also prevents effective T-cell–mediated antitumor responses.[20,78] IDO-expressing tumor cells were shown to enhance tumor progression and associate with immunotherapy resistance through the recruitment and activation of MDSCs. In human melanoma tumors, the expression of IDO is associated with infiltration of MDSCs, that in turn induced immunosuppression.[79] Moreover, patients with melanoma with IDO-positive sentinel have higher IDO-expressing PBMCs, particularly in monocytic MDSCs and DCs.[80] In addition, polymorphonuclear MDSCs secrete immunosuppressive molecule IL-1β that induce infiltration of these polymorphonuclear MDSCs into tumors to promote tumorigenesis.[81] Apart from the immunosuppressive role of MDSCs, these cells are also proangiogenic through secretion of VEGF, IL-10, arginase I, matrix metalloproteinase members, and proinflammatory S100 family members.[82–84] In sum, MDSCs play key roles in immunosuppression and proangiogenic processes through the induction and secretion of numerous factors including cytokines, proangiogenic, and immunoinhibitory molecules.

Conventionally, CD8[+] and CD4[+] T cells are considered the prominent effector lymphocytes capable of eradicating tumor cells.[20,55] The efficiency of both CD8[+] and CD4[+] effector T cells in modulating immune responses is highly dependent on the specificity of T-cell receptor signaling. During cell-mediated immune responses, their cytotoxic function is fueled by production of the IFN-γ and tumor necrosis factor-α produced after T-cell receptor–MHC/tumor peptide interactions.[16] However, molecules generated within the TME are capable of transforming CD8[+] and CD4[+] T cells into inhibitory T cells (eg, CD8[+] exhausted T cells and CD4[+] Treg) that lose their ability to kill tumor cells.[20,55,78] Tumor infiltrating CD4[+]FOXP3[+] Treg have recently found to be significantly associated with unfavorable overall survival rates in 17 different types of cancer, including melanoma and cervical, renal, and breast cancers. In contrast, expression of CD4[+]FOXP3[+] Tregs is associated with better overall survival rates in colorectal, head and neck, and esophageal cancers,[20,85] suggesting that there is some heterogeneity of the CD4[+]FOXP3[+] Treg subpopulation in the TME. Two distinct nonsuppressive CD4[+]FOXP3[lo]–infiltrating Treg subsets were discovered in colorectal cancer: (1) a low frequency FOXP3[lo] Treg (<9.8%), and (2) a high frequency FOXP3[lo] Treg (>9.8%) with elevated messenger RNA expression of IL-12A and TGF-β1, which have improved disease free survival.[20,86] Thus, given the high heterogeneity of TILs, a single prognostic marker may not accurately predict successful antitumor immune responses. Instead, perhaps a combination of prognostic and predictive markers might provide a better prediction value for antitumor immunity.

Classically, cytotoxic CD8 T cells are known to be critical in immunotherapy effectiveness; improving tumor eradication. Until recently, CD8 T cells with high expression of checkpoints such as programmed cell death 1 (PD-1) and T-cell immunoglobulin and mucin-domain containing-3 (TIM-3) are functionally exhausted.[87–90] However, numerous studies using advanced transcriptome analysis have identified significant heterogeneity within CD3[+]CD8[+]PD-1[+] T cells, which previously were thought to be dogmatically exhausted. In fact, a unique and highly proliferative subset of CD8 T cells were identified in these exhausted T cells.[91–94] There have been conflicting reports on the role of these CD8 T cells in the response to immunotherapy in melanoma.[93–96] Interestingly,

exhausted CD8[+]PD-1[+]TIM-3[+] T cells from tumor are capable of suppressing healthy T cells and are associated with ICI resistance.[97–100] These findings suggest that exhausted CD8 T cells are highly heterogenous, proliferative, functionally suppressive and associated with ICI resistance.

In addition to T cells, ongoing studies are currently examining the roles of B cells in the TME. Reports indicate that increased numbers of CD20[+] B cells among melanoma TILs predict better patient survival.[20,101] Some studies also demonstrated the possibility that putative regulatory B cells exist that can secrete immunosuppressive IL-10 and TGF-β.[102]

There are multiple mechanisms mediating the immune regulation of TILs in the TME that could be potential targets of immunotherapies. However, there are also numerous redundant pathways facilitating immune escape, resulting in the failure to eradicate tumor cells. Thus, there is a pressing need to explore novel immunotherapeutic and combinatorial interventions that are not solely dependent on T cells. Such therapies might also include other subpopulations such as NK cells, tumor-associated macrophages, and tumor-infiltrating DC, which collectively could lead to greater antitumor efficacy.

Dendritic Cells

DCs are purportedly the most efficient cell type capable of stimulating naïve antigen-specific CD8[+] T cells to becoming fully activated, cytotoxic effectors. For mature DCs to effectively activate a naïve T cell, an number of cell–cell interactions are required to ensure full maturation and proper cross-priming. These mechanisms include (1) the binding of a T cell's T-cell receptor with an antigen-presenting cell's MHC/peptide complexes (2) costimulatory signaling via the binding of CD80/CD86 on DCs with CD28 expressed on T cells, (3) induction of cytokine signaling, and (4) the expression of tumor-derived chemokines to traffic the now activated T cells from the lymph nodes to the TME.[16,103–106] In cancer, interference with any of these interactions would prevent an effective T-cell–mediated antitumor responses.

In contrast, tumor-infiltrating DC are more commonly immunosuppressive owing to their loss of costimulatory molecules CD80 and CD86, and hence their inefficiency at presenting antigens.[20,107,108] As with TIL, immunosuppressive factors within the TME such as VEGF, TGFβ, and IDO can transform tumor-infiltrating DC into immunosuppressive cells. Additionally, the increased expression of immune checkpoint receptors including PD-1 and TIM-3 diminishes the ability to DCs to activate immune responses.[20,107] These tumor-infiltrating DC-derived immunosuppressive molecules can in turn stimulate the synthesis of inhibitory cytokines such as IL-10 and/or TGFβ, which feedback to further induce the suppressive effects of tumor-infiltrating DC. The regulatory tumor-infiltrating DC mediate immunosuppression in the TME through either inhibition of T-cell proliferation, the generation of Treg, the production of anergic T cells and the activation of PD-1/PD-L1 pathway.[109–111] Despite numerous studies demonstrating that tumor-infiltrating DC are able to mediate their immunosuppressive effects via multiple mechanisms, the ability to distinguish conventional DC from immunosuppressive DC in patients with melanoma remains a challenge.[110,112–117] For that reason antimelanoma interventions based on targeting tumor-infiltrating DC have not been thoroughly explored, leaving that as an area of potential future investigation.

Although studies have also demonstrated the ability of DCs to suppress immune responses under specific circumstances, the mechanism by which occurs is still largely unexplored. The key function of DCs is to process and present antigen to T cells, and they do so by placing the peptides from extracellular antigens on MHC class II molecules, and peptides from intracellular antigens on MHC class I molecules. DCs also have the capacity to present extracellular antigens on MHC class I molecules to activate CD8[+] cytotoxic T cells by a process known as cross-presentation.[20,118–120] Numerous in vitro and in vivo studies have demonstrated the ability of DC vaccine to induce tumor-specific T-cell immunity.[121–124] These reports highlight the vital role of DC-based vaccines in cancer treatment. In fact, in the 1990s, DC-based immunotherapies have entered into clinical trials to treat various cancers, including melanoma, colorectal cancer, and lymphoma.[125–128] Despite showing a good safety profile and improved antitumor immunity, the clinical responses are not too promising, with tumor response rates of approximately 15%.[129] Emerging paradigms of combinations of DC vaccines with other cancer therapies, such as adoptive T-cell transfer and ICI, has shown great potential in improving clinical responses.[130–133] For example, ICI-resistant metastatic patients with melanoma treated with combination of tumor-infiltrating lymphocyte adoptive T-cell transfer and DC vaccination showed complete and sustained clinical responses. These recent findings represent and pave the next key strategy of DC-based combinatorial treatment modalities in treating patients with cancer.

Natural Killer Cells

NK cells are innate lymphocytes that mediate protective responses against both pathogens and cancer cells.[20,134] Depending on the surface markers expressed by their potential targets, NK cells can either be activated or suppressed. Human NK cells are characterized by being CD3[−]CD56[+] and expressing NKp46 surface receptors. They can be further subdivided by their differential expression of CD16 and CD56 surface markers, that is, subpopulations that are either CD16[+]CD56[dim] or CD16[−]CD56[bright]. In addition to CD3-CD56+ NK cells, there is also a subset of CD3[+]CD56[+] NK cells known as NKT cells. Canonical NK cells recognize tumor cells that have downregulated MHC class I molecule expression, whereas others can bind to antibody-expressing tumor cells.[20,134] NK cells induce their cytotoxic effects through the production of granzymes, perforin, FasL, and tumor necrosis factor-related apoptosis inducing ligand. After activation, NK cells secrete proinflammatory cytokines and IFN-γ that subsequently attract more immune cell subsets into the inflammatory site.[20,134] Thus, it is not surprising that some studies reported that infiltrating NK cells seems to have positive prognostic value in numerous cancers.[135]

In vitro studies indicate that melanoma cell lines express elevated levels of ligands that are known to activate antitumor responses by NK cells by binding the NK "activating receptors" NKG2D, DNAM1, and NKp30.[20,136] Melanoma cells are known to downregulate their MHC class I expression in an attempt to circumvent CD8[+] CTL defenses, leaving them open to attack by NK cells based on both their low MHC class I expression and the capacity of melanoma surface molecules to bind NK cell activating receptors.[136] However, melanoma still seems capable of escaping NK cell attack by multiple mechanisms. Through the process of immunoediting, metastatic melanoma cells can either gain more MHC class I expression or downregulate NK ligands by decreasing MICA expression.[136] Melanoma cells also inhibit NK cells by upregulating TIGIT, IDO and/or prostaglandin E2. Some melanomas and other cancers, including breast and colon cancer, are found to be infiltrated by a regulatory CD56[bright] NK cell subpopulation.[20,137]

Despite these inconsistent findings, NK cells are still considered a vital target for antitumor immunotherapy. In fact, autologous and allogeneic NK cell adoptive therapy has been used to treat advanced melanoma started from as early as the 1980s, and is still being tested in clinical trials.[20,136,138–140] Importantly, 2 monoclonal antibodies used for NK cell blockade (lirilumab, anti-KIR and monalizumab (IPH2201), anti-NKG2A/CD94) have been developed and are currently being investigated in clinical trials either as monotherapy or combinatorial therapy.[141–144] For example, lirilumab is being used in combination with anti–PD-1 and anti–CTLA-4 for treating advanced solid tumors (NCT03203876, NCT01714739) and monalizumab is being used with cetuximab (anti-epidermal growth factor receptor) in metastatic head and neck cancers (NCT04590963, NCT02643550) or with durvalumab (a human IgGκ monoclonal antibody blocking interaction of PD-L1 with PD-1) for the therapy of advanced solid tumors (NCT02671435). Nevertheless, further study of NK cells as anticancer agents, particularly in melanoma, is required to better understand the underlying mechanism involved in effective NK immunity. It is crucial to discover NK cell subpopulations that might be able to mediate sustained antitumor responses.

Cytokines

The melanoma TME is characterized by a diverse cytokine and chemokine composition. Some cytokines exert proinflammatory effects such as tumor necrosis factor-α, IL-16, IL-17, IL-21, IL-22, and IL-23, and are often associated with tumorigenesis, although cytokines such as IFN-γ and IL-12 are instead associated with cytolytic immune responses and antitumor activity.[70,145–149] In contrast, immunosuppressive cytokines including IL-10 and TGF-β are secreted by regulatory T cells and are known to inhibit antitumor immune responses.[145,146,150–152] Melanoma cells themselves also produce a set of cytokines, including basic fibroblast growth factor, platelet-derived growth factor, melanoma growth stimulatory activity, IL-1, IL-6, IL-8, and granulocyte–macrophage colony-stimulating factor[34] that, when secreted into the TME, regulate immune responses by multiple mechanisms. Although melanoma-derived IL-6 mostly inhibits the immune response, the granulocyte-macrophage colony-stimulating factor secreted by melanomas can both downregulate antitumor responses,[34,153,154] or promote them by recruiting DCs to the tumor to facilitate the presentation of tumor antigens.[34,155]

The discovery of cytokines led to several preclinical and clinical trials using cytokine-based therapy to treat numerous type of diseases in the 1980s and 1990s.[156–164] Two cytokines, IL-2 and IFN-γ, were approved by the FDA for treatment of several cancers. Based on durability of treatment responses, high-dose IL-2 therapy was approved for treatment of patients with metastatic renal cancer in 1992 and for metastatic melanoma in 1998.[160,165] IFN-γ was first granted FDA approval in 1995 as an adjuvant therapy for patients with advanced melanoma after surgery.[166] Then, in 2011, pegylated interferon was approved by the FDA to treat resected node-positive melanoma.[166] Since then, other cytokines also have entered into clinical trials, including IL-7, IL-10, IL-15, IL-21, and IL-10.[156,167–172] The clinical application of these cytokines represents an important milestone in cancer immunotherapy, demonstrating favorable regulation of antitumor immune responses. However, many of these high-dose cytokine-based immunotherapies have intolerable high toxicity and low antitumor efficacy.[156] Despite these setbacks, cytokine-based immunotherapy continues to revolutionize to better enhance clinical response with minimal toxicity. At present, cytokine-based therapy is used to treat cancers in combination with ICI immunotherapy.[156,167,173,174] These combinatorial therapies are rapidly entering into clinical trial, investigating the safety and effectiveness of these treatments.[156,173,175,176] Finding synergistic combinations of cytokine-based therapies with other cancer immunotherapy modalities, such as ICIs, TIL therapies, will mark the next milestone in cancer immunotherapy.

SUMMARY

There is compelling evidence to implicate the cells and molecules of the immune system in the development of melanoma. Understanding how elements of the immune system interact with tumor cells in the TME has also provided insight into the role of immunosurveillance in both eradicating tumor cells and selecting for variants capable of immune escape.[16] Most significantly, understanding the cellular and molecular events that govern either tumor destruction or tumor progression have led to novel treatment strategies and new targets for immunotherapy. Indeed, more durable clinical responses are now being achieved with recently developed mono- and combo-immunotherapies.[12,31,32,177] In fact, immunotherapy is currently one of the first line treatment strategies for numerous forms of metastatic malignancies including head and neck cancer, colorectal cancer and non-small cell lung cancer.[16,178–180] However, despite recent advances in immunotherapy, there remains a large subset of patients that fail to benefit or achieve a sustained and durable clinical response,[12] which requires additional research to understand the complex cellular and molecular interactions of immune effectors that occur in the TME. For example, what individual or combinatorial immunologic interventions will overcome the resistance that different tumors display for current therapies, and what is the optimal treatment sequence that will enhance their effectiveness?

The next meaningful achievement in the realm of cancer treatment will be a personalized form of precision medicine. To make personalized immunotherapies a reality, continuous and collaborative efforts are required to comprehensively interrogate the tumor–host relationship. Leveraging the current state-of-the-art technologies such as single cell RNA sequencing, spatial multiomics, and humanized mouse models provides us with more sensitive and precise methods to elucidate exactly how the immune system can be manipulated to more potently mediate antitumor responses. Understanding the immunobiology of melanoma will be an important step in developing personalized immunotherapies in the near future.

CLINICS CARE POINTS

- Advances in understanding immunobiology have greatly improved current immunotherapeutic interventions for patients with cancer.

- However, there remains a subset of patients with melanoma that fails to sustain durable antitumor responses.

- Despite improved efficacy using various ICI combinations, there are challenges that remain unanswered:

  o Identification of predictive markers identifying refractory patients,

  o Deciphering mechanistic networks and pathways that contribute to treatment failure, and

  o Discovery of novel, targetable drugs for refractory patients.

- Efforts to address these challenges are hampered by the vast immune diversity that characterizes different TME, a phenomenon that is still largely understudied.

- A better understanding of the immunobiology of melanoma holds great promise for the development of precision and personalized immunotherapy, which will significantly improve patient care.

DISCLOSURE

The authors have no conflicts of interest to declare.

REFERENCES

1. About melanoma skin cancer. Available at: https://www.cancer.org/cancer/melanoma-skin-cancer/about/key-statistics.html.

2. Coricovac D, Dehelean C, Moaca EA, et al. Cutaneous melanoma-a long road from experimental models to clinical outcome: a review. Int J Mol Sci 2018;19(6):1566.

3. Cancer facts & figures 2020. Atlanta: American Cancer Society; 2020.

4. Cancer facts & figures 2010. Atlanta: American Cancer Society; 2010.

5. Siegel RL, Miller KD, Jemal A. Cancer statistics, 2020. CA Cancer J Clin 2020;70(1):7–30.

6. Medler TR, Coussens LM. Duality of the immune response in cancer: lessons learned from skin. J Invest Dermatol 2014;134(e1):E23–8.

7. Dunn GP, Bruce AT, Ikeda H, et al. Cancer immunoediting: from immunosurveillance to tumor escape. Nat Immunol 2002;3(11):991–8.

8. Dunn GP, Old LJ, Schreiber RD. The immunobiology of cancer immunosurveillance and immunoediting. Immunity 2004;21(2):137–48.

9. Dunn GP, Old LJ, Schreiber RD. The three Es of cancer immunoediting. Annu Rev Immunol 2004; 22:329–60.

10. Swann JB, Smyth MJ. Immune surveillance of tumors. J Clin Invest 2007;117(5):1137–46.

11. Alva A, Daniels GA, Wong MK, et al. Contemporary experience with high-dose interleukin-2 therapy and impact on survival in patients with metastatic melanoma and metastatic renal cell carcinoma. Cancer Immunol Immunother 2016;65(12):1533–44.

12. Larkin J, Chiarion-Sileni V, Gonzalez R, et al. Five-year survival with combined nivolumab and ipilimumab in advanced melanoma. N Engl J Med 2019; 381(16):1535–46.

13. Doherty M, Robertson MJ. Some early trends in immunology. Trends Immunol 2004;25(12):623–31.

14. Galon J, Bruni D. Tumor immunology and tumor evolution: intertwined histories. Immunity 2020; 52(1):55–81.

15. McCarthy EF. The toxins of William B. Coley and the treatment of bone and soft-tissue sarcomas. Iowa Orthop J 2006;26:154–8.

16. Passarelli A, Mannavola F, Stucci LS, et al. Immune system and melanoma biology: a balance between immunosurveillance and immune escape. Oncotarget 2017;8(62):106132–42.

17. Palmieri G, Ombra M, Colombino M, et al. Multiple molecular pathways in melanomagenesis: characterization of therapeutic targets. Front Oncol 2015;5:183.

18. Smyth MJ, Godfrey DI, Trapani JA. A fresh look at tumor immunosurveillance and immunotherapy. Nat Immunol 2001;2(4):293–9.

19. Shankaran V, Ikeda H, Bruce AT, et al. IFNgamma and lymphocytes prevent primary tumour development and shape tumour immunogenicity. Nature 2001;410(6832):1107–11.

20. Sadozai H, Gruber T, Hunger RE, et al. Recent successes and future directions in immunotherapy of cutaneous melanoma. Front Immunol 2017;8:1617.

21. Mittal D, Gubin MM, Schreiber RD, et al. New insights into cancer immunoediting and its three component phases–elimination, equilibrium and escape. Curr Opin Immunol 2014;27:16–25.

22. Herrera-Gonzalez NE. Interaction between the immune system and melanoma. In: Davids LM, editor. Recent advances in the biology, therapy and management of melanoma. IntechOpen; 2013.

23. Cali B, Molon B, Viola A. Tuning cancer fate: the unremitting role of host immunity. Open Biol 2017; 7(4):170006.

24. Mahmoud F, Shields B, Makhoul I, et al. Immune surveillance in melanoma: from immune attack to melanoma escape and even counterattack. Cancer Biol Ther 2017;18:451–69.

25. Vesely MD, Kershaw MH, Schreiber RD, et al. Natural innate and adaptive immunity to cancer. Annu Rev Immunol 2011;29:235–71.

26. Algarra I, Cabrera T, Garrido F. The HLA crossroad in tumor immunology. Hum Immunol 2000;61(1): 65–73.

27. Marincola FM, Jaffee EM, Hicklin DJ, et al. Escape of human solid tumors from T-cell recognition: molecular mechanisms and functional significance. Adv Immunol 2000;74:181–273.

28. Terabe M, Berzofsky JA. Immunoregulatory T cells in tumor immunity. Curr Opin Immunol 2004;16(2): 157–62.

29. Diaz-Montero CM, Salem ML, Nishimura MI, et al. Increased circulating myeloid-derived suppressor cells correlate with clinical cancer stage, metastatic tumor burden, and doxorubicin-cyclophosphamide chemotherapy. Cancer Immunol Immunother 2009; 58(1):49–59.

30. Khong HT, Restifo NP. Natural selection of tumor variants in the generation of "tumor escape" phenotypes. Nat Immunol 2002;3(11):999–1005.

31. Hodi FS, Chiarion-Sileni V, Gonzalez R, et al. Nivolumab plus ipilimumab or nivolumab alone versus ipilimumab alone in advanced melanoma (CheckMate 067): 4-year outcomes of a multicentre, randomised, phase 3 trial. Lancet Oncol 2018;19(11): 1480–92.

32. Larkin J, Chiarion-Sileni V, Gonzalez R, et al. Combined nivolumab and ipilimumab or monotherapy in untreated melanoma. N Engl J Med 2015; 373(1):23–34.

33. Chen DS, Mellman I. Oncology meets immunology: the cancer-immunity cycle. Immunity 2013;39(1): 1–10.

34. Armstrong CA, Ansel JC. Immunology of malignant melanoma. Photochem Photobiol 1996;63(4): 418–20.

35. van der Bruggen P, Traversari C, Chomez P, et al. A gene encoding an antigen recognized by cytolytic T lymphocytes on a human melanoma. Science 1991;254(5038):1643–7.

36. Coulie PG, Brichard V, Van Pel A, et al. A new gene coding for a differentiation antigen recognized by autologous cytolytic T lymphocytes on HLA-A2 melanomas. J Exp Med 1994;180(1):35–42.

37. Kawakami Y, Eliyahu S, Delgado CH, et al. Cloning of the gene coding for a shared human melanoma antigen recognized by autologous T cells infiltrating into tumor. Proc Natl Acad Sci U S A 1994;91(9): 3515–9.

38. Kawakami Y, Eliyahu S, Delgado CH, et al. Identification of a human melanoma antigen recognized by tumor-infiltrating lymphocytes associated with in vivo tumor rejection. Proc Natl Acad Sci U S A 1994;91(14):6458–62.

39. Kawakami Y, Eliyahu S, Sakaguchi K, et al. Identification of the immunodominant peptides of the MART-1 human melanoma antigen recognized by the majority of HLA-A2-restricted tumor infiltrating lymphocytes. J Exp Med 1994;180(1):347–52.

40. Kawakami Y, Eliyahu S, Jennings C, et al. Recognition of multiple epitopes in the human melanoma antigen gp100 by tumor-infiltrating T lymphocytes associated with in vivo tumor regression. J Immunol 1995;154(8):3961–8.

41. Topalian SL, Rivoltini L, Mancini M, et al. Human CD4+ T cells specifically recognize a shared melanoma-associated antigen encoded by the tyrosinase gene. Proc Natl Acad Sci U S A 1994; 91(20):9461–5.

42. Ferrone S, Marincola FM. Loss of HLA class I antigens by melanoma cells: molecular mechanisms, functional significance and clinical relevance. Immunol Today 1995;16(10):487–94.

43. Townsend SE, Allison JP. Tumor rejection after direct costimulation of CD8+ T cells by B7-transfected melanoma cells. Science 1993; 259(5093):368–70.

44. Chen L, McGowan P, Ashe S, et al. Tumor immunogenicity determines the effect of B7 costimulation on T cell-mediated tumor immunity. J Exp Med 1994;179(2):523–32.

45. De Plaen E, Lurquin C, Van Pel A, et al. Immunogenic (tum-) variants of mouse tumor P815: cloning of the gene of tum- antigen P91A and identification of the tum- mutation. Proc Natl Acad Sci U S A 1988;85(7):2274–8.

46. Weon JL, Potts PR. The MAGE protein family and cancer. Curr Opin Cell Biol 2015;37:1–8.

47. Coulie PG, Van den Eynde BJ, van der Bruggen P, et al. Tumour antigens recognized by T

lymphocytes: at the core of cancer immunotherapy. Nat Rev Cancer 2014;14(2):135–46.

48. Vigneron N. Human tumor antigens and cancer immunotherapy. Biomed Res Int 2015;2015: 948501.

49. Yarchoan M, Johnson BA 3rd, Lutz ER, et al. Targeting neoantigens to augment antitumour immunity. Nat Rev Cancer 2017;17(9):569.

50. Epping MT, Bernards R. A causal role for the human tumor antigen preferentially expressed antigen of melanoma in cancer. Cancer Res 2006; 66(22):10639–42.

51. Pitcovski J, Shahar E, Aizenshtein E, et al. Melanoma antigens and related immunological markers. Crit Rev Oncol Hematol 2017;115:36–49.

52. Wong KK, Li WA, Mooney DJ, et al. Advances in therapeutic cancer vaccines. Adv Immunol 2016; 130:191–249.

53. Maverakis E, Cornelius LA, Bowen GM, et al. Metastatic melanoma - a review of current and future treatment options. Acta Derm Venereol 2015; 95(5):516–24.

54. Hinrichs CS, Restifo NP. Reassessing target antigens for adoptive T-cell therapy. Nat Biotechnol 2013;31(11):999–1008.

55. Hadrup S, Donia M, Thor Straten P. Effector CD4 and CD8 T cells and their role in the tumor microenvironment. Cancer Microenviron 2013;6(2):123–33.

56. Ramirez-Montagut T, Turk MJ, Wolchok JD, et al. Immunity to melanoma: unraveling the relation of tumor immunity and autoimmunity. Oncogene 2003;22(20):3180–7.

57. Saiag P, Gutzmer R, Ascierto PA, et al. Prospective assessment of a gene signature potentially predictive of clinical benefit in metastatic melanoma patients following MAGE-A3 immunotherapeutic (PREDICT). Ann Oncol 2016;27(10):1947–53.

58. Adams S, O'Neill DW, Nonaka D, et al. Immunization of malignant melanoma patients with full-length NY-ESO-1 protein using TLR7 agonist imiquimod as vaccine adjuvant. J Immunol 2008; 181(1):776–84.

59. Robbins PF, Kassim SH, Tran TL, et al. A pilot trial using lymphocytes genetically engineered with an NY-ESO-1-reactive T-cell receptor: long-term follow-up and correlates with response. Clin Cancer Res 2015;21(5):1019–27.

60. Thomas R, Al-Khadairi G, Roelands J, et al. NY-ESO-1 based immunotherapy of cancer: current perspectives. Front Immunol 2018;9:947.

61. Gutzmer R, Rivoltini L, Levchenko E, et al. Safety and immunogenicity of the PRAME cancer immunotherapeutic in metastatic melanoma: results of a phase I dose escalation study. ESMO Open 2016;1(4):e000068.

62. Dohms JE, Saif YM. Criteria for evaluating immunosuppression. Avian Dis 1984;28(2):305–10.

63. Speiser DE, Utzschneider DT, Oberle SG, et al. T cell differentiation in chronic infection and cancer: functional adaptation or exhaustion? Nat Rev Immunol 2014;14(11):768–74.

64. Jiang Y, Li Y, Zhu B. T-cell exhaustion in the tumor microenvironment. Cell Death Dis 2015;6:e1792.

65. Uppaluri R, Dunn GP, Lewis JS Jr. Focus on TILs: prognostic significance of tumor infiltrating lymphocytes in head and neck cancers. Cancer Immun 2008;8:16.

66. Fridman WH, Pages F, Sautes-Fridman C, et al. The immune contexture in human tumours: impact on clinical outcome. Nat Rev Cancer 2012;12(4): 298–306.

67. Takenaka M, Seki N, Toh U, et al. FOXP3 expression in tumor cells and tumor-infiltrating lymphocytes is associated with breast cancer prognosis. Mol Clin Oncol 2013;1(4):625–32.

68. Huang Y, Liao H, Zhang Y, et al. Prognostic value of tumor-infiltrating FoxP3+ T cells in gastrointestinal cancers: a meta analysis. PLoS One 2014;9(5): e94376.

69. Lee N, Zakka LR, Mihm MC Jr, et al. Tumour-infiltrating lymphocytes in melanoma prognosis and cancer immunotherapy. Pathology 2016;48(2): 177–87.

70. Weiss SA, Han SW, Lui K, et al. Immunologic heterogeneity of tumor-infiltrating lymphocyte composition in primary melanoma. Hum Pathol 2016;57: 116–25.

71. Galon J, Pages F, Marincola FM, et al. Cancer classification using the Immunoscore: a worldwide task force. J Transl Med 2012;10:205.

72. Jones GW, Hill DG, Jones SA. Understanding immune cells in tertiary lymphoid organ development: it is all starting to come together. Front Immunol 2016;7:401.

73. Sautes-Fridman C, Lawand M, Giraldo NA, et al. Tertiary lymphoid structures in cancers: prognostic value, regulation, and manipulation for therapeutic intervention. Front Immunol 2016;7:407.

74. Li Q, Liu X, Wang D, et al. Prognostic value of tertiary lymphoid structure and tumour infiltrating lymphocytes in oral squamous cell carcinoma. Int J Oral Sci 2020;12(1):24.

75. Engelhard VH, Rodriguez AB, Mauldin IS, et al. Immune cell infiltration and tertiary lymphoid structures as determinants of antitumor immunity. J Immunol 2018;200(2):432–42.

76. Messina JL, Fenstermacher DA, Eschrich S, et al. 12-Chemokine gene signature identifies lymph node-like structures in melanoma: potential for patient selection for immunotherapy? Sci Rep 2012;2:765.

77. Melero I, Rouzaut A, Motz GT, et al. T-cell and NK-cell infiltration into solid tumors: a key limiting factor for efficacious cancer immunotherapy. Cancer Discov 2014;4(5):522–6.

78. Speiser DE, Ho PC, Verdeil G. Regulatory circuits of T cell function in cancer. Nat Rev Immunol 2016;16(10):599–611.

79. Holmgaard RB, Zamarin D, Li Y, et al. Tumor-expressed Ido recruits and activates MDSCs in a treg-dependent manner. Cell Rep 2015;13(2):412–24.

80. Chevolet I, Speeckaert R, Schreuer M, et al. Characterization of the in vivo immune network of Ido, tryptophan metabolism, PD-L1, and CTLA-4 in circulating immune cells in melanoma. Oncoimmunology 2015;4(3):e982382.

81. Tannenbaum CS, Rayman PA, Pavicic PG, et al. Mediators of inflammation-driven expansion, trafficking, and function of tumor-infiltrating MDSCs. Cancer Immunol Res 2019;7(10):1687–99.

82. Albini A, Bruno A, Noonan DM, et al. Contribution to tumor angiogenesis from innate immune cells within the tumor microenvironment: implications for immunotherapy. Front Immunol 2018;9:527.

83. Sinha P, Okoro C, Foell D, et al. Proinflammatory S100 proteins regulate the accumulation of myeloid-derived suppressor cells. J Immunol 2008;181(7):4666–75.

84. Ye XZ, Yu SC, Bian XW. Contribution of myeloid-derived suppressor cells to tumor-induced immune suppression, angiogenesis, invasion and metastasis. J Genet Genomics 2010;37(7):423–30.

85. Shang B, Liu Y, Jiang SJ, et al. Prognostic value of tumor-infiltrating FoxP3+ regulatory T cells in cancers: a systematic review and meta-analysis. Sci Rep 2015;5:15179.

86. Saito T, Nishikawa H, Wada H, et al. Two FOXP3(+) CD4(+) T cell subpopulations distinctly control the prognosis of colorectal cancers. Nat Med 2016;22(6):679–84.

87. Gallimore A, Glithero A, Godkin A, et al. Induction and exhaustion of lymphocytic choriomeningitis virus-specific cytotoxic T lymphocytes visualized using soluble tetrameric major histocompatibility complex class I-peptide complexes. J Exp Med 1998;187(9):1383–93.

88. Zajac AJ, Blattman JN, Murali-Krishna K, et al. Viral immune evasion due to persistence of activated T cells without effector function. J Exp Med 1998;188(12):2205–13.

89. Wherry EJ. T cell exhaustion. Nat Immunol 2011;12(6):492–9.

90. Hashimoto M, Kamphorst AO, Im SJ, et al. CD8 T cell exhaustion in chronic infection and cancer: opportunities for interventions. Annu Rev Med 2018;69:301–18.

91. Thommen DS, Schumacher TN. T Cell dysfunction in cancer. Cancer Cell 2018;33(4):547–62.

92. Thommen DS, Koelzer VH, Herzig P, et al. A transcriptionally and functionally distinct pd-1 + cd8 + t cell pool with predictive potential in non-small-cell lung cancer treated with pd-1 blockade. Nat Med 2018;24:994–1004.

93. Auslander N, Zhang G, Lee JS, et al. Robust prediction of response to immune checkpoint blockade therapy in metastatic melanoma. Nat Med 2018;24(10):1545–9.

94. Sade-Feldman M, Yizhak K, Bjorgaard SL, et al. Defining T cell states associated with response to checkpoint immunotherapy in melanoma. Cell 2018;175:998–1013.e20.

95. Thommen DS, Koelzer VH, Herzig P, et al. A transcriptionally and functionally distinct PD-1(+) CD8(+) T cell pool with predictive potential in non-small-cell lung cancer treated with PD-1 blockade. Nat Med 2018;24(7):994–1004.

96. Li H, van der Leun AM, Yofe I, et al. Dysfunctional CD8 T cells form a proliferative, dynamically regulated compartment within human melanoma. Cell 2019;176(4):775–89.e8.

97. Montes CL, Chapoval AI, Nelson J, et al. Tumor-induced senescent T cells with suppressor function: a potential form of tumor immune evasion. Cancer Res 2008;68:870–9.

98. Maybruck BT, Pfannenstiel LW, Diaz-Montero M, et al. Tumor-derived exosomes induce CD8(+) T cell suppressors. J Immunother Cancer 2017;5(1):65.

99. Pfannenstiel LW, Diaz-Montero CM, Tian YF, et al. Immune-checkpoint blockade opposes CD8(+) T-cell suppression in human and murine cancer. Cancer Immunol Res 2019;3(3):510–25.

100. Zhang Y, Pfannenstiel LW, Bolesta E, et al. Interleukin-7 inhibits tumor-induced CD27-CD28- suppressor T cells: implications for cancer immunotherapy. Clin Cancer Res 2011;17(15):4975–86.

101. Chiaruttini G, Mele S, Opzoomer J, et al. B cells and the humoral response in melanoma: the overlooked players of the tumor microenvironment. Oncoimmunology 2017;6(4):e1294296.

102. Mauri C, Menon M. The expanding family of regulatory B cells. Int Immunol 2015;27(10):479–86.

103. Liu K, Nussenzweig MC. Development and homeostasis of dendritic cells. Eur J Immunol 2010;40(8):2099–102.

104. Liu K, Nussenzweig MC. Origin and development of dendritic cells. Immunol Rev 2010;234(1):45–54.

105. Tucci M, Stucci S, Passarelli A, et al. The immune escape in melanoma: role of the impaired dendritic cell function. Expert Rev Clin Immunol 2014;10(10):1395–404.

106. Schwartz RH. Costimulation of T lymphocytes: the role of CD28, CTLA-4, and B7/BB1 in interleukin-2 production and immunotherapy. Cell 1992;71(7):1065–8.

107. Tran Janco JM, Lamichhane P, Karyampudi L, et al. Tumor-infiltrating dendritic cells in cancer pathogenesis. J Immunol 2015;194(7):2985–91.

108. Ma Y, Shurin GV, Peiyuan Z, et al. Dendritic cells in the cancer microenvironment. J Cancer 2013;4(1): 36–44.

109. Zhao ZG, Xu W, Sun L, et al. The characteristics and immunoregulatory functions of regulatory dendritic cells induced by mesenchymal stem cells derived from bone marrow of patient with chronic myeloid leukaemia. Eur J Cancer 2012;48(12): 1884–95.

110. Shurin GV, Ma Y, Shurin MR. Immunosuppressive mechanisms of regulatory dendritic cells in cancer. Cancer Microenviron 2013;6(2):159–67.

111. Huang H, Dawicki W, Zhang X, et al. Tolerogenic dendritic cells induce CD4+CD25hiFoxp3+ regulatory T cell differentiation from CD4+CD25-/loFoxp3- effector T cells. J Immunol 2010;185(9):5003–10.

112. Norian LA, Rodriguez PC, O'Mara LA, et al. Tumor-infiltrating regulatory dendritic cells inhibit CD8+ T cell function via L-arginine metabolism. Cancer Res 2009;69(7):3086–94.

113. Fallarino F, Grohmann U, Vacca C, et al. T cell apoptosis by kynurenines. Adv Exp Med Biol 2003;527:183–90.

114. Mellor AL, Munn DH. Ido expression by dendritic cells: tolerance and tryptophan catabolism. Nat Rev Immunol 2004;4(10):762–74.

115. Muller AJ, Prendergast GC. Indoleamine 2,3-dioxygenase in immune suppression and cancer. Curr Cancer Drug Targets 2007;7(1):31–40.

116. Keir ME, Francisco LM, Sharpe AH. PD-1 and its ligands in T-cell immunity. Curr Opin Immunol 2007; 19(3):309–14.

117. Latchman YE, Liang SC, Wu Y, et al. PD-L1-deficient mice show that PD-L1 on T cells, antigen-presenting cells, and host tissues negatively regulates T cells. Proc Natl Acad Sci U S A 2004; 101(29):10691–6.

118. Vyas JM, Van der Veen AG, Ploegh HL. The known unknowns of antigen processing and presentation. Nat Rev Immunol 2008;8(8):607–18.

119. Joffre OP, Segura E, Savina A, et al. Cross-presentation by dendritic cells. Nat Rev Immunol 2012; 12(8):557–69.

120. Segura E, Amigorena S. Cross-presentation in mouse and human dendritic cells. Adv Immunol 2015;127:1–31.

121. Bender A, Sapp M, Feldman M, et al. Dendritic cells as immunogens for human CTL responses. Adv Exp Med Biol 1997;417:383–7.

122. Schuler G, Steinman RM. Dendritic cells as adjuvants for immune-mediated resistance to tumors. J Exp Med 1997;186(8):1183–7.

123. Schuler G, Schuler-Thurner B, Steinman RM. The use of dendritic cells in cancer immunotherapy. Curr Opin Immunol 2003;15(2):138–47.

124. Gong J, Chen D, Kashiwaba M, et al. Induction of antitumor activity by immunization with fusions of dendritic and carcinoma cells. Nat Med 1997; 3(5):558–61.

125. Escudier B, Dorval T, Chaput N, et al. Vaccination of metastatic melanoma patients with autologous dendritic cell (DC) derived-exosomes: results of the first phase I clinical trial. J Transl Med 2005; 3(1):10.

126. Carreno BM, Magrini V, Becker-Hapak M, et al. Cancer immunotherapy. A dendritic cell vaccine increases the breadth and diversity of melanoma neoantigen-specific T cells. Science 2015; 348(6236):803–8.

127. Reinhard G, Marten A, Kiske SM, et al. Generation of dendritic cell-based vaccines for cancer therapy. Br J Cancer 2002;86(10):1529–33.

128. Toh HC, Wang WW, Chia WK, et al. Clinical benefit of allogeneic melanoma cell Lysate-pulsed autologous dendritic cell vaccine in MAGE-positive colorectal cancer patients. Clin Cancer Res 2009; 15(24):7726–36.

129. Anguille S, Smits EL, Lion E, et al. Clinical use of dendritic cells for cancer therapy. Lancet Oncol 2014;15(7):e257–67.

130. Lovgren T, Wolodarski M, Wickstrom S, et al. Complete and long-lasting clinical responses in immune checkpoint inhibitor-resistant, metastasized melanoma treated with adoptive T cell transfer combined with DC vaccination. Oncoimmunology 2020;9(1):1792058.

131. Saberian C, Amaria RN, Najjar AM, et al. Randomized phase II trial of lymphodepletion plus adoptive cell transfer of tumor-infiltrating lymphocytes, with or without dendritic cell vaccination, in patients with metastatic melanoma. J Immunother Cancer 2021;9(5).

132. Santos PM, Adamik J, Howes TR, et al. Impact of checkpoint blockade on cancer vaccine-activated CD8+ T cell responses. J Exp Med 2020;217(7): e20191369.

133. Nowicki TS, Berent-Maoz B, Cheung-Lau G, et al. A pilot trial of the combination of transgenic NY-ESO-1-reactive adoptive cellular therapy with dendritic cell vaccination with or without ipilimumab. Clin Cancer Res 2019;25(7):2096–108.

134. Morvan MG, Lanier LL. NK cells and cancer: you can teach innate cells new tricks. Nat Rev Cancer 2016;16(1):7–19.

135. Larsen SK, Gao Y, Basse PH. NK cells in the tumor microenvironment. Crit Rev Oncog 2014;19(1–2): 91–105.

136. Tarazona R, Duran E, Solana R. Natural killer cell recognition of melanoma: new clues for a more effective immunotherapy. Front Immunol 2015;6: 649.

137. Levi I, Amsalem H, Nissan A, et al. Characterization of tumor infiltrating natural killer cell subset. Oncotarget 2015;6(15):13835–43.

138. van der Burg SH, Arens R, Ossendorp F, et al. Vaccines for established cancer: overcoming the challenges posed by immune evasion. Nat Rev Cancer 2016;16(4):219–33.

139. Besser MJ, Shoham T, Harari-Steinberg O, et al. Development of allogeneic NK cell adoptive transfer therapy in metastatic melanoma patients: in vitro preclinical optimization studies. PLoS One 2013;8(3):e57922.

140. Exley MA, Friedlander P, Alatrakchi N, et al. Adoptive transfer of invariant NKT cells as immunotherapy for advanced melanoma: a phase I clinical trial. Clin Cancer Res 2017;23(14):3510–9.

141. van Hall T, Andre P, Horowitz A, et al. Monalizumab: inhibiting the novel immune checkpoint NKG2A. J Immunother Cancer 2019;7(1):263.

142. Vey N, Karlin L, Sadot-Lebouvier S, et al. A phase 1 study of lirilumab (antibody against killer immunoglobulin-like receptor antibody KIR2D; IPH2102) in patients with solid tumors and hematologic malignancies. Oncotarget 2018;9(25):17675–88.

143. Tinker AV, Hirte HW, Provencher D, et al. Dose-ranging and cohort-expansion study of monalizumab (IPH2201) in patients with advanced gynecologic malignancies: a trial of the Canadian Cancer Trials Group (CCTG): IND221. Clin Cancer Res 2019; 25(20):6052–60.

144. Andre P, Denis C, Soulas C, et al. Anti-NKG2A mAb is a checkpoint inhibitor that promotes anti-tumor immunity by unleashing both T and NK cells. Cell 2018;175(7):1731–43.e3.

145. Bridge JA, Lee JC, Daud A, et al. Cytokines, chemokines, and other biomarkers of response for checkpoint inhibitor therapy in skin cancer. Front Med (Lausanne) 2018;5:351.

146. Tang L, Wang K. Chronic inflammation in skin malignancies. J Mol Signal 2016;11:2.

147. Pegram HJ, Lee JC, Hayman EG, et al. Tumor-targeted T cells modified to secrete IL-12 eradicate systemic tumors without need for prior conditioning. Blood 2012;119(18):4133–41.

148. Nicholas C, Lesinski GB. Immunomodulatory cytokines as therapeutic agents for melanoma. Immunotherapy 2011;3(5):673–90.

149. Weiss JM, Subleski JJ, Wigginton JM, et al. Immunotherapy of cancer by IL-12-based cytokine combinations. Expert Opin Biol Ther 2007;7(11):1705–21.

150. Teng MW, Darcy PK, Smyth MJ. Stable IL-10: a new therapeutic that promotes tumor immunity. Cancer Cell 2011;20(6):691–3.

151. Perrot CY, Javelaud D, Mauviel A. Insights into the transforming growth factor-beta signaling pathway in cutaneous melanoma. Ann Dermatol 2013;25(2):135–44.

152. Nonomura Y, Otsuka A, Nakashima C, et al. Peripheral blood Th9 cells are a possible pharmacodynamic biomarker of nivolumab treatment efficacy in metastatic melanoma patients. Oncoimmunology 2016;5(12):e1248327.

153. Armstrong CA, Murray N, Kennedy M, et al. Melanoma-derived interleukin 6 inhibits in vivo melanoma growth. J Invest Dermatol 1994;102(3):278–84.

154. Armstrong CA, Botella R, Galloway TH, et al. Antitumor effects of granulocyte-macrophage colony-stimulating factor production by melanoma cells. Cancer Res 1996;56(9):2191–8.

155. Dranoff G, Jaffee E, Lazenby A, et al. Vaccination with irradiated tumor cells engineered to secrete murine granulocyte-macrophage colony-stimulating factor stimulates potent, specific, and long-lasting anti-tumor immunity. Proc Natl Acad Sci U S A 1993;90(8):3539–43.

156. Berraondo P, Sanmamed MF, Ochoa MC, et al. Cytokines in clinical cancer immunotherapy. Br J Cancer 2019;120(1):6–15.

157. Rosenberg SA, Lotze MT, Muul LM, et al. Observations on the systemic administration of autologous lymphokine-activated killer cells and recombinant interleukin-2 to patients with metastatic cancer. N Engl J Med 1985;313(23):1485–92.

158. Rosenberg SA, Lotze MT, Muul LM, et al. A progress report on the treatment of 157 patients with advanced cancer using lymphokine-activated killer cells and interleukin-2 or high-dose interleukin-2 alone. N Engl J Med 1987;316(15):889–97.

159. Rosenberg SA. IL-2: the first effective immunotherapy for human cancer. J Immunol 2014; 192(12):5451–8.

160. Fyfe G, Fisher RI, Rosenberg SA, et al. Results of treatment of 255 patients with metastatic renal cell carcinoma who received high-dose recombinant interleukin-2 therapy. J Clin Oncol 1995; 13(3):688–96.

161. Fyfe GA, Fisher RI, Rosenberg SA, et al. Long-term response data for 255 patients with metastatic renal cell carcinoma treated with high-dose recombinant interleukin-2 therapy. J Clin Oncol 1996; 14(8):2410–1.

162. Kirkwood JM, Strawderman MH, Ernstoff MS, et al. Interferon alfa-2b adjuvant therapy of high-risk resected cutaneous melanoma: the Eastern Cooperative Oncology Group Trial EST 1684. J Clin Oncol 1996;14(1):7–17.

163. Solal-Celigny P, Lepage E, Brousse N, et al. Recombinant interferon alfa-2b combined with a regimen containing doxorubicin in patients with advanced follicular lymphoma. Groupe d'Etude des Lymphomes de l'Adulte. N Engl J Med 1993; 329(22):1608–14.

164. Golomb HM, Jacobs A, Fefer A, et al. Alpha-2 interferon therapy of hairy-cell leukemia: a multicenter study of 64 patients. J Clin Oncol 1986;4(6):900–5.

165. Atkins MB, Lotze MT, Dutcher JP, et al. High-dose recombinant interleukin 2 therapy for patients with metastatic melanoma: analysis of 270 patients treated between 1985 and 1993. J Clin Oncol 1999;17(7):2105–16.

166. Sondak VK, Kudchadkar R. Pegylated interferon for the adjuvant treatment of melanoma: FDA approved, but what is its role? Oncologist 2012; 17(10):1223–4.

167. Conlon KC, Lugli E, Welles HC, et al. Redistribution, hyperproliferation, activation of natural killer cells and CD8 T cells, and cytokine production during first-in-human clinical trial of recombinant human interleukin-15 in patients with cancer. J Clin Oncol 2015;33(1):74–82.

168. Schmidt H, Brown J, Mouritzen U, et al. Safety and clinical effect of subcutaneous human interleukin-21 in patients with metastatic melanoma or renal cell carcinoma: a phase I trial. Clin Cancer Res 2010;16(21):5312–9.

169. Naing A, Papadopoulos KP, Autio KA, et al. Safety, antitumor activity, and immune activation of pegylated recombinant human interleukin-10 (AM0010) in patients with advanced solid tumors. J Clin Oncol 2016;34(29):3562–9.

170. Leonard JP, Sherman ML, Fisher GL, et al. Effects of single-dose interleukin-12 exposure on interleukin-12-associated toxicity and interferon-gamma production. Blood 1997;90(7):2541–8.

171. Sportes C, Babb RR, Krumlauf MC, et al. Phase I study of recombinant human interleukin-7 administration in subjects with refractory malignancy. Clin Cancer Res 2010;16(2):727–35.

172. Donnelly RP, Young HA, Rosenberg AS. An overview of cytokines and cytokine antagonists as therapeutic agents. Ann N Y Acad Sci 2009;1182:1–13.

173. Minn AJ, Wherry EJ. Combination cancer therapies with immune checkpoint blockade: convergence on interferon signaling. Cell 2016;165(2):272–5.

174. Kleef R, Nagy R, Baierl A, et al. Low-dose ipilimumab plus nivolumab combined with IL-2 and hyperthermia in cancer patients with advanced disease: exploratory findings of a case series of 131 stage IV cancers - a retrospective study of a single institution. Cancer Immunol Immunother 2021;70(5):1393–403.

175. Zibelman M, Plimack ER. Pembrolizumab plus ipilimumab or pegylated interferon alfa-2b for patients with melanoma or renal cell carcinoma: take new drugs but keep the old? Ann Transl Med 2019; 7(Suppl 3):S95.

176. Atkins MB, Hodi FS, Thompson JA, et al. Pembrolizumab plus pegylated interferon alfa-2b or ipilimumab for advanced melanoma or renal cell carcinoma: dose-finding results from the phase ib KEYNOTE-029 study. Clin Cancer Res 2018; 24(8):1805–15.

177. Wolchok JD, Chiarion-Sileni V, Gonzalez R, et al. Overall survival with combined nivolumab and ipilimumab in advanced melanoma. N Engl J Med 2017;377(14):1345–56.

178. Reck M, Rodriguez-Abreu D, Robinson AG, et al. Pembrolizumab versus chemotherapy for PD-L1-positive non-small-cell lung cancer. N Engl J Med 2016;375(19):1823–33.

179. Kaufman HL, Russell J, Hamid O, et al. Avelumab in patients with chemotherapy-refractory metastatic Merkel cell carcinoma: a multicentre, single-group, open-label, phase 2 trial. Lancet Oncol 2016;17(10):1374–85.

180. Motzer RJ, Escudier B, McDermott DF, et al. Nivolumab versus everolimus in advanced renal-cell carcinoma. N Engl J Med 2015;373(19):1803–13.

Clinical Diagnosis and Classification
Including Biopsy Techniques and Noninvasive Imaging

Kavita T. Vakharia, MD, MS

KEYWORDS

• Melanoma • Biopsy • Imaging • Lymph node examination • Laboratory testing

KEY POINTS

- The diagnosis of melanoma begins by obtaining a complete history of the lesion, including changes in appearance, and the patient, including sun exposure, family history, and personal history of other skin cancers or dysplastic nevi.
- Melanomas often conform to the ABCDE rule: asymmetry, border irregularity, color variegation, diameter, and evolution.
- The physical examination should include an evaluation of the lesion, surrounding skin to note for satellite lesions or in-transit metastases, and palpation of lymph node basins.
- A biopsy is required to establish a diagnosis, and an excisional biopsy of the entire lesion with a 1- to 2-mm margin of normal skin and some subcutaneous fat is the preferred method.
- Imaging is needed for staging in patients with proven or high risk of metastatic disease, and these are done with computed tomography (CT), MRI, and PET/CT.

INTRODUCTION

The clinical diagnosis of melanoma begins with a thorough history and physical examination. The history often elicits particular risk factors for melanoma, which may alert the clinician to include the diagnosis within the differential for a suspicious lesion. Demographic factors, comorbidities, family history, and social history can help to determine if a diagnosis of melanoma should be considered. These factors can impact the type of biopsy that is then used to further investigate the lesion. Concerning lesions should undergo a biopsy to determine the histologic characteristics. These characteristics in melanoma serve as prognostic indicators and are also used to determine the appropriate treatment plan. Finally, different imaging modalities may be required to assist in staging and during follow-up treatment.

HISTORY

Patients with melanoma may present with a mole that is concerning to them or that they notice has been changing over time in shape, color, or surface texture. Itching and burning can be associated with a suspicious lesion in addition to pain, although painful lesions are unusual in melanoma. Patients may also report for a routine skin examination or for a different reason, and the suspicious nevus is noted on subsequent physical examination. Approximately 13% to 17% of melanomas are diagnosed from lymph node biopsies without an identifiable primary site.[1] A history of a congenital melanocytic nevus is significant, as risk of malignant transformation is high during childhood for lesions larger than 40 cm and during adulthood for lesions smaller than 40 cm.[2] Patients often have a personal history of atypical nevi and other types of skin cancer, squamous cell carcinoma, and basal

The author have nothing to disclose.
Department of Plastic Surgery, Cleveland Clinic, 9500 Euclid Avenue, A51, Cleveland, OH 44195, USA
E-mail address: vakhark@ccf.org

Clin Plastic Surg 48 (2021) 577–585
https://doi.org/10.1016/j.cps.2021.06.006
0094-1298/21/© 2021 Elsevier Inc. All rights reserved.

cell carcinoma. Questions in their personal history should also be documented regarding recreational or occupational intense and chronic sun exposure, tanning bed use, and tendency for blistering sunburns. It is important to note that melanomas can occur on non-sun-exposed areas. Around 10% of patients report a family history of melanoma, and these may be related to genetic mutations in BRCA2 and P16(CDKN2A).[3]

PHYSICAL EXAMINATION

Melanoma can arise as a new mole or as malignant transformation of a previously existing nevus. They can be flat or nodular, can bleed and have different pigments, or may be amelanotic and erythematous. A suspected melanoma lesion should be differentiated from similarly appearing lesions, such as atypical (dysplastic) nevus, seborrheic keratosis, pyogenic granuloma, and pigmented basal cell carcinoma.[4] Histologically, melanoma in situ is characterized by atypical melanocytes migrating above the dermal-epidermal junction and appearing within the adnexal structures. When the atypical melanocytes invade the dermis, the diagnosis becomes melanoma.[4,5]

Atypical (Dysplastic) Nevus

Atypical nevus is a clinical term used to describe a nevus with melanocytes within the epidermis and dermis that has features concerning for malignancy. These features include a larger size (usually >5 mm), asymmetry, border irregularities, and variegated pigmentation. The term dysplastic nevus is the histologic diagnosis used to describe the architectural and cytologic atypia seen microscopically.[6] The molecular profile of a dysplastic nevus is different, however, than that of melanoma, and studies have shown that there is a higher burden of mutation compared with benign nevi, but less than seen in melanoma lesions.[7] There is an overall consensus that patients with numerous nevi and the presence of large atypical nevi do have an increased risk of melanoma, up to 15-fold, but the probability of progression to melanoma in a single dysplastic nevus is similar or only slightly higher than that of a benign nevus.[6] Most dermatologists still believe in excising dysplastic nevi to negative margins if a positive margin is present on biopsy.[8]

ABCDEs OF MELANOMA

The American Cancer Society has established the ABCDE guidelines of clinical features of pigmented lesions that can aid in identifying a melanoma.[9–11]

A: Asymmetry: benign lesions are often round and symmetric. As a melanoma develops, the lesion can change shape and become asymmetric, going from round to oval.

B: Border Irregularity: the margins of benign lesions are regular and smooth, but early melanomas acquire irregular margins as the lesion grows resulting from variable growth rates from within different portions of the lesion.

C: Color Variegation: a benign nevus usually has a uniform color. A hallmark of concern for a malignant lesion is a nevus with several different colors within it, and possibly changes color over time. Malignant lesions often darken and can have a mixture of tan, brown, and black. Occasionally, there is some red and white intermingled with the darker colors.

D: Diameter: most benign nevi have a small diameter, 6 mm or less. Pigmented lesions larger than 6 mm are concerning for malignancy, in addition to seeing an increase in size over time.

E: Evolving: skin malignancy often has a dynamic course with the appearance changing over time. This criterion takes note of changes that have occurred in the lesion with respect to size, shape, color, elevation, and development of symptoms of itching, tenderness, or bleeding,

These criteria have served to be useful in screening for melanoma and can be used by both patients as well as clinicians.

CLASSIFICATION

Melanoma can be characterized histologically in cutaneous and noncutaneous forms. Cutaneous melanoma is the most common, and it begins at the dermoepidermal junction with invasion of melanocytes vertically into the dermis. The depth of invasion is an important prognostic indicator for recurrent and metastatic disease. Noncutaneous melanoma occurs in other areas of the body where melanocytes are present, mucous membranes and the uveal tract in eyes.

Mucosal melanoma comprises about 1% of primary melanoma diagnoses and can occur in the nasopharynx, gastrointestinal tract, and genitourinary tract. They often arise at the mucocutaneous junction of squamous and columnar epithelia. These tumors can often be amelanotic, and because of this and the location, often present in advanced stages.[12] Mucosal melanomas are genetically distinct from cutaneous melanomas, harboring different subsets of mutations. Often, mucosal melanomas have activating *KIT* mutations, which can make the tumor susceptible to KIT-inhibiting drugs.[13]

About 5% of melanomas are primary ocular melanomas, and these can be divided into conjunctival and uveal. The uveal melanomas can occur in the iris, ciliary body, and choroid. Choroidal melanoma is the most common location and often is discovered on routine eye examination. Many patients do not experience symptoms, but those with symptoms can note visual loss, flashing lights, floaters, or visual field defects. Uveal melanomas can appear as brown pigmented masses. Melanomas in the iris can grow into the anterior chamber leading to secondary glaucoma.[14] Indirect ophthalmoscopy is the most reliable way to make the diagnosis, and fine needle aspiration biopsy can be a helpful adjunct. Cytogenetic analysis of ocular melanomas often reveal mutations in chromosomes 1, 3, 6, and 8 with mutations in chromosome 3 having the worst prognosis.[15]

Cutaneous melanoma subtypes include superficial spreading, nodular, lentigo maligna melanoma (LMM), acral lentiginous, and desmoplastic.

Lentigo Maligna

Lentigo maligna (LM) is a type of melanoma in situ, historically known as the melanotic freckle of Hutchinson.[16] It is most commonly found in chronically sun-damaged skin in the middle aged and elderly and usually presents as a tan or brown macule that progressively enlarges over time. The growth is centrifugal, and the pigmentation often changes to include shades of dark brown or black.[17] The growth pattern histologically is often radial and confined to the dermal-epidermal junction, but if a dermal component is acquired, it is reclassified as LMM. LMM is one of the major subtypes of melanoma and comprises an estimated 4% to 15% of invasive melanomas.[17] It is unknown the percentage of LM that develops into LMM, or the timeframe in which this development occurs. The risk of LMM may be proportional to the size of the lesion, and large LM lesions can have small foci of invasive melanoma. Increasing color variation, expanding lesion, increasing border irregularity, elevation, and white macular areas signaling regression are changes considered suspicious for malignant transformation.[18] The histology of LM shows a proliferation of atypical melanocytes along the dermal-epidermal junction with bridging of the rete pegs, epidermal atrophy, extension down adnexal structures, and a background of solar elastosis. There is also a characteristic dermal lymphocytic infiltrate.[16,17] The clinical examination for LM may be complicated by prior intervention; therefore, a low threshold for biopsy should be present for pigmented facial lesions and especially those that might be changing over time.

Superficial Spreading Melanoma

Superficial spreading melanoma is the most common subtype, accounting for about 70% of all melanoma diagnoses (**Fig. 1**). The histology is characterized by pagetoid spread of atypical melanocytes upward from the basal cell layer into the epidermis. There is often a radial growth pattern present for several years before a vertical growth phase. Two-thirds of these can exhibit regression, which is the interaction of the human immune system with the growing tumor. This regression can be seen as hypopigmented or depigmented portions within the lesion.[19] This subtype also harbors BRAF mutations more frequently than other subtypes.[20]

Nodular Melanoma

Nodular melanoma accounts for approximately 20% to 30% of cases and is the second most common type. They most frequently occur on the trunk and head and neck areas and more often in men than women. They are blue or black and often raised, but can also present as amelanotic, sometimes a pink or red papule that could be ulcerated or bleeding. Nodular melanomas are known to skip the horizontal growth phase and enter into a vertical growth phase for tumorigenesis. Patients with nodular melanomas often present late in thicker or more advanced stages and tend to have a poorer prognosis.[21]

Acral Lentiginous Melanoma

Acral lentiginous melanoma occurs typically on the palms of hands, on the soles of feet, and in nail beds (**Fig. 2**). It is the least common subtype,

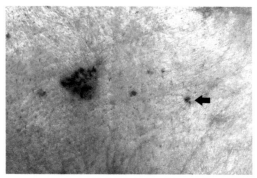

Fig. 1. Cutaneous melanoma, superficial spreading type within transit metastasis (*arrow*).

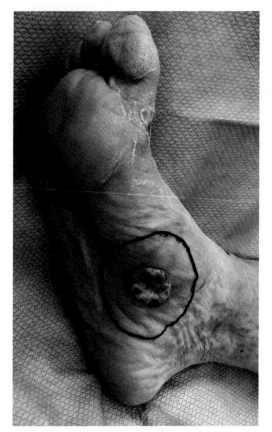

Fig. 2. Acral lentiginous melanoma on the foot.

superficial biopsies of this lesion can make it appear to be fibrosis rather than malignancy. Half of desmoplastic melanomas are characterized as pure with 100% spindle cells or mixed with spindle cells and another melanoma subtype. Desmoplastic melanomas can also exhibit a neural transforming type of neurotropism whereby there is de novo formation of nervelike structures distinct from preexisting nerves in the tumor.[23] In pure desmoplastic melanomas, the rates of sentinel lymph node metastasis are lower than for other subtypes.[24]

Primary Dermal Melanoma

A rare but distinct type of melanoma, primary dermal melanoma usually presents as a skin-colored or bluish-red firm nodule. It can be histologically similar to cutaneous melanoma but does not have an epidermal or in situ component. The tumor resides within the dermis and can have nodular or multinodular architecture. There is also no evidence of ulceration, preexisting nevus, or regression. It can be confused with a cutaneous metastasis, so if a patient presents with no prior history of melanoma and diagnosis of primary dermal melanoma is considered, a metastatic workup is warranted to search for other areas of disease as well as a full skin examination to search for the primary tumor. The conventional parameters for prognosis used for melanoma may not be as equally applicable for primary dermal melanoma.[25]

accounting for 4% to 10% of cases, but it is the most common subtype among those with Asian or African descent. These melanomas usually present at advanced stages, also bringing a poor prognosis. Almost one-third of acral lentiginous melanomas are incorrectly diagnosed when they are first evaluated, and this diagnosis should be included in the differential for nonhealing ulcers on the foot.[22] Melanoma of the nail matrix should be considered for darkly pigmented, or irregularly pigmented bands in the nail as well as lesions within the nail having a width greater than 3 mm. Similar to mucosal melanomas, acral lentiginous melanomas have more and distinct genetic mutation profiles, and many display activating mutations in *KIT*.[13,20]

Desmoplastic Melanoma

Desmoplastic melanomas can appear on the surface of the skin as a scar in an area where the patient has not had a previous injury. It often does not have pigment and is a rare subtype of melanoma. Histologically, the lesion has cicatricial growth with malignant spindle cells, collagen deposition, and chronic inflammatory cells. Because of this,

IN-TRANSIT METASTASES

Melanoma may metastasize through lymphatic channels, which is the most common, or hematogenous spread. Skin or subcutaneous metastases that appear more than 2 cm away from the primary lesion are defined as microscopic satellitosis, or in-transit metastases. These metastases indicate intralymphatic spread of melanoma in the skin. Approximately 30% of melanomas thicker than 3 mm have microscopic satellitosis on pathology.[4] Similar to the presence of regional lymph node metastasis, lesions with microscopic satellitosis and in-transit disease predict poorer disease-free and overall survival, and the patients are upstaged in the current guidelines of treatment.[26,27]

LYMPH NODE EXAMINATION

A complete physical examination also includes examination of the draining lymph node basins. All major lymph node basins, bilaterally, should be examined regardless of the location of the primary melanoma, but particular focus should be given to the areas of potential drainage from the lesion. In part, this is because the closest nodal basin may not be the location of the first draining node of the region, and multiple nodal basins can equally drain a cutaneous area.[28,29] In the head and neck region, the parotid, cervical, and supraclavicular areas should be palpated. For extremity lesions, the epitrochlear and axillary for upper extremity lesions, and popliteal and inguinal for lower extremity lesions should be palpated. Lesions on the trunk may drain to either side and can drain to the axilla or inguinal regions. Occasionally, patients will present with lymph node metastasis without an identifiable primary site. When lymph node metastases are suspected, further evaluation with imaging and a biopsy, and often a fine needle aspiration, is warranted to establish a diagnosis. In clinically node-negative patients, up to 20% have metastatic involvement; the characteristics of the primary tumor may designate that a sentinel lymph node biopsy is indicated at the time of wide excision.[30]

DERMOSCOPY EXAMINATION

Dermoscopy involves the use of a hand-held device with a magnifying lens and a lighting source. With the higher-power magnification, certain morphologic structures of the lesion within the epidermis and dermis can help identify malignant lesions. Diagnostic sensitivity is significantly improved with the use of dermoscopy; however, it does require a skilled examiner.[31] The use of dermoscopy often includes a 2-step algorithm. The first step is to identify if a lesion is of a melanocytic origin. If it is, then the second step is to differentiate the lesion between benign melanocytic nevi and melanoma.[32]

REFLECTANCE CONFOCAL MICROSCOPY

Reflectance confocal microscopy (RCM) is a noninvasive imaging technique that allows for imaging of the epidermis and dermis at the cellular level. It can be performed both at the bedside (in vivo) and in the laboratory (ex vivo) on excised skin. It serves as an important adjunct to clinical examination, dermoscopy, and histopathologic assessment when evaluating and managing a pigmented skin lesion. A light source is focused on the skin and is then reflected by melanin, collagen, and keratin at varying refractive indices. The reflected light enters the RCM detector and is processed by software to produce a 2-dimensional grayscale image of the skin. The RCM depth is up to 250 μm corresponding to the papillary dermis or upper dermis.[33] It has found to be more sensitive (0.93) and specific (0.89) when compared with dermoscopy (0.73 and 0.84, respectively) for the diagnosis of LM.[34] It is also particularly useful in the head and neck region and over curved surfaces. A scoring system has been developed to distinguish LM from benign lesions of the face. Some of the criteria include the presence of round, large pagetoid cells and the presence of more than 3 atypical cells at the dermoepidermal junction in 5 images.[35] Subsequent additions to the scoring include seeing a single large round or dendritic cell, or atypical dendritic cells continuing from the LM trailing edge.[36,37] The use of this algorithm was also effective in identifying amelanotic lesions.[35] The limitations of its use include some anatomic areas that might have a thickened epidermis (palm of hands, plantar surface of feet), crusting or ulceration of the lesion, a limited depth of imaging, difficulty in detecting dendritic melanocytes in pagetoid spread from Langerhans cells mimicking pagetoid spread, which can relate to operator experience.[33,38] Overall, however, RCM is useful for the diagnosis of lesions, assessment of lesions in cosmetically sensitive areas, identifying margins before surgery or biopsy, and detecting treatment response or recurrence.[39]

COMPUTER-BASED TECHNOLOGY

One advancement of the use of technology in health care is the increasing use of artificial intelligence and machine learning to help with the diagnosis and management of disease. Computer-based learning algorithms can be used to improve efficiency and accuracy of diagnosis as well as TO predict prognosis.[40] In dermatology, computer-based learning is being used to improve noninvasive methods of skin cancer detection. Several different algorithms have been developed, but the convolutional neural network system has been shown to be most beneficial. It is used for classifying images, for assembling input images, and in image recognition.[41] Neural networks have been shown to be more specific and sensitive than visual physical examination, and it can allow for early detection and therefore early treatment.[42] The need for large data sets, across different populations, extensive training, expensive equipment, and applicability for ease of use by the patient are some of the limitations that exist for widespread use of machine based diagnosis.[41,43]

BIOPSY

Excisional biopsy is the most accurate sampling method for the diagnosis of melanoma. The biopsy specimen should include 1 to 2 mm of normal skin and some subcutaneous fat. The full-thickness nature of the biopsy is important in order to obtain a true assessment of the thickness of the lesion and architecture, which is required for patient staging and determination of subsequent treatment. An incisional biopsy can have sampling error but may be needed if the lesion is too large for complete excision. An incisional biopsy may be needed in cosmetically sensitive areas or in areas where primary closure after an excisional biopsy may not be possible. For incisional biopsies, the location should include the suspected deepest part of the lesion, keeping in mind future treatment may be necessary. A punch biopsy uses a circular blade and can be either excisional or incisional depending on the size of the lesion. Incisional punch biopsies have been shown to be associated with a false negative rate of 23.3% compared with 1.7% for excisional biopsy.[44] Shave biopsies are the most commonly used technique owing to how quickly they can be done, the simplicity of wound care, and cost-effectiveness. Shave biopsies have a false negative rate of 4.5%.[44] It can be difficult to discern the depth of a melanocytic lesion, so the true thickness of the melanoma may never be able to be determined if a shave biopsy is performed, making staging inaccurate in up to 19% of cases.[44,45] Superficial shave biopsies are contraindicated if melanoma is suspected or clinically if there is diagnostic uncertainty. If a shave biopsy is pursued, it is best reserved for suspected superficial lesions (in situ disease) and performed by clinicians with experience in biopsy of superficial lesions who know to access the deeper dermal layers. A deep saucerization biopsy may be performed if the lesion is flat, covers a large surface area, and is suspected to be thin, such as a melanoma in situ; however, sampling error for this type of biopsy can occur. As many as 35% to 60% of shave biopsies have a transected base, which can lead to an underestimation of tumor thickness and inaccurate staging.[46]

LABORATORY TESTING

Some biomarkers for metastatic melanoma can be detected in the serum. Lactate dehydrogenase (LDH) is a catalyst for the conversion of pyruvate into lactate in anoxic conditions. A melanoma tumor microenvironment is often oxygen depleted; therefore, LDH can be elevated in patients with metastatic disease. Serum LDH levels have been shown to be one of the strongest prognostic indicators for patients with stage IV disease, with elevated levels indicating a lower chance of survival.[47] Elevated LDH levels can also be a negative predictor of response to drug treatment.[48] Another marker with high diagnostic sensitivity is protein S100B levels. In patients with high-risk melanoma that has been surgically resected, an elevated baseline S100B or increasing S100B serum level was shown to be an independent prognostic marker for mortality. These levels are often obtained in European countries at the time of staging and during surveillance examinations in patients in whom there is concern for an elevated risk of recurrence.[49] Concerns related to differences in assay used in different studies, the presence of S100B in other disease conditions, and heterogeneity of disease stages in the several studies have limited its routine use in the United States.[47]

IMAGING

There are several imaging modalities that are used to assist in diagnosing metastatic disease. If a patient with a history of melanoma presents with a suspicious palpable mass, located within the excision scar, surrounding subcutaneous tissues, or lymph node basin, an ultrasound may be the first imaging modality selected for further evaluation. Ultrasound can be paired with a fine needle aspiration of the mass, using ultrasound guidance, so that a sample can be obtained for pathologic analysis and diagnosis. Patients with stage III or IV disease should have initial and continued surveillance with advanced radiologic imaging. Distant organ metastases can be detected with computed tomographic (CT) scans of the chest, abdomen, and pelvis.[50] A CT or MRI scan of the brain should also be performed to evaluate for brain metastases (Fig. 3). Whole-body MRIs can also be highly sensitive in detecting liver and bone metastases.[51] Where available, a PET/CT should also be considered. A PET scan uses an 18F-flurodeoxyglucose (FDG) dye that becomes concentrated in areas of higher metabolic activity. Melanoma metastases can be the focus of higher metabolic rates compared with normal tissue, and whole-body PET/CT has become the most sensitive method of detecting melanoma metastases (Fig. 4). An MRI is superior in detecting lesions in the central nervous system, liver, and bone marrow, whereas the PET/CT scan is preferred for evaluating for metastases in the lymph nodes and any other organ system.[51]

DISCUSSION

The diagnosis of melanoma begins with a thorough history and physical examination. In the

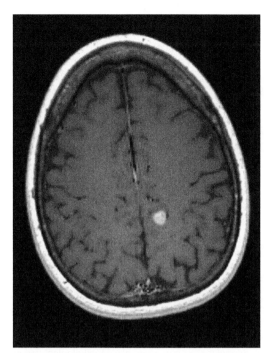

Fig. 3. MRI T1 sequence imaging of brain showing an enhancing left parietal melanoma metastasis.

history, information about lifelong sun exposure, prior skin cancers, family history of melanoma, in addition to the details of changes in the lesion can be useful in considering melanoma as a diagnosis. Melanomas often have characteristic features of asymmetry, border irregularity, color variegation, a larger diameter, and often some change that occurred over a period of time. They are usually pigmented, but amelanotic lesions can also occur. Lymph node basins should be palpated during the examination to evaluate for lymphadenopathy at the time of presentation. If a melanoma is included in the differential diagnosis for a lesion, an excisional biopsy is recommended, as a full-thickness sample can provide the most accurate information needed to determine staging and subsequent treatment. If a sentinel lymph node biopsy is indicated and performed, the results can help further determine the stage of a patient. For stage III and IV patients, further investigation may be needed with laboratory tests and imaging. The laboratory testing should include a complete blood count, blood chemistry, an LDH level, and possibly hepatic function tests. Imaging modalities that are used in patient surveillance and metastatic workup include ultrasound, CT, MRI, and PET/CT. The imaging can be used to detect widespread disease, but further biopsies, core or needle, may be required to confirm the diagnosis. In addition, serial imaging scans are obtained

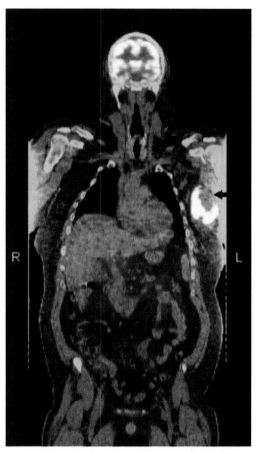

Fig. 4. PET/CT scan showing an FDG-avid mass in the left axilla with central necrosis (*arrow*). This was a biopsy-proven metastatic melanoma.

when patients are on medical treatment to assess for treatment response.

CLINICS CARE POINTS

- The ABCDE's of melanoma is a validated tool for the clinical diagnosis of melanoma.
- The gold standard of histopathologic diagnosis continues to be biopsy; an excisional biopsy is the most accurate.
- The specificity and sensitivity of diagnosis of pigmented lesions are increased with the use of dermoscopy and confocal reflectance microscopy compared with physical examination alone.
- Imaging may be needed to diagnose metastatic disease; PET/CTs in particular have a high sensitivity in detecting metastatic melanoma.

REFERENCES

1. Sondak VK, Messina JL. Unusual presentations of melanoma. Melanoma of unknown primary site, melanoma arising in childhood, and melanoma arising in the eye and on mucosal surfaces. Surg Clin North Am 2014;94(5):1059–73.
2. Tracy ET, Aldrink JH. Pediatric melanoma. Semin Pediatr Surg 2016;25(5):290–8.
3. LM S. Melanoma and nonmelanoma skin cancers. In: Goldman L, Schafer AI, Cecil RL, editors. Goldman-cecil medicine. 26th edition. Philadelphia: Elsevier Inc; 2020.
4. Ariyan S, Berger A. Melanoma, plastic surgery: volume 1: principles. 4th edition. Philadelphia: Elsevier Inc; 2018.
5. Ackerman AB. Macular and patch lesions of malignant melanoma: malignant melanoma in situ. J Dermatol Surg Oncol 1983;9(8):615–8.
6. Ardakani NM. Dysplastic/Clark naevus in the era of molecular pathology. Australas J Dermatol 2019; 60(3):186–91.
7. Melamed RD, Aydin IT, Rajan GS, et al. Genomic characterization of dysplastic nevi unveils implications for diagnosis of melanoma. J Invest Dermatol 2017;137(4):905–9.
8. Winkelmann RR, Rigel DS. Management of dysplastic nevi: a 14-year follow-up survey assessing practice trends among US dermatologists. J Am Acad Dermatol 2015;73(6):1056–9.
9. Friedman RJ, Rigel DS, Kopf AW. Early detection of malignant melanoma: the role of physician examination and self-examination of the skin. CA Cancer J Clin 1985;35(3):130–51.
10. Rigel DS, Friedman RJ. The rationale of the ABCDs of early melanoma. J Am Acad Dermatol 1993; 29(6):1060–1.
11. Abbasi NR, Shaw HM, Rigel DS, et al. Early diagnosis of cutaneous melanoma: revisiting the ABCD criteria. J Am Med Assoc 2004;292(22):2771–6.
12. Tomicic J, Wanebo HJ. Mucosal melanomas. Surg Clin North Am 2003;83(2):237–52.
13. Torres-Cabala CA, Wang WL, Trent J, et al. Correlation between KIT expression and KIT mutation in melanoma: a study of 173 cases with emphasis on the acral-lentiginous/mucosal type. Mod Pathol 2009;22(11):1446–56.
14. Shields CL, Shields JA. Ocular melanoma: relatively rare but requiring respect. Clin Dermatol 2009;27(1): 122–33.
15. Prescher G, Bornfeld N, Hirche H, et al. Prognostic implications of monosomy 3 in uveal melanoma. Lancet 1996;347(9010):1222–5.
16. Wayte DM, Helwig EB. Melanotic freckle of Hutchinson. Cancer 1968;21(5):893–911.
17. McKenna JK, Florell SR, Goldman GD. Lentigo maligna/lentigo maligna melanoma. Dermatol Surg 2006;32(4):493–504.
18. Cohen LM. Lentigo maligna and lentigo maligna melanoma. J Am Acad Dermatol 1995;33(6):923–36.
19. Garbe C, Bauer J. Melanoma. In: Bolognia JL, Schaffer JV, Cerroni L, editors. Dermatology. 4th edition. Philadelphia: Elsevier; 2018.
20. Curtin JA, Fridlyand J, Kageshita T, et al. Distinct sets of genetic alterations in melanoma. N Engl J Med 2005;353(20):2135–47.
21. Demierre MF, Chung C, Miller DR, et al. Early detection of thick melanomas in the United States: beware of the nodular subtype. Arch Dermatol 2005;141(6):745–50.
22. Liu XK, Li J. Acral lentiginous melanoma. Lancet 2018;391(10137):e21.
23. Bruijn JA, Mihm MC, Barnhill RL. Desmoplastic melanoma. Histopathology 1992;20(3):197–205.
24. Broer PN, Walker ME, Goldberg C, et al. Desmoplastic melanoma: a 12-year experience with sentinel lymph node biopsy. Eur J Surg Oncol 2013;39(7):681–5.
25. Simonetti O, Molinelli E, Brisigotti V, et al. Primary dermal melanoma: a rare clinicopathological variant mimicking metastatic melanoma. Dermatopathology 2021;8(1):29–32.
26. León P, Daly JM, Synnestvedt M, et al. The prognostic implications of microscopic satellites in patients with clinical stage I melanoma. Arch Surg 1991;126(12):1461–8.
27. Edge SB, Compton CC. The American Joint Committee on Cancer: the 7th edition of the AJCC Cancer Staging Manual and the future of TNM. Ann Surg Oncol 2010;17(6):1471–4.
28. McHugh JB, Su L, Griffith KA, et al. Significance of multiple lymphatic basin drainage in truncal melanoma patients undergoing sentinel lymph node biopsy. Ann Surg Oncol 2006;13(9):1216–23.
29. Leong SPL, Marita ET, Südmeyer M, et al. Heterogeneous patterns of lymphatic drainage to sentinel lymph nodes by primary melanoma from different anatomic sites. Clin Nucl Med 2005;30(3):150–8.
30. Evaluation and treatment of regional lymph nodes in melanoma - UpToDate. Available at: https://www-uptodate-com.ccmain.ohionet.org/contents/evaluation-and-treatment-of-regional-lymph-nodes-in-melanoma?search=Evaluation and treatment of regional lymph nodes in melanoma&source=search_result&selectedTitle=1~150&usage_type=default&display_rank=1. Accessed March 26, 2021.
31. Jaimes N, Marghoob AA. The morphologic universe of melanoma. Dermatol Clin 2013;31(4):599–613.
32. Argenziano G, Soyer HP, Chimenti S, et al. Dermoscopy of pigmented skin lesions: results of a consensus meeting via the internet. J Am Acad Dermatol 2003;48(5):679–93.

33. Ahlgrimm-Siess V, Laimer M, Rabinovitz HS, et al. Confocal microscopy in skin cancer. Curr Dermatol Rep 2018;7(2):105–18.

34. Cinotti E, Fiorani D, Labeille B, et al. The integration of dermoscopy and reflectance confocal microscopy improves the diagnosis of lentigo maligna. J Eur Acad Dermatol Venereol 2019;33(10):e372–4.

35. Guitera P, Pellacani G, Crotty KA, et al. The impact of in vivo reflectance confocal microscopy on the diagnostic accuracy of lentigo maligna and equivocal pigmented and nonpigmented macules of the face. J Invest Dermatol 2010;130(8):2080–91.

36. Champin J, Perrot JL, Cinotti E, et al. In vivo reflectance confocal microscopy to optimize the spaghetti technique for defining surgical margins of lentigo maligna. Dermatol Surg 2014;40(3):247–56.

37. Yélamos O, Cordova M, Blank N, et al. Correlation of handheld reflectance confocal microscopy with radial video mosaicing for margin mapping of lentigo maligna and lentigo maligna melanoma. JAMA Dermatol 2017;153(12):1278–84.

38. Serban ED, Farnetani F, Pellacani G, et al. Role of in vivo reflectance confocal microscopy in the analysis of melanocytic lesions. Acta Dermatovenerol Croat 2018;26(1):64–7.

39. Farnetani F, Manfredini M, Chester J, et al. Reflectance confocal microscopy in the diagnosis of pigmented macules of the face: differential diagnosis and margin definition. Photochem Photobiol Sci 2019;18(5):963–9.

40. Alix-Panabieres C, Magliocco A, Cortes-Hernandez LE, et al. Detection of cancer metastasis: past, present and future. Clin Exp Metastasis 2021; 1–8. https://doi.org/10.1007/s10585-021-10088-w.

41. Dildar M, Akram S, Irfan M, et al. Skin cancer detection: a review using deep learning techniques. Int J Environ Res Public Health 2021;18(10):5479.

42. Efimenko M, Ignatev A, Koshechkin K. Review of medical image recognition technologies to detect melanomas using neural networks. BMC Bioinformatics 2020;21(11):270.

43. Pai VV, Pai RB. Artificial intelligence in dermatology and healthcare: an overview. Indian J Dermatol Venereol Leprol 2021;87(4):457–67.

44. Ng JC, Swain S, Dowling JP, et al. The impact of partial biopsy on histopathologic diagnosis of cutaneous melanoma: experience of an Australian tertiary referral service. Arch Dermatol 2010;146(3): 234–9.

45. Mills JK, White I, Diggs B, et al. Effect of biopsy type on outcomes in the treatment of primary cutaneous melanoma. Am J Surg 2013;205(5):585–90.

46. Menezes SL, Kelly JW, Wolfe R, et al. The increasing use of shave biopsy for diagnosing invasive melanoma in Australia. Med J Aust 2019;211:213–8.

47. Palmer SR, Erickson LA, Ichetovkin I, et al. Circulating serologic and molecular biomarkers in malignant melanoma. Mayo Clin Proc 2011;86(10): 981–90.

48. Agarwala SS, Keilholz U, Gilles E, et al. LDH correlation with survival in advanced melanoma from two large, randomised trials (Oblimersen GM301 and EORTC 18951). Eur J Cancer 2009;45(10):1807–14.

49. Tarhini AA, Stuckert J, Lee S, et al. Prognostic significance of serum s100b protein in high-risk surgically resected melanoma patients participating in intergroup trial ECOG 1694. J Clin Oncol 2009;27(1): 38–44.

50. Müller-Horvat C, Radny P, Eigentler TK, et al. Prospective comparison of the impact on treatment decisions of whole-body magnetic resonance imaging and computed tomography in patients with metastatic malignant melanoma. Eur J Cancer 2006;42(3): 342–50.

51. Pfannenberg C, Aschoff P, Schanz S, et al. Prospective comparison of 18F-fluorodeoxyglucose positron emission tomography/computed tomography and whole-body magnetic resonance imaging in staging of advanced malignant melanoma. Eur J Cancer 2007;43(3):557–64.

Histopathologic and Molecular Diagnosis of Melanoma

Morgan L. Wilson, MD

KEYWORDS

• Melanoma • Diagnosis • Histopathology • Pathology • Plastic surgery • Report

KEY POINTS

- Histopathology is the mainstay of diagnosis for melanocytic neoplasms.
- The melanoma pathology report includes multiple prognostic indicators that inform surgical and medical management.
- Diagnostic accuracy is optimized when the pathologist is provided with key clinical information regarding the history, physical examination, prior biopsy findings, method of sampling, and orientation of the specimen.
- Immunohistochemistry and molecular testing may assist with diagnosis.

INTRODUCTION

Conventional histopathology is the primary method of melanoma diagnosis. A melanoma pathology report contains multiple prognostic indicators; understanding of these facilitates an appropriate management plan. Ancillary stains and molecular techniques are available to assist in the diagnosis of challenging cases.

HISTOPATHOLOGY OF MELANOMA

Benign melanocytic nevi and melanoma occur in an array of morphologic variants, and can show considerable overlap in histopathologic features. On average, melanomas are less symmetric and less circumscribed than nevi. The intraepidermal portion of a melanoma may show confluent proliferation of melanocytes at the dermal-epidermal junction (**Fig. 1**A), pagetoid scatter of melanocytes into the suprabasilar epidermis, and effacement of the overlying epidermis. Melanomas often show cytologic atypia (see **Fig. 1**B), and within the invasive component, the melanocytes are less likely to mature (decrease in size with depth) than those of a nevus. Mitotic figures in nevi are infrequent, and typically confined to the superficial portion of the lesion. Frequent, deep, or atypical mitoses raise concern for melanoma.

THE MELANOMA REPORT

The melanoma pathology report includes a synopsis of features relevant to prognosis and management. Several of the more important and/or problematic areas will be discussed. A sample melanoma report is provided (**Box 1**). If a melanoma report lacks essential information, this should be discussed with the interpreting pathologist. If indicated, review by a dermatopathologist may be requested.

Histologic Type

Lentigo maligna (LM) is a type of melanoma in situ that occurs on chronically sun-damaged skin. It often presents as an irregular brown patch on the head or neck of elderly patients, and histologically shows an increase in singly dispersed and irregularly nested junctional melanocytes (**Fig. 2**A) with underlying solar elastosis. When invasion occurs, the term "lentigo maligna melanoma" is used. In many instances, there is a long, indolent in situ

Division of Dermatology, Southern Illinois University School of Medicine, PO Box 19644, Springfield, IL 62794-9644, USA
E-mail address: mwilson3@siumed.edu

Clin Plastic Surg 48 (2021) 587–598
https://doi.org/10.1016/j.cps.2021.05.003

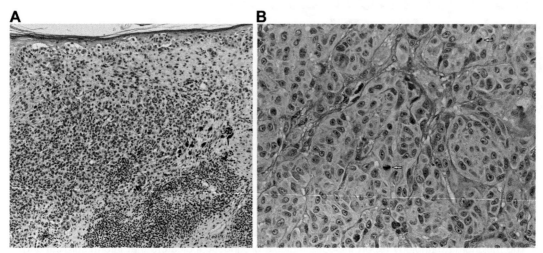

Fig. 1. (*A*) Melanoma with confluent nests of melanocytes at the dermoepidermal junction. Melanoma cells invade the superficial dermis; the smaller cells in the lower right corner represent associated nevus. (H&E ×100). (*B*) Invasive melanoma with large nuclei, prominent nucleoli, and mitotic figures (*arrows*). (H&E × 400).

phase prior to the occurrence of invasion.[1] Unfortunately, there is no way to predict which cases of lentigo maligna will progress to invasion and aggressive behavior. Delineation of margins is often challenging, as will be discussed.

Acral lentiginous melanoma shows an increase in atypical and (initially) predominantly singly dispersed junctional melanocytes (**Fig. 2**B), with subsequent formation of irregular junctional nests and suprabasilar scatter. It occurs on the palms, soles, and digits, including subungually, where it may clinically manifest as longitudinal melanonychia. Although rare in all populations, it proportionally constitutes a higher percentage of melanomas in individuals with dark skin because of the rarity of other types of melanoma in these patients.[2] Because of a less conspicuous location and a reluctance to perform biopsies in acral and subungual sites, acral lentiginous melanoma presents on average at a later stage than other cutaneous melanomas, and in some studies has shown a slightly worse prognosis when controlled for stage.[2]

Superficial spreading melanoma is the most common type on the trunk and proximal extremities, and it is histologically characterized by irregular nests, increased singly dispersed junctional melanocytes, and prominent pagetoid scatter of melanocytes into the suprabasilar epidermis (**Fig. 2**C).

Nodular melanoma is uncommon, and it shows a prominent and typically deep nodular proliferation of malignant melanocytes within the dermis. Unlike the aforementioned variants, it appears to grow in a vertical/invasive phase from its inception, and has only a small intraepidermal component.

Desmoplastic melanoma clinically presents as a firm plaque, often on the face or scalp of an elderly person. Many lesions are amelanotic. It is histopathologically characterized by a dermal and subcutaneous proliferation of spindled melanocytes within a scar-like collagenous stroma (**Fig. 2**D). It can occur as pure desmoplastic melanoma, defined as more than 80% to 90% spindle cells with stromal fibrosis, or can be mixed with conventional melanoma. The neoplastic spindle cells may be deceptively bland, and the diagnosis is easily missed. The presence of scattered lymphocytic aggregates and a focal overlying atypical junctional component are helpful clues. The tumor stroma can blend with scar from a prior procedure, making margin assessment difficult. Approximately half of cases show neurotropism, and a recent study showed a local recurrence rate of 13%.[3] Pure desmoplastic melanoma has a higher average Breslow thickness compared with superficial spreading melanoma, but when controlled for depth, has a lower rate of sentinel lymph node (SLN) positivity and lower melanoma-specific mortality.[3]

The histologic type of melanoma can help to predict the genetic characteristics of the tumor. A subset of acral lentiginous, mucosal, and lentigo maligna melanomas harbors aberrations in *KIT*,[4] some of which confer susceptibility to treatment with imatinib.[5] In contrast, superficial spreading melanomas on the trunk and extremities rarely contain *KIT* aberrations, but frequently have BRAF V600 mutations,[4] which may confer susceptibility to BRAF and MEK inhibitors.

Breslow Thickness

The Breslow thickness is measured using a micrometer in the ocular lens of the microscope. It is the

Box 1
Sample melanoma synoptic report

Sample Melanoma Pathology Report with Synoptic Data

Final Pathologic Diagnosis

Skin and subcutaneous tissue, right upper arm, excision: Melanoma, Breslow thickness 1.8 mm, ulcerated, see synoptic data

Sentinel lymph node, right axilla #1, excision:

One sentinel lymph node positive for metastatic melanoma (1/1), see synoptic data

Maximum diameter of largest discrete melanoma deposit: 0.2 mm

No extranodal extension is identified

A single subcapsular tumor deposit is highlighted with stains for SOX10 and HMB45

Sentinel lymph node, right axilla #2, excision:

1 lymph node with no evidence of malignancy (0/1)

Immunohistochemical stains for SOX10 and HMB45 are negative

Melanoma of the Skin: Synoptic Data

Procedure: excision and sentinel lymph node biopsy

Specimen laterality: right

Tumor

Tumor site: right upper arm

Tumor size: 1 cm (based on gross examination)

Macroscopic satellite nodules: not identified

Histologic type: superficial spreading melanoma

Maximum tumor (Breslow) thickness: 1.8 mm

Anatomic (Clark) level: IV (melanoma invades reticular dermis)

Ulceration: present (extent of ulceration: 1 mm)

Peripheral margins: positive for melanoma in situ; negative for invasive melanoma

Invasive melanoma is 3.2 mm from the nearest peripheral margin

Deep margin: negative for invasive melanoma; negative for melanoma in situ

Invasive melanoma is 7.5 mm from the nearest deep margin

Mitotic rate: 3 mitoses/mm^2

Microsatellitosis: not identified

Lymph-vascular invasion: not identified

Neurotropism: not identified

Tumor-infiltrating lymphocytes: present, not brisk

Tumor regression: present, involving less than 75% of the lesion

Associated nevus: not identified

Lymph nodes

Site: right axilla

Number of lymph nodes examined: 2

Number of sentinel lymph nodes examined: 2

Number of sentinel lymph nodes involved: 1

Size of largest metastatic deposit in sentinel lymph node: 0.2 mm

Location of metastatic deposit: subcapsular

Extranodal extension: not identified

Matted nodes: not identified

Pathologic stage classification (pTNM, AJCC 8th edition)

Primary tumor (pT): pT2b (melanoma >1.0–2.0 mm in thickness, with ulceration)

Regional lymph nodes (pN): pN1a (1 clinically occult, tumor-involved node (ie, detected by sentinel lymph node biopsy) with no in-transit, satellite, and/or microsatellite metastases

---

distance from the top of the granular layer of the epidermis to the deepest aspect of the invasive primary tumor.[6] If the tumor is ulcerated, it is measured from the base of the ulcer to the deepest extent of the tumor. Periadnexal extension to a depth greater than that of the main tumor has been shown not to worsen overall clinical outcomes, and it has therefore been suggested that such foci of deeper periadnexal extension should not be included in measurement of tumor thickness.[7] Breslow thickness is correlated with risk of metastasis and death, and it is therefore a primary determinant of tumor stage.[8]

Clark (Anatomic) Level

Clark level is a designation of the histologic level of tumor invasion, defined as[6]

- Level I: melanoma confined to the epidermis (melanoma in situ)
- Level II: melanoma invades the papillary dermis
- Level III: melanoma fills and expands the papillary dermis
- Level IV: melanoma invades the reticular dermis

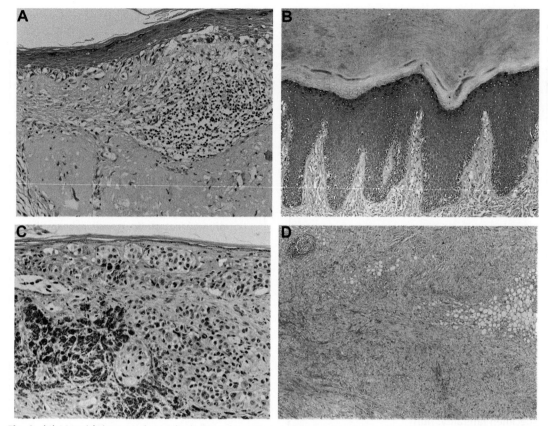

Fig. 2. (*A*) LM with increase in singly dispersed junctional melanocytes and underlying blue-gray solar elastosis. (H&E × 200). (*B*) Acral lentiginous melanoma in situ, with increased singly dispersed junctional melanocytes. The thick epidermis is characteristic of the acral site. (H&E × 100). (*C*) Superficial spreading melanoma with upward scatter of melanocytes into the epidermis. (H&E, × 200). (*D*) Desmoplastic melanoma shows a scar-like increase in collagen density with spindled melanocytes. (H&E × 40).

- Level V: melanoma invades the subcutaneous tissue

Prognosis worsens with increasing Clark level. The Clark level is less objective and less reproducible among pathologists than the Breslow depth, and is not consistently identified as an independent prognostic factor in multivariate analysis[9]; it is therefore no longer used as a determinant of tumor stage.[6]

Ulceration

Ulceration is defined as full-thickness loss of epidermis overlying any portion of the tumor, together with crust and/or inflammation. A lack of the latter features indicates that the epidermal disruption may have occurred artifactually during processing. Likewise, if the ulceration is secondary to a prior biopsy, it is not counted.[6] Ulceration is a negative prognostic indicator, and together with Breslow thickness, is a determinant of tumor stage.

Margins

A melanoma pathology report includes the status of the deep and peripheral margins. In some synoptic reports, the distance in millimeters from the nearest margin (as measured histologically) is provided, and this is sometimes a source of confusion for clinicians. It must be understood that standard recommendations for surgical margins refer to a clinical measurement (ie, the margin of clinically uninvolved tissue resected at the time of surgery) and do not imply a necessity of achieving a particular marginal clearance as measured histologically.

For example, suppose that a melanoma of Breslow thickness 0.5 mm is excised with the recommended 1 cm clinical margin. The pathology report indicates that the deep and peripheral margins are negative, and that the tumor is 4 mm from the closest peripheral margin. It is not necessary to perform additional surgery to achieve a histologic margin of 1 cm. There is no standard guideline as to the necessary histologic clearance; the goal is typically to achieve an unequivocally negative margin, regardless of the histologically measured distance.

Mitotic Index

Mitotic index is the number of mitotic figures in 1 mm^2 of the invasive component of the tumor, using a routine hematoxylin and eosin (H&E) stain. The count is started in the area in with the most mitotic activity. Mitotic rate is an independent predictor of melanoma survival in multivariate analysis.[9] Current guidelines[10] suggest discussing and considering SLN biopsy in the uncommon scenario of a melanoma ≤0.8 mm with a mitotic index of at least 2/mm.[2]

Microsatellitosis

Three distinct terms are used to describe local/regional metastases in the skin and subcutis, which presumably arise because of lymphatic or other vascular spread[6]:

- A microsatellite metastasis is a focus of metastatic tumor in the dermis or subcutis that is adjacent to but discontinuous with the primary melanoma, and is identified during histopathologic assessment of the primary tumor excision.
- A satellite metastasis is a clinically evident cutaneous or subcutaneous metastasis that is within 2 cm of, but discontinuous with, the primary tumor.
- An in transit metastasis is a clinically evident cutaneous or subcutaneous metastasis greater than 2 cm from the primary melanoma, and typically situated between the primary melanoma and the regional lymph node basin.

Examination of multiple sections is helpful in ensuring that a possible microsatellite is truly separate from the primary tumor. Microsatellites are a poor prognostic indicator,[11] and when identified, mandate a designation of at least stage III.[6]

Tumor Regression

Regression is histologically identified as an area within a melanoma in which there is dermal fibrosis, lymphocytic inflammation, and partial or complete loss of tumor cells, which has occurred naturally, and not as a result of a prior procedure. Melanophages are often noted within the dermis in the area of regression. Regression can sometimes be visualized clinically as an area of depigmentation or hypopigmentation within an otherwise pigmented lesion. Regression is thought to result

from an immune response against the tumor cells. Although once regarded as a negative prognostic sign, several recent studies have found histologic regression to be a neutral to favorable prognostic indicator.[12–14] When there is extensive regression, there may be a reduction in certainty regarding the validity of the measured Breslow depth.

PROBLEM AREAS
Pathology Requisition Form

The optimal diagnosis of melanocytic neoplasms occurs via the integration of clinical and histopathologic information. The pathology requisition form ideally provides the pathologist with clinical information critical to best interpretation of the specimen. Unfortunately, pathology requisitions are often submitted with only incomplete and vague information, such as "lesion" or "rule out atypia." The provision of sufficient clinical information with requisition forms has been shown to increase the probability of a correct diagnosis[15,16] and appears not to adversely bias the pathologist when evaluating melanocytic lesions.[17] Recommended information for submission with cutaneous pathology specimens[18] is shown in **Box 2**.

The value of verbal communication between the clinician and pathologist cannot be overemphasized. Review of slides with a pathologist can help the clinician to better visualize the tumor and understand areas of concern. Multidisciplinary tumor boards are a commonly employed forum for this purpose.

Nail Unit Specimens

When melanoma produces longitudinal melanonychia, the responsible tumor is most often located in the nail matrix, and representation of this area is essential to an adequate biopsy specimen. Assessment of the nail plate alone does not permit

---

Box 2
Key information to submit with dermatopathology specimens

- Clinical history of lesion (duration, change, trauma)
- Description of lesion (size, color, symmetry, solitary vs multiple)
- Partial versus complete sampling
- History of prior biopsies at this site (include copy of prior pathology reports)
- Clinical photograph
- Clinical differential diagnosis

adequate assessment for a melanocytic neoplasm.

Surgical specimens from the nail unit pose a unique challenge, as they lack the epidermal surface and subcutaneous adipose tissue, which are helpful in orienting cutaneous specimens from other sites. Therefore, it can be difficult to understand and orient nail unit specimens at the time of grossing and embedding. Improper orientation can result in loss of the most critical portions of the specimen during sectioning. It is recommended that nail unit specimens be photographed and labeled, with communication of the correct orientation to the individual who will be grossing the specimen in the pathology laboratory. One method for achieving this is to place the specimen in its correct orientation on a diagram of the nail unit, and then to place this between sponges in a tissue cassette prior to immersion in a formalin bottle, as illustrated in a review of the handling of nail specimens.[19]

Lentigo Maligna Margins

Lentigo maligna is often poorly circumscribed, both clinically and histopathologically. Even when the microscopic findings are definitive in the center of the lesion, the proliferation of junctional melanocytes often gradually diminishes at the periphery, and blends with adjacent melanocytic hyperplasia (MH), making it difficult to define the boundary of the LM (**Fig. 3**). Although an increased density of junctional melanocytes can be observed in either LM or MH, nesting is not expected in MH, and pagetoid scatter is rare; therefore, when present, these features favor a diagnosis of LM.[20,21]

Routine sectioning (breadloafing) of tissue specimens results in histologic visualization of only a small percentage of the total peripheral margin;

therefore, methods of more comprehensive assessment have been utilized for lentigo maligna specimens. Mohs micrographic surgery with MART-1 immunostaining has been associated with a recurrence rate of 0.3%, with 5- and 10-year melanoma-specific survival of 99.5% and 99.2%, respectively.[22] As the availability of this procedure is limited, staged excision with permanent section evaluation of circumferential en face margins has also been utilized, with a 5-year recurrence rate of 1.4%.[23] If permanent sections with en face margins are desired, it is essential to communicate with the pathology laboratory in advance so that the marginal tissue is processed in the appropriate manner.

In cases in which the clinically visible and histopathologically definitive LM has been completely excised, but histologically equivocal findings persist at the margins, topical imiquimod may be considered, particularly if further surgery would be associated with unacceptable morbidity.[10]

Spitz Nevi and Atypical Spitz Tumors

A Spitz nevus is a form of benign melanocytic nevus occurring most commonly in children and young adults. Histopathologically, Spitz nevi can show considerable architectural disorder and cytologic atypia, and therefore can be difficult to distinguish from melanoma. As the size, circumscription, and symmetry are important in the histopathologic diagnosis of Spitz nevi, partial biopsies can limit assessment; therefore, when a Spitz nevus is suspected, the biopsy should include the entire lesion when feasible. Melanoma is rare in children younger than 10 years[24]; therefore, a lesion suspicious for melanoma in this age group should prompt dermatopathology review with a low threshold for second opinion.

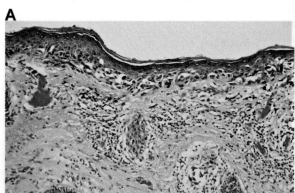 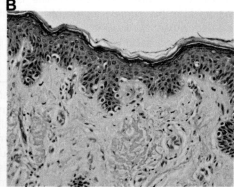

Fig. 3. Lentigo maligna. (*A*) Center of lesion with unequivocal LM: confluent proliferation of melanocytes at the dermoepidermal junction. (H&E ×200). (*B*) Periphery of the same lesion with scattered junctional melanocytes; it is difficult to distinguish benign melanocytic hyperplasia from the tapering edge of LM. (H&E × 400).

Molecular testing can provide useful adjunctive information[25,26]; unfortunately, such testing does not always provide a definitive answer in histopathologically ambiguous spitzoid tumors.[27] In some instances, spitzoid lesions show atypical features, but do not meet criteria for melanoma, leading to designation as atypical Spitz tumor. Complete excision of such lesions is recommended.[28] Although SLN biopsies in such patients are commonly positive, most patients have excellent outcomes regardless of SLN status, leading to uncertainty as to the role of SLN biopsy in these patients.[28,29]

Second Opinions

Accuracy of diagnosis in melanocytic lesions may be improved by obtaining a second opinion.[30] Many melanoma referral centers routinely perform a review of outside pathology slides before finalizing a treatment plan; this practice leads to a change in diagnosis in 1.8% to 5.1% of patients,[31,32] change in tumor staging in 12% to 22% of patients,[31,32] change in excision margin in 4.3% to 11.2% of patients,[32,33] and change in SLN recommendation in 5.9% to 8.6% of patients.[32,33]

IMMUNOHISTOCHEMISTRY

Multiple immunohistochemical stains are available for staining melanocytes. Those most commonly employed include S100, SOX10, Melan-A, MART1, HMB45, MITF, and tyrosinase. Such stains can be helpful in visualizing morphologically subtle melanocytic proliferations (**Fig. 4**), as well as those obscured by inflammation. These stains vary in specificity; for example, S100 also stains Langerhans cells, histiocytes, adipocytes, and nerve. Reduced sensitivity is a problem in desmoplastic melanoma, in which S100 and SOX10 are usually positive, while other melanocytic markers are commonly lost.

Although the aforementioned stains are useful for highlighting melanocytes, they do not distinguish benign from malignant melanocytes. The proliferation marker Ki67 stains a higher percentage of nuclei in melanoma than in nevi,[34] but considerable overlap exists. An immunohistochemical stain for PRAME has been reported to have 75% sensitivity and 98.8% specificity for the diagnosis of melanoma in histologically challenging lesions[35] and was able to consistently differentiate nodal melanoma metastasis from benign nodal nevus.[36] Although this stain will be increasingly used as an aid in distinction of nevi from melanoma, additional data are needed to characterize its reliability and limitations; for instance, it has been noted that PRAME does not diffusely stain most desmoplastic melanomas.[37]

MOLECULAR TESTING

An increasing number of molecular tests have become available to assist in establishing the diagnosis, prognosis, and susceptibility to targeted therapy of melanocytic neoplasms. These should be interpreted in the context of the clinical and histopathologic findings.

Comparative Genomic Hybridization

Comparative genomic hybridization (CGH) is a technique used to detect chromosomal copy number abnormalities in a tumor sample. Most melanomas (96.2%) have such abnormalities, while they are rare in benign nevi.[38] A key advantage is that CGH assesses the entire chromosomal complement in 1 study. Disadvantages include expense, long turnaround time, limited availability, and the need for a relatively pure tumor sample.

Fluorescence In Situ Hybridization

Fluorescence in situ hybridization (FISH) is used to detect chromosomal copy number alterations at specific genomic loci. It has a sensitivity of 86.7% and specificity of 95.4% when applied to a group of melanomas and benign nevi[39]; however, when applied to a group of histologically ambiguous lesions with long-term clinical follow up, lower sensitivity and specificity rates were

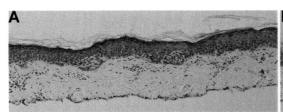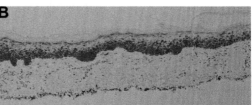

Fig. 4. Melanoma in situ. (*A*) Routinely stained sections show only subtle findings, with rare nests of melanocytes at the dermoepidermal junction. (H&E ×100). (*B*) A Melan-A stain on the same specimen highlights a confluent proliferation of junctional melanocytes with suprabasilar scatter, consistent with melanoma in situ. (× 100).

reported.[40] Advantages include greater availability, lower cost, and faster turnaround time than for CGH, as well as the potential to study a specific morphologic population within a heterogeneous tumor. A disadvantage is that only a small number of chromosomes are assessed in a given assay, which may compromise sensitivity. The test is operator dependent, and is best performed by an experienced laboratory. Like CGH, FISH detects chromosomal copy number alterations, but does not detect mutations.

Next-Generation Sequencing

Next-generation sequencing (NGS) is a technique for sequencing many genes simultaneously, providing much greater speed than previous methodologies. NGS can detect not only chromosomal copy number alterations, but also point mutations, insertions, deletions, and rearrangements. It can be used to sequence the entire genome or a set of specifically targeted genes.

NGS is currently used to assess melanoma specimens for therapeutically actionable mutations; for example, a BRAF V600E or V600K mutation would suggest candidacy for therapy with BRAF and MEK inhibitors, if clinically indicated. Because NGS also has the ability to more broadly characterize the mutational profile of melanocytic neoplasms, it will likely play an increasingly important role in establishing diagnosis[41] and prognosis. Its potential in this regard should be increasingly realized as data sets are established with correlation of mutational profile, histopathologic findings, and clinical outcomes.

Gene Expression Profiling

A 23-gene expression profile (23-GEP) is available for assistance in classifying melanocytic neoplasms as either benign or malignant. This assay had a sensitivity of 72% and specificity of 94% in 189 cases with an unequivocal histopathologic diagnosis of either nevus or melanoma; in histologically ambiguous lesions, the sensitivity and specificity were 50% and 96%, respectively.[42] The assay performs best with a specimen in which tumor cells comprise at least 10% of the sample volume.[43]

For tumors in which a diagnosis of melanoma has already been established, a prognostic 31-gene expression profile (31-GEP) is available; this categorizes lesions as having either a projected low risk (class 1) or high risk (class 2) of recurrence and metastasis.[44] The sensitivity and positive predictive value are low in stage I melanoma, limiting utility in this group.[45] It remains unclear whether patient outcomes improve as a result of management changes driven by a 31-GEP; NCCN guidelines recommend that additional studies be performed prior to routine implementation of this test.[10] A recent study showed that patients greater than 65 years of age with T1 and T2 melanoma and a low risk (class 1A) 31-GEP score had a very low frequency of SLN positivity (1.6%).[46] If these results are reproducible, this assay could find utility in identifying a group of patients in whom SLN biopsy has a low anticipated yield.

SENTINEL LYMPH NODE PATHOLOGY

Sentinel lymph node pathology (SLN) biopsy is commonly performed for staging of melanoma of at least 0.8 mm in thickness, and may also be considered in tumors of lower thickness when other high-risk features are present (mitotic index $\geq 2/mm^2$, lymphatic invasion, ulceration).[10] There is currently no standard protocol for the handling and processing of melanoma SLN specimens by pathology laboratories, and practices vary widely.[47,48] In a survey of multiple institutions, commonly employed practices included: (1) submission of all SLN tissue for histopathologic examination, (2) gross dissection of lymph nodes by cutting along the longitudinal axis, (3) examination of multiple tissue sections, and (4) use of immunohistochemical stains.[47]

Immunohistochemical stains commonly employed to detect melanocytes within an SLN include S100, SOX10, Melan-A, HMB45, and tyrosinase. S100 is highly sensitive, but challenging to interpret because of staining of normal nodal dendritic cells. SOX10 and Melan-A provide high sensitivity[49,50] and improved specificity. Occasional small, SOX10-positive perivascular cells may be observed, and should not be misinterpreted as melanoma.[51]

Melanocytic deposits in lymph nodes may be benign (nodal nevus) or malignant (metastatic melanoma), and this histopathologic distinction can be difficult, particularly when deposits are small. Comparison of the cellular morphology with the primary tumor can be helpful, with morphologic similarity to a previously biopsied melanoma favoring a diagnosis of metastatic melanoma. Nodal nevi most often consist of small, bland melanocytes within the fibrous capsule or trabeculae,[52] while melanoma cells are more likely to show cytologic atypia and a subcapsular or intraparenchymal location (**Fig. 5**).[53] Reticulin staining is noted around individual cells in most nevi, and around groups of cells in melanomas.[54] Most melanoma metastases stain for HMB45, while nodal nevi often show little to no staining for this marker.[52,53] Staining for PRAME

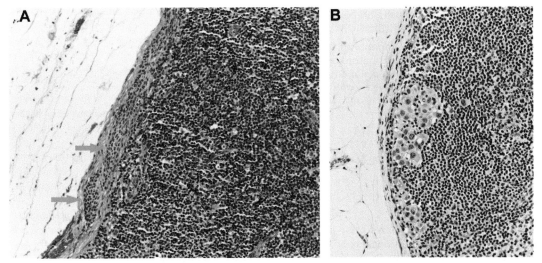

Fig. 5. Sentinel lymph nodes. (*A*) Nodal nevus: within the fibrous capsule, there is a deposit of small, bland melanocytes (*arrows*). (H&E ×200). (*B*) Metastatic melanoma: within the nodal parenchyma, there is a deposit of large, atypical melanocytes. (H&E ×200).

in most of the melanocytes favors melanoma over nodal nevus.[36,55] Although these stains can be a useful adjunct, they are not always feasible, as small melanocytic deposits may no longer be present if additional sections must be obtained for further immunohistochemistry.

A SLN is considered to be positive if any melanoma cells are identified, regardless of the number of cells, or how they are detected (H&E vs immunohistochemistry).[6] It is important to note that cells detected immunohistochemically must have morphologic characteristics of melanoma to be considered as malignant; if isolated cells are positive on immunohistochemistry, but do not show morphologic features of melanoma, they should not prompt designation as a positive sentinel lymph node.[56]

To assess tumor burden in a positive SLN, the maximum dimension of the largest discrete melanoma deposit is histologically measured.[6] Larger deposits have been associated with increased risk of positive non-SLNs and poorer melanoma-specific survival.[57,58] Extranodal extension, defined as nodal metastasis extending through the lymph node capsule into adjacent tissues, is associated with reduced relapse-free survival and melanoma-specific survival.[6,58]

SUMMARY

Most melanocytic neoplasms can be accurately classified on the basis of conventional histopathology. Good communication between the clinician, pathologist, and laboratory staff is necessary to optimize the accuracy of histopathologic

diagnosis. For diagnostically challenging lesions, immunohistochemical stains and molecular tests are available, but must be interpreted in the context of the clinical history, examination findings, and histomorphology.

CLINICS CARE POINTS

- Breslow thickness and ulceration are major determinants of melanoma prognosis.

- Recommended surgical margins for melanoma refer to a clinical measurement; there is not a standard recommendation for the necessary distance from the margin as measured histologically.

- Providing clinical information on a pathology requisition form increases the chances of obtaining an accurate histopathologic diagnosis.

- Nail unit specimens are often difficult to orient in the laboratory; special care and communication with laboratory staff are necessary to ensure proper handling.

- Lentigo maligna is often poorly circumscribed histologically, and assessment of margins is consequently challenging.

- Spitz nevi can mimic melanoma histologically; a diagnosis of melanoma in a child should be questioned to ensure veracity.

- Melanocytic deposits in lymph nodes can be either benign (nodal nevus) or malignant (melanoma); when deposits are very small, the distinction can be difficult.

- An increasing array of immunohistochemical stains and molecular assays is becoming available to assist in establishing melanoma diagnosis, prognosis, and therapeutic options.

DISCLOSURE

The author has no financial conflicts of interest to disclose.

REFERENCES

1. Weinstock MA, Sober AJ. The risk of progression of lentigo maligna to lentigo maligna melanoma. Br J Dermatol 1987;116(3):303–10.
2. Huang K, Fan J, Misra S. Acral lentiginous melanoma: incidence and survival in the United States, 2006-2015, an analysis of the SEER registry. J Surg Res 2020;251:329–39.
3. Howard MD, Wee E, Wolfe R, et al. Differences between pure desmoplastic melanoma and superficial spreading melanoma in terms of survival, distribution and other clinicopathologic features. J Eur Acad Dermatol Venereol 2019;33(10):1899–906.
4. Curtin JA, Busam K, Pinkel D, et al. Somatic activation of KIT in distinct subtypes of melanoma. J Clin Oncol 2006;24(26):4340–6.
5. Hodi FS, Corless CL, Giobbie-Hurder A, et al. Imatinib for melanomas harboring mutationally activated or amplified KIT arising on mucosal, acral, and chronically sun-damaged skin. J Clin Oncol 2013; 31(26):3182–90.
6. Gershenwald JE, Scolyer RA, Hess KR, et al. Melanoma of the skin. In: Amin MD, Edge SB, Greene FL, et al, editors. AJCC cancer staging manual. 8th edition. New York: Springer; 2017. p. 563–85.
7. Dodds TJ, Lo S, Jackett L, et al. Prognostic significance of periadnexal extension in cutaneous melanoma and its implications for pathologic reporting and staging. Am J Surg Pathol 2018;42(3):359–66.
8. Gershenwald JE, Scolyer RA, Hess KR, et al. Melanoma staging: evidence-based changes in the American Joint Committee on Cancer 8th edition cancer staging manual. CA Cancer J Clin 2017; 67(6):472–92.
9. Thompson JF, Soong SJ, Balch CM, et al. Prognostic significance of mitotic rate in localized primary cutaneous melanoma: an analysis of patients in the multi-institutional American Joint Committee on Cancer melanoma staging database. J Clin Oncol 2011; 29(16):2199–205.
10. NCCN clinical practice guidelines in oncology: cutaneous melanoma. Version 4.2020. Available at: https://www.nccn.org/professionals/physician_gls/pdf/cutaneous_melanoma.pdf.   Accessed September 8, 2020.
11. Read RL, Haydu L, Saw RP, et al. In-transit melanoma metastases: incidence, prognosis, and the role of lymphadenectomy. Ann Surg Oncol 2015; 22(2):475–81.
12. Kaur C, Thomas RJ, Desai N, et al. The correlation of regression in primary melanoma with sentinel lymph node status. J Clin Pathol 2008;61(3): 297–300.
13. Gualano MR, Osella-Abate S, Scaioli G, et al. Prognostic role of histological regression in primary cutaneous melanoma: a systematic review and meta-analysis. Br J Dermatol 2018;178(2):357–62.
14. Ribero S, Galli F, Osella-Abate S, et al. Prognostic impact of regression in patients with primary cutaneous melanoma >1 mm in thickness. J Am Acad Dermatol 2019;80(1):99–105.
15. Cerroni L, Argenyi Z, Cerio R, et al. Influence of evaluation of clinical pictures on the histopathologic diagnosis of inflammatory skin disorders. J Am Acad Dermatol 2010;63(4):647–52.
16. Aslan C, Göktay F, Mansur AT, et al. Clinicopathological consistency in skin disorders: a retrospective study of 3949 pathological reports. J Am Acad Dermatol 2012;66(3):393–400.
17. Ferrara G, Annessi G, Argenyi Z, et al. Prior knowledge of the clinical picture does not introduce bias in the histopathologic diagnosis of melanocytic skin lesions. J Cutan Pathol 2015;42(12): 953–8.
18. Wong C, Peters M, Tilburt J, et al. Dermatopathologists' opinions about the quality of clinical information in the skin biopsy requisition form and the skin biopsy care process: a semiqualitative assessment. Am J Clin Pathol 2015;143(4):593–7.
19. Reinig E, Rich P, Thompson CT. How to submit a nail specimen. Dermatol Clin 2015;33(2):303–7.
20. Hendi A, Brodland DG, Zitelli JA. Melanocytes in long-standing sun-exposed skin: quantitative analysis using the MART-1 immunostain. Arch Dermatol 2006;142(7):871–6.
21. Hendi A, Wada DA, Jacobs MA, et al. Melanocytes in nonlesional sun-exposed skin: a multicenter comparative study. J Am Acad Dermatol 2011; 65(6):1186–93.
22. Kunishige JH, Brodland DG, Zitelli JA. Surgical margins for melanoma in situ. J Am Acad Dermatol 2012;66(3):438–44.
23. Liu A, Botkin A, Murray C, et al. Outcomes of staged excision with circumferential en face margin control for lentigo maligna of the head and neck. J Cutan Med Surg 2020;10. 1203475420952425.
24. Campbell LB, Kreicher KL, Gittleman HR, et al. Melanoma incidence in children and adolescents: decreasing trends in the United States. J Pediatr 2015;166(6):1505–13.

25. Zedek DC, McCalmont TH. Spitz nevi, atypical spitzoid neoplasms, and spitzoid melanoma. Clin Lab Med 2011;31(2):311–20.

26. Ritter A, Tronnier M, Vaske B, et al. Reevaluation of established and new criteria in differential diagnosis of Spitz nevus and melanoma. Arch Dermatol Res 2018;310(4):329–42.

27. Wiesner T, Kutzner H, Cerroni L, et al. Genomic aberrations in spitzoid melanocytic tumours and their implications for diagnosis, prognosis and therapy. Pathology 2016;48(2):113–31.

28. Massi D, De Giorgi V, Mandalà M. The complex management of atypical Spitz tumours. Pathology 2016;48(2):132–41.

29. Ludgate MW, Fullen DR, Lee J, et al. The atypical Spitz tumor of uncertain biologic potential: a series of 67 patients from a single institution. Cancer 2009;115(3):631–41.

30. Piepkorn MW, Longton GM, Reisch LM, et al. Assessment of second-opinion strategies for diagnoses of cutaneous melanocytic lesions. JAMA Netw Open 2019;2(10):e1912597.

31. Beatson M, Eleryan MG, Reserva J, et al. Importance of pathology review to complement clinical management of melanoma. J Am Acad Dermatol 2020;83(6):1784–6.

32. Niebling MG, Haydu LE, Karim RZ, et al. Pathology review significantly affects diagnosis and treatment of melanoma patients: an analysis of 5011 patients treated at a melanoma treatment center. Ann Surg Oncol 2014;21(7):2245–51.

33. Isom C, Hooks M, Kauffmann RM. Internal pathology review of invasive melanoma: an academic institution experience. J Surg Res 2020;250:97–101.

34. Rudolph P, Schubert C, Schubert B, et al. Proliferation marker Ki-S5 as a diagnostic tool in melanocytic lesions. J Am Acad Dermatol 1997;37(2 Pt 1): 169–78.

35. Lezcano C, Jungbluth AA, Busam KJ. Comparison of immunohistochemistry for PRAME with cytogenetic test results in the evaluation of challenging melanocytic tumors. Am J Surg Pathol 2020;44(7): 893–900.

36. Lezcano C, Pulitzer M, Moy AP, et al. Immunohistochemistry for PRAME in the distinction of nodal nevi from metastatic melanoma. Am J Surg Pathol 2020;44(4):503–8.

37. Lezcano C, Jungbluth AA, Nehal KS, et al. PRAME expression in melanocytic tumors. Am J Surg Pathol 2018;42(11):1456–65.

38. Bastian BC, Olshen AB, LeBoit PE, et al. Classifying melanocytic tumors based on DNA copy number changes. Am J Pathol 2003;163(5):1765–70.

39. Gerami P, Jewell SS, Morrison LE, et al. Fluorescence in situ hybridization (FISH) as an ancillary diagnostic tool in the diagnosis of melanoma. Am J Surg Pathol 2009;33(8):1146–56.

40. Gaiser T, Kutzner H, Palmedo G, et al. Classifying ambiguous melanocytic lesions with FISH and correlation with clinical long-term follow up. Mod Pathol 2010;23(3):413–9.

41. Jackett LA, Colebatch AJ, Rawson RV, et al. Molecular profiling of noncoding mutations distinguishes nevoid melanomas from mitotically active nevi in pregnancy. Am J Surg Pathol 2020;44(3):357–67.

42. Reimann JDR, Salim S, Velazquez EF, et al. Comparison of melanoma gene expression score with histopathology, fluorescence in situ hybridization, and SNP array for the classification of melanocytic neoplasms. Mod Pathol 2018;31(11):1733–43.

43. Clarke LE, Flake DD 2nd, Busam K, et al. An independent validation of a gene expression signature to differentiate malignant melanoma from benign melanocytic nevi. Cancer 2017;123(4):617–28.

44. Zager JS, Gastman BR, Leachman S, et al. Performance of a prognostic 31-gene expression profile in an independent cohort of 523 cutaneous melanoma patients. BMC Cancer 2018;18(1):130.

45. Fried L, Tan A, Bajaj S, et al. Technological advances for the detection of melanoma: advances in molecular techniques. J Am Acad Dermatol 2020; 83(4):996–1004.

46. Vetto JT, Hsueh EC, Gastman BR, et al. Guidance of sentinel lymph node biopsy decisions in patients with T1-T2 melanoma using gene expression profiling. Future Oncol 2019;15(11):1207–17.

47. Dekker J, Duncan LM. Lack of standards for the detection of melanoma in sentinel lymph nodes: a survey and recommendations. Arch Pathol Lab Med 2013;137(11):1603–9.

48. Cole CM, Ferringer T. Histopathologic evaluation of the sentinel lymph node for malignant melanoma: the unstandardized process. Am J Dermatopathol 2014;36(1):80–7.

49. Karimipour DJ, Lowe L, Su L, et al. Standard immunostains for melanoma in sentinel lymph node specimens: which ones are most useful? J Am Acad Dermatol 2004;50(5):759–64.

50. Szumera-Ciećkiewicz A, Bosisio F, Teterycz P, et al, EORTC Melanoma Group. SOX10 is as specific as S100 protein in detecting metastases of melanoma in lymph nodes and is recommended for sentinel lymph node assessment. Eur J Cancer 2020;137: 175–82.

51. Merelo Alcocer V, Flamm A, Chen G, et al. SOX10 Immunostaining in granulomatous dermatoses and benign reactive lymph nodes. J Cutan Pathol 2019; 46(8):586–90.

52. Carson KF, Wen DR, Li PX, et al. Nodal nevi and cutaneous melanomas. Am J Surg Pathol 1996; 20(7):834–40.

53. Murray CA, Leong WL, McCready DR, et al. Histopathological patterns of melanoma metastases in sentinel lymph nodes. J Clin Pathol 2004;57(1):64–7.

54. Kanner WA, Barry CI, Smart CN, et al. Reticulin and NM23 staining in the interpretation of lymph nodal nevus rests. Am J Dermatopathol 2013;35(4): 452–7.

55. See SHC, Finkelman BS, Yeldandi AV. The diagnostic utility of PRAME and p16 in distinguishing nodal nevi from nodal metastatic melanoma. Pathol Res Pract 2020;216(9):153105.

56. Scolyer RA, Gershenwald JE, Thompson JF. Isolated immunohistochemistry-positive cells without morphologic characteristics of melanoma should not result in designation as a positive sentinel lymph node according to the AJCC 8th edition staging system. Am J Surg Pathol 2019;43(10):1442–4.

57. van der Ploeg AP, van Akkooi AC, Haydu LE, et al. The prognostic significance of sentinel node tumour burden in melanoma patients: an international, multicenter study of 1539 sentinel node-positive melanoma patients. Eur J Cancer 2014;50(1):111–20.

58. Namikawa K, Aung PP, Milton DR, et al. Correlation of tumor burden in sentinel lymph nodes with tumor burden in nonsentinel lymph nodes and survival in cutaneous melanoma. Clin Cancer Res 2019; 25(24):7585–93.

American Joint Committee on Cancer Staging and Other Platforms to Assess Prognosis and Risk

Paola Barriera-Silvestrini, MD[a], Julie Iacullo, MD[a],
Thomas J. Knackstedt, MD[a,b],*

KEYWORDS

- Melanoma • Staging • Prognosis • Sentinel lymph node biopsy • Survival

KEY POINTS

- Patients with stages I and II melanoma have localized disease, while those with stages III and IV melanoma have regional and distant metastatic disease, respectively.
- With more accurate nodal staging, survival outcomes for patients with similar stage groups were generally greater in the eighth edition than in the seventh edition.
- A number of clinical and pathologic parameters excluded from the staging system are independent predictors of outcome, such as advancing age and female gender, among others.
- Regional lymph nodes represent the most common first site of metastasis in melanoma patients.

INTRODUCTION

An effective staging system must be simple, intuitive, and practical while accurately determining the prognosis of the patients to whom it is being applied. Formal staging of cancer is fundamental in developing treatment strategies, facilitating centralized registry reporting, and designing, conducting, and analyzing clinical trials.

Over 4 decades ago, the first multivariate analysis of prognostic factors for melanoma was published, and several reports have subsequently promoted our understanding of relevant prognostic indicators for this disease.[1–3] It later became apparent that a unified melanoma staging system applicable to both clinical practice and research was needed.[4–6] In 1998, the American Joint Committee on Cancer (AJCC) Melanoma Staging Committee developed the AJCC melanoma staging database, an international compilation of prospectively accumulated melanoma outcome data from several centers and clinical trials.[7] This system relies on assessments of the primary tumor (T), regional lymph nodes (N), and distant metastatic sites (M).

Recently, the progressive refinement of the staging system, based on an international contemporary cohort of 43,792 patients, led to revisions adopted in the AJCC eighth edition. This update has improved risk stratification, introduced new staging categories, and resulted in stage migration of patients with improved outcomes (**Fig. 1**).[8]

EIGHTH EDITION AMERICAN JOINT COMMITTEE ON CANCER STAGING SYSTEM

Melanoma staging in AJCC eighth edition shows greater reproducibility and higher concordance

Disclosures: The authors have nothing to disclose.
Funding sources: none.
This work has not been previously presented or published.
a Department of Dermatology, MetroHealth System, 2500 Metrohealth Drive, Cleveland, OH 44109, USA;
b Case Western Reserve University, School of Medicine, Cleveland, OH, USA
* Corresponding author. 2500 Metrohealth Drive, Cleveland, OH 44109.
E-mail address: thomas.j.knackstedt@gmail.com

Clin Plastic Surg 48 (2021) 599–606
https://doi.org/10.1016/j.cps.2021.05.004

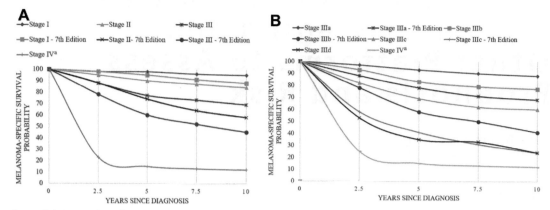

Fig. 1. (*A*) Composite of 10-year melanoma survival data based on comparing American Joint Committee on Cancer Seventh and Eighth Editions Stages I-IV. (*B*) Composite of 10-year melanoma survival data based on comparing American Joint Committee on Cancer Seventh and Eighth Editions Stages III-IV. [a]*The survival curve for stage IV melanoma remains unchanged in the eighth edition. (Data from* Gershenwald JE, Scolyer RA, Hess KR, et al. Melanoma staging: Evidence-based changes in the American Joint Committee on Cancer eighth edition cancer staging manual. *CA Cancer J Clin.* 2017;67:472–492 and Balch CM, Gershenwald JE, Soong SJ, et al. Final version of 2009 AJCC melanoma staging and classification. *J Clin Oncol.* 2009;27:6199–6206.)

with a reference standard. For T1a diagnoses, concordance with the consensus reference diagnosis increased from 44% (95% confidence interval [CI], 41%-48%) to 54% (95% CI, 51%-57%) using AJCC 7 and AJCC 8 criteria, respectively. For cases of T1b or greater, the concordance increased from 72% (95% CI, 68%-75%) to 78% (95% CI, 75%-80%). Intraobserver reproducibility of diagnoses also improved, increasing from 59% (95% CI, 56%-63%) to 64% (95% CI, 62%-67%) for T1a invasive melanoma, and from 74% (95% CI, 71%-76%) to 77% (95% CI, 74%-79%) for T1b or greater invasive melanoma cases.[9] In view of the clinical ramifications, even modest changes suggest a positive impact on patients.

T CATEGORY

In the eighth edition of AJCC staging system, the T-category thresholds of melanoma Breslow thickness continue to be defined at 1-, 2-, and 4-mm intervals. Patients are stratified into 8 T subcategories (T1a through T4b).[5,10] Letters "a" and "b" note the respective absence or presence of tumor ulceration.

Evaluation of the entire tumor from an excisional biopsy is recommended to ensure measurement of the thickest part of the lesion. The maximal tumor thickness is measured perpendicular to the surface of the skin over the tumor mass. The upper reference point is the superficial aspect of the granular cell layer of the epidermis, or the base of the lesion if the tumor is ulcerated. The lower reference point is the deepest point of invasion and may be represented by "detached" cell

clusters beneath the mass.[11] In prior editions of the AJCC Cancer Staging Manual, primary melanoma tumor thickness was recorded to the nearest 0.01 mm. In the eighth edition, the second decimal point was omitted in accordance with the recommendations by the International Collaboration on Cancer Reporting and the International Melanoma Pathology Study Group.[10,12,13]

T1 tumors are defined as ≤1 mm, with T1a being less than 0.8 mm without ulceration and T1b being less than 0.8 mm with ulceration or 0.8 to 1.0 mm with or without ulceration. The subdivision of T1 tumors is based on an analysis of factors predicting melanoma-specific survival (MSS) among 7568 patients with T1N0 melanoma from the International Melanoma Database and Discovery Platform database.[10] In a multivariate analysis, MSS was worse for patients with a melanoma of thickness ≥0.8 mm compared with less than 0.8 mm (hazard ratio [HR], 1.7; $P = .057$) and for those with ulceration compared with those with nonulcerated melanoma (HR, 2.6; $P = .035$). Moreover, the subcategorization of T1 melanomas using the 0.8-mm threshold is predictive of sentinel lymph node (SNL) metastasis. Overall, a positive SLN biopsy occurs in less than 5% of those with a melanoma of thickness 0.8 mm compared with 5% to 12% in those with 0.8- to 1.0-mm-thick melanoma. SNL biopsy can be considered in the latter group.[14–17]

The remaining T-categories are T0, Tis, TX, T2, T3, and T4.[8] T0 melanomas have a completely regressed or unknown primary tumor (eg, in a patient who presents with nodal or visceral metastasis and no known primary tumor). Tis is used for melanoma *in situ* (restricted to the epidermis) even if it represents the remainder of a tumor after complete regression of its invasive component. TX tumors are those in which the tumor thickness cannot be assessed (eg, curettage specimens). T2 is used for tumors of thickness greater than 1.0 to 2.0 mm, T3 for greater than 2.0 to 4.0 mm, and T4 for greater than 4.0 mm; these are subdivided into a or b based on the absence or presence of ulceration, respectively. Ulceration, defined as the absence of an intact epithelium over the melanoma, is an important prognostic factor and T-category criterion associated with worse outcomes.[1,8,18–20] In partially regressed invasive melanomas, the thickness should be measured in standard technique to the deepest viable tumor which will determine the appropriate T category.

The role of mitotic rate in the development of clinical assessment tools remains under exploration. The AJCC Cancer Staging Manual recommends using the "hot-spot" approach to determine the mitotic rate, whereby it is reported as the maximum dermal mitotic figures identified per square millimeter.[8] Challenges to standard reporting include interobserver variability, irregular distribution of mitotic figures throughout the tumor sections, and factors that may obscure mitotic figures such as heavy pigmentation, high cellularity, pyknotic debris, and necrosis.[21] As a dichotomous variable comparing less than 1 mitosis/mm^2 with greater than 1 mitosis/mm^2, mitotic rate was not an independent factor for predicting MSS among 7568 T1 N0 melanoma patients (HR, 0.85; $P = .57$). Nevertheless, increasing mitotic rate was significantly associated with decreasing MSS in univariate analyses among T1 to T4 melanomas of the eighth edition database.[10] Therefore, the significance of mitotic rate remains under investigation, and the AJCC Melanoma Expert Panel strongly recommends that mitotic rate be assessed and recorded for all primary melanomas eventhough the mitotic rate was not incorporated into the AJCC eighth edition.[8]

N CATEGORY

The N category serves to record metastatic disease, both in regional lymph nodes (LNs) and in nonnodal locoregional sites (ie, microsatellites, satellites, and in-transit metastases).

In the eighth edition, regional LN involvement is classified as clinically occult or clinically detected. Clinically occult nodal metastasis (formerly known as microscopic nodal metastasis) describes patients with microscopically identified regional node metastasis via SLN biopsy. LNs are also considered as tumor-involved if melanoma cells are found in a lymphatic channel within or immediately adjacent to them. Clinically detected nodal metastasis (formerly known as macroscopic nodal metastasis) describes patients with regional node metastasis identified by clinical, radiographic, or ultrasound examination.[22] When two or more nodes are found adhering to one another through metastatic disease during macroscopic evaluation of pathology specimens, they are regarded as matted nodes.[10]

Furthermore, the N category documents nonnodal locoregional metastases: microsatellite, satellite, and in-transit metastases.[8] These are thought to represent intralymphatic or angiotrophic tumor spread. Microsatellites are defined histopathologically as microscopic cutaneous and/or subcutaneous metastases adjacent to or deep to and completely discontinuous from a primary melanoma with unaffected stroma occupying the space between.[23] Satellites are defined as clinically evident cutaneous and/or subcutaneous metastases occurring within 2 cm of the primary melanoma; however, they are regarded as in-transit metastases if found at a distance beyond 2 cm.[22,23]

As a general rule, the total number of tumor-involved regional LNs determines the N categories. N0 is used when regional metastases are not detected; N1 refers to one involved LN, or in transit, satellite, and/or microsatellite metastases with no tumor-involved nodes; N2 documents two or three tumor-involved nodes, or in transit, satellite, and/or microsatellite metastases with one tumor-involved node; and N3 identifies four or more tumor-involved nodes, in transit, satellite, and/or microsatellite metastases with two or more tumor-involved nodes, or any number of matted nodes with or without in transit, satellite, and/or microsatellite metastases. All the N categories are subdivided into a (clinically occult nodal metastasis), b (clinically detected nodal metastasis), and c (presence of nonnodal locoregional metastases). When regional nodes are not assessed (eg, SNL biopsy not performed, previously resected nodes for other reasons), the NX designation is used.[8]

Extranodal extension (ENE) is defined as nodal metastasis extending through the LN capsule and into adjacent tissue on microscopic examination.[8] A multicenter retrospective cohort study of 515 patients with nodal metastases comprehensively analyzed the clinical relevance of extracapsular extension (ECS), which is synonymous with ENE. Data analysis revealed that ECS was significantly associated with worse overall survival (OS), disease-specific survival, and progression-free survival (Kaplan–Meier log-rank test $P<.0001$, all instances).[24] Although ENE is not formally included as an N criterion, it is recommended that this factor be recorded for future investigations.[25] LN ratio—the number of metastatic LNs over the number of excised LNs after lymphadenectomy—has become more prevalent as a prognostic factor in patients with LN-positive cancer. In 2010, Balch and colleagues conducted a research on 2313 melanoma patients with metastatic LNs.[26] Results suggested that the number of metastatic LNs had the most significant impact on OS when compared with age, ulceration, tumor thickness, and nodal tumor burden.[26] In addition, when these patients were stratified according to tumor burden, microscopic nodal metastases had a more heterogeneous range in 5-year survival (between 23% and 87%) than the narrower range of 5-year survival among patients with nodal macrometastases (between 29% and 51.6%). Data from other studies further support that clinically occult regional node disease portends better outcomes than clinically macroscopic disease.[27–29]

M CATEGORY

In the eighth edition of AJCC melanoma staging system, patients are assigned to an M subcategory based on the anatomic site of metastasis.[8] M1a is used for metastasis to skin, subcutaneous tissue, muscle, or distant LN; M1b categorizes lung metastasis; M1c designates metastasis to other visceral sites (exclusive of the central nervous system [CNS]); and M1d identifies CNS metastasis. The latter is a new addition to the staging system and reflects the associated poor overall survival outcome for patient with CNS metastases.

Serum lactate dehydrogenase (LDH) is an important independent prognostic factor.[30,31] A meta-analysis of 52 studies found that elevated LDH levels were associated with an HR for OS of 1.72 (95% CI, 1.6–1.85; $P<.0001$) and an HR for progression-free survival of 1.83 (95% CI, 1.53–2.2; $P<.0001$).[32] In the seventh edition, an elevated LDH would automatically place patients in the M1c category.[18] The current edition has been modified to include a designation for LDH status: (0) for nonelevated LDH and (1) for elevated LDH. For example, M1b(1) would depict a patient with lung metastasis and elevated serum LDH.

PROGNOSTIC STAGE GROUPS

Tumor size, the number of involved LNs, and metastases of melanoma contribute toward its stage group. As in prior editions, there is a distinction between clinical and pathologic staging. Clinical

staging (cTNM) is based on physical examination and imaging results, whereas pathologic staging (pTNM) combines the clinical information with details derived from surgical procedures (wide excision of primary tumor and regional LN assessment).[8]

Stage 0 melanoma is reserved for melanoma in situ (Tis).

Stage I melanoma is considered a localized tumor, meaning there is no evidence of spread beyond the primary tumor (ie, regional or distant metastases). It is divided into the subgroups IA and IB which include melanomas less than 1 mm in thickness with or without ulceration and those up to 2 mm in thickness without ulceration (T1a, T1b, and T2a). With appropriate treatment, stage I melanoma is highly curable. It is in association with a low risk for recurrence or metastasis. The 5-year relative survival rate for stage I disease is 99%.[33]

Stage II melanoma is also considered a localized tumor of higher recurrence risk either due to depth of tumor or presence of ulceration. It is divided into the subgroups IIA, IIB, and IIC which include tumors beyond 1 mm in thickness with ulceration and those beyond 2 mm with or without ulceration (T2b, T3a, T3b, T4a, and T4b). The 5-year survival rate for stage II disease ranges from 63% to 82%.[10,34]

Stage III melanomas are tumors that have spread to regional LNs or have developed in-transit or satellite metastases (N1, N2, and N3) but have no evidence of distant metastasis. Stage III is known as regional melanoma, meaning it has spread beyond the primary tumor to the closest LNs but not distant sites. It is subclassified as IIIa, IIIb, IIIc, and IIId based on the extent of lymphatic disease. Stages IIIa and IIIb were formerly (AJCC seventh edition) only defined by the status of regional LNs and primary tumor ulceration. In the eighth edition, survival in these stages has improved, as they are now restricted to thinner primary tumors. The addition of stage IIId, newly created for T4bN3M0 tumors, has allowed for further separation of the survival curves and stratification of patients. The 5-year MSS rate according to stage III subgroups ranges from 93% in patients with stage IIIa disease to 32% for those with stage IIId disease.[31]

Stage IV melanomas are tumors that have spread beyond the regional LNs to distant sites (M1a to M1d). There are no subgroups for stage IV melanoma because the survival differences among patients within this stage group were historically narrow. With the increasing armamentarium of contemporary treatment modalities for advanced disease, stage IV survival outcomes are expected to improve. The 5-year relative survival rate for stage IV disease is 25%.[33]

OTHER PROGNOSTIC FACTORS

Many other factors not directly related to the tumor also affect the outcome. Some prognostic factors are essential to decisions about the goals and treatment choice.

- Age—A large multi-institutional study investigated patient age as an independent predictor of survival outcome.[35] The study included 11,088 cases of stage I, II, and III melanoma in the AJCC Melanoma Staging Database used for the seventh edition. Multivariate analyses found that age was independently associated with survival among all stage groups. Furthermore, they found that melanoma in patients younger than 20 years tended to have more aggressive features yet a more favorable outcome than all other age groups. Patients older than 70 years had melanomas with the most aggressive prognostic features and higher lethality than all other age groups. Finally, patients aged 20 to 70 years had few discernible differences in the natural history of their disease.
- Gender—Female gender appears to be consistently associated with better prognosis. In a multivariate analysis of 10,233 patients in the seventh edition of AJCC Melanoma Staging Database, female gender was an independent factor for survival ($\chi^2 = 33.9$; $P<.001$).[36] An analysis of 2672 patients with stage I/II melanoma included in the European Organisation for Research and Treatment of Cancer (EORTC) showed that female gender had a higher independent advantage in overall survival (adjusted HR, 0.70; 95% CI, 0.59–0.83), disease-specific survival (adjusted HR, 0.74; 95% CI, 0.62–0.88), time to LN metastasis (adjusted HR, 0.70; 95% CI, 0.51–0.96), and time to distant metastasis (adjusted HR, 0.69; 95% CI, 0.59–0.81).[37] A pooled analysis of five randomized trials conducted by the EORTC which included 2734 stage III and 1306 stage IV melanoma patients showed that females had a superior disease-specific and relapse-free survivals.[38]
- Anatomic location—Additional analyses have demonstrated that cutaneous melanomas arising on the head neck area and trunk have a worse prognosis.[36,39,40]
- Tumor burden within a SNL—A retrospective, multicenter cohort study noted that larger tumor burden within a positive LN (eg, size >1 mm, nonsubcapsular location, increasing tumor penetrative depth) appears to be associated with poorer melanoma-specific and disease-free survivals.[41]

- Histologic subtype—An observational study of roughly 120,000 patients suggested that nodular melanoma subtype is an independent risk factor for death.[42]
- Amelanotic melanoma—Amelanotic melanomas (AMs) are difficult to diagnose, as primary lesions not only lack the pigment typical of melanoma but also lack other features associated with these tumors. As a result, a delay in the implementation of treatment may contribute to a worse prognosis. Using cross-sectional, prospective data from 18 Surveillance, Epidemiology, and End Results registries, investigators found that AMs are significantly more likely to present with regional or distant metastases, as well as other unfavorable prognostic factors, than melanotic melanoma (MM). In addition, 5-year MSS was significantly lower in patients with AM than in patients with MM (72.3 vs 91.1%, $P<.001$).[43] Finally, in one series, patients with AM were more likely to have *BRAF* or *KIT* mutations, which may have consequences for implementation of the novel targeted therapies to treat this life-threatening disease.[44]
- Nevus association—Data from a retrospective analysis of two cohorts suggested that de novo melanomas are more aggressive than nevus-associated melanomas.[45]
- Circulating melanoma cells—Detection of circulating melanoma cells in the peripheral blood using reverse transcriptase polymerase chain reaction for tyrosinase and other markers such as Mart-1/Melan-A, MAGE-A3, and GalNAc-T might have a clinically valuable prognostic utility in patients with melanoma. However, caution is warranted given the heterogeneity of the studies published thus far.[46–49]

APPROACH TO STAGING PATIENTS WITH MULTIPLE PRIMARY MELANOMAS

As stated by the eighth edition of AJCC Principles of Cancer Staging, when patients present with multiple primary cutaneous melanomas, each is considered a different primary site and categorized accordingly. In patients with multiple primary melanomas draining to the same regional node basin who happen to harbor regional node metastases, the primary tumor with the highest T category should be regarded as the origin of the nodal metastases. If distant metastases are present, the primary tumor with the highest N category (or the highest T category if N0) should be designated as the origin.[22]

The stage used will be the highest of the primary tumors. One of two suffixes is added to indicate the presence of multiple primary tumors: the m suffix or the number of primary tumors.[22]

APPROACH TO STAGING PATIENTS AFTER NEOADJUVANT THERAPY

Effective systemic therapies have broadened the treatment approaches for patients with unresectable and regionally advanced melanoma. A staging schema for patients after treatment has been proposed in the eight edition of Principles of Cancer Staging chapter. Patients who receive radiation or systemic therapy as definitive treatment are classified as ycTNM after completion. Those who undergo neoadjuvant therapy followed by surgical resection are categorized as ypTNM.[22] This classification, although considered likely useful, is rarely used, and future studies are required for refinement.

APPROACH TO STAGING PATIENTS AFTER RECURRENCE/RETREATMENT

Clinical and pathologic classification according to the AJCC staging system occurs at the time of initial melanoma presentation. The eighth edition of Principles of Cancer Staging chapter also includes an additional classification schema for patients who experience recurrence, namely rTNM, which is further divided into "r-clinical" (rcTNM) and "r-pathological" (rpTNM) stages.[8] Nonetheless, this schema is relatively unknown, and future analyses will likely eventuate in revisions.

SUMMARY

A contemporary and accurate cancer staging system systematically guides treatment plans and allows meaningful comparisons to be made across patient populations. The landscape of melanoma staging and care will continue to evolve as new prognostic factors and evidence-based approaches are developed and validated.

CLINICS CARE POINTS

- Mitotic rate is no longer used to subcategorize T1 melanomas but should still be reported as it can impact prognosis for patients with stages I to III melanomas.
- Patients with stage II melanoma with high-risk features (such as greater tumor thickness and presence of ulceration) may have a worse prognosis than patients with primary melanoma with more favorable features and limited occult regional metastatic (stage IIIA) disease.
- The risk of sentinel lymph node metastasis is very uncommon among patients with T1a melanomas but rises with increasing primary melanoma thickness.
- Sentinel lymph node biopsy is recommended for patients with primary melanomas of thickness greater than 1.0 mm.

REFERENCES

1. Balch CM, Murad TM, Soong SJ, et al. A multifactorial analysis of melanoma: prognostic histopathological features comparing Clark's and Breslow's staging methods. Ann Surg 1978;188:732.
2. Eldh J, Boeryd B, Peterson LE. Prognostic factors in cutaneous malignant melanoma in stage I. A clinical, morphological and multivariate analysis. Scand J Plast Reconstr Surg 1978;12:243.
3. Van Der Esch EP, Cascinelli N, Preda F, et al. Stage I melanoma of the skin: evaluation of prognosis according to histologic characteristics. Cancer 1981; 48:1668.
4. Buzaid AC, Ross MI, Balch CM, et al. Critical analysis of the current American Joint Committee on Cancer staging system for cutaneous melanoma and proposal of a new staging system. J Clin Oncol 1997;15:1039.
5. Gershenwald JE, Buzaid AC, Ross MI. Classification and staging of melanoma. Hematol Oncol Clin North Am 1998;12:737.
6. Ross M. Modifying the criteria of the American Joint Commission on Cancer staging system in melanoma. Curr Opin Oncol 1998;10:153.
7. Thompson JF, Shaw HM, Hersey P, et al. The history and future of melanoma staging. J Surg Oncol 2004; 86:224.
8. Gershenwald JE, Scolyer RA, Hess KR, et al. Melanoma of the skin. In: Amin MB, Edge SB, Greene FL, et al, editors. AJCC cancer staging manual. 8. New York: Springer International Publishing; 2017. p. 563–85.
9. Elmore JG, Elder DE, Barnhill RL, et al. Concordance and reproducibility of melanoma staging according to the 7th vs 8th edition of the *AJCC cancer staging manual.* JAMA Netw Open 2018; 1(1):e180083.
10. Gershenwald JE, Scolyer RA, Hess KR, et al. For members of the American Joint Committee on cancer melanoma Expert Panel and the international melanoma database and Discovery Platform. Melanoma staging: evidence-based changes in the American Joint Committee on cancer eighth edition

cancer staging manual. CA Cancer J Clin 2017; 67(6):472–92.

11. Scolyer RA, Judge MJ, Evans A, et al. Data set for pathology reporting of cutaneous invasive melanoma: recommendations from the International Collaboration on Cancer Reporting (ICCR). Am J Surg Pathol 2013;37:1797–814.

12. Ge L, Vilain RE, Lo S, et al. Breslow thickness measurements of melanomas around American Joint Committee on cancer staging Cut-off points: imprecision and terminal digit bias have important implications for staging and patient management. Ann Surg Oncol 2016;23(8):2658–63.

13. Knackstedt T, Knackstedt RW, Couto R, et al. Malignant melanoma: diagnostic and management update. Plast Reconstr Surg 2018;142(2):202e–16e.

14. Andtbacka RH, Gershenwald JE. Role of sentinel lymph node biopsy in patients with thin melanoma. J Natl Compr Canc Netw 2009;7(3):308–17.

15. Cordeiro E, Gervais MK, Shah PS, et al. Sentinel lymph node biopsy in thin cutaneous melanoma: a systematic review and meta-analysis. Ann Surg Oncol 2016;23(13):4178–88.

16. Han D, Zager JS, Shyr Y, et al. Clinicopathologic predictors of sentinel lymph node metastasis in thin melanoma. J Clin Oncol 2013;31(35): 4387–93.

17. Murali R, Haydu LE, Quinn MJ, et al. Sentinel lymph node biopsy in patients with thin primary cutaneous melanoma. Ann Surg 2012;255(1):128–33.

18. Balch CM, Gershenwald JE, Atkins MB, et al. Melanoma of the skin. In: Edge SB, Byrd DR, Compton CC, et al, editors. AJCC cancer staging manual. 7. New York: Springer International Publishing; 2010. p. 325–46.

19. Balch CM, Gershenwald JE, Soong SJ, et al. Final version of 2009 AJCC melanoma staging and classification. J Clin Oncol 2009;27:6199–206.

20. In 't Hout FE, Haydu LE, Murali R, et al. Prognostic importance of the extent of ulceration in patients with clinically localized cutaneous melanoma. Ann Surg 2012;255:1165–70.

21. Hale CS, Qian M, Ma MW, et al. Mitotic rate in melanoma: prognostic value of immunostaining and computer-assisted image analysis. Am J Surg Pathol 2013;37(6):882–9.

22. Gress DM, Edge SB, Greene FL, et al. Principles of cancer staging. In: Amin MB, Edge SB, Greene FL, et al, editors. AJCC cancer staging manual. 8. New York: Springer International Publishing; 2017. p. 3–30.

23. Greene FL, Compton CC, Fritz AG, et al, editors. AJCC cancer staging Atlas. 6. New York: Springer; 2006. p. 207–16. Melanoma of the skin.

24. Lo M, Robinson A, Wade R, et al. Extracapsular spread in melanoma Lymphadenopathy: prognostic implications, classification, and management. Ann

Surg Oncol 2020. https://doi.org/10.1245/s10434-020-09099-w.

25. Crookes TR, Scolyer RA, Lo S, et al. Extra-nodal spread is associated with recurrence and poor survival in stage III cutaneous melanoma patients. Ann Surg Oncol 2017;4:1378–85.

26. Balch CM, Gershenwald JE, Soong SJ, et al. Multivariate analysis of prognostic factors among 2,313 patients with stage III melanoma: comparison of nodal micrometastases versus macrometastases. J Clin Oncol 2010;28:2452–9.

27. Balch CM, Buzaid AC, Soong SJ, et al. Final version of the American Joint Committee on Cancer staging system for cutaneous melanoma. J Clin Oncol 2001; 19:3635–48.

28. Balch CM, Soong S, Ross MI, et al. Long-term results of a multi-institutional randomized trial comparing prognostic factors and surgical results for intermediate thickness melanomas (1.0 to 4.0 mm). Intergroup Melanoma Surgical Trial. Ann Surg Oncol 2000;7:87–97.

29. Cascinelli N, Belli F, Santinami M, et al. Sentinel lymph node biopsy in cutaneous melanoma: the WHO Melanoma Program experience. Ann Surg Oncol 2000;7:469–74.

30. Kelderman S, Heemskerk B, van Tinteren H, et al. Lactate dehydrogenase as a selection criterion for ipilimumab treatment in metastatic melanoma. Cancer Immunol Immunother 2014;63:449–58.

31. Long GV, Grob JJ, Nathan P, et al. Factors predictive of response, disease progression, and overall survival after dabrafenib and trametinib combination treatment: a pooled analysis of individual patient data from randomised trials. Lancet Oncol 2016; 17:1743–54.

32. Petrelli F, Ardito R, Merelli B, et al. Prognostic and predictive role of elevated lactate dehydrogenase in patients with melanoma treated with immunotherapy and BRAF inhibitors: a systematic review and meta-analysis. Melanoma Res 2019;29(1):1–12.

33. Howlader N, Noone AM, Krapcho M, et al, editors. SEER cancer Statistics Review, 1975-2016. Bethesda, MD: National Cancer Institute; 2019. Available at: https://seer.cancer.gov/csr/1975_2016/. based on November 2018 SEER data submission, posted to the SEER website.

34. Miller R, Walker S, Shui I, et al. Epidemiology and survival outcomes in stages II and III cutaneous melanoma: a systematic review. Melanoma Manag 2020;7(1):MMT39.

35. Balch CM, Soong SJ, Gershenwald JE, et al. Age as a prognostic factor in patients with localized melanoma and regional metastases. Ann Surg Oncol 2013;20(12):3961–8.

36. Thompson JF, Soong SJ, Balch CM, et al. Prognostic significance of mitotic rate in localized primary cutaneous melanoma: an analysis of patients in the

multi-institutional American Joint Committee on Cancer melanoma staging database. J Clin Oncol 2011; 29(16):2199–205.

37. Joosse A, Collette S, Suciu S, et al. Superior outcome of women with stage I/II cutaneous melanoma: pooled analysis of four European Organisation for Research and Treatment of Cancer phase III trials. J Clin Oncol 2012;30(18):2240.

38. Joosse A, Collette S, Suciu S, et al. Sex is an independent prognostic indicator for survival and relapse/progression-free survival in metastasized stage III to IV melanoma: a pooled analysis of five European organisation for research and treatment of cancer randomized controlled trials. J Clin Oncol 2013;31(18):2337.

39. Balch CM, Soong SJ, Gershenwald JE, et al. Prognostic factors analysis of 17,600 melanoma patients: validation of the American Joint Committee on Cancer melanoma staging system. J Clin Oncol 2001; 19(16):3622–34.

40. Callender GG, Egger ME, Burton AL, et al. Prognostic implications of anatomic location of primary cutaneous melanoma of 1 mm or thicker. Am J Surg 2011;202(6):659–64 [discussion: 664–5].

41. van der Ploeg AP, van Akkooi AC, Haydu LE, et al. The prognostic significance of sentinel node tumour burden in melanoma patients: an international, multicenter study of 1539 sentinel node-positive melanoma patients. Eur J Cancer 2014;50(1):111–20.

42. Lattanzi M, Lee Y, Simpson D, et al. Primary melanoma histologic subtype: impact on survival and response to therapy. J Natl Cancer Inst 2019; 111(2):180–8.

43. Moreau JF, Weissfeld JL, Ferris LK. Characteristics and survival of patients with invasive amelanotic melanoma in the USA. Melanoma Res 2013;23(5): 408–13.

44. Massi D, Pinzani P, Simi L, et al. BRAF and KIT somatic mutations are present in amelanotic melanoma. Melanoma Res 2013;23(5):414–9.

45. Cymerman RM, Shao Y, Wang K, et al. De novo vs nevus-associated melanomas: differences in associations with prognostic indicators and survival. J Natl Cancer Inst 2016;108(10):djw121.

46. Koyanagi K, O'Day SJ, Gonzalez R, et al. Serial monitoring of circulating melanoma cells during neoadjuvant biochemotherapy for stage III melanoma: outcome prediction in a multicenter trial. J Clin Oncol 2005;23(31):8057–64.

47. Mocellin S, Hoon D, Ambrosi A, et al. The prognostic value of circulating tumor cells in patients with melanoma: a systematic review and meta-analysis. Clin Cancer Res 2006;12(15):4605–13.

48. Fusi A, Collette S, Busse A, et al. Circulating melanoma cells and distant metastasis-free survival in stage III melanoma patients with or without adjuvant interferon treatment (EORTC 18991 side study). Eur J Cancer 2009;45(18):3189–97.

49. Hoshimoto S, Shingai T, Morton DL, et al. Association between circulating tumor cells and prognosis in patients with stage III melanoma with sentinel lymph node metastasis in a phase III international multicenter trial. J Clin Oncol 2012;30(31):3819–26.

Sentinel Lymph Node Biopsy, Lymph Node Dissection, and Lymphedema Management Options in Melanoma

Brian A. Mailey, MD[a],*, Ghaith Alrahawan, MS[b], Amanda Brown, BS[c], Maki Yamamoto, MD[d], Aladdin H. Hassanein, MD, MMSc[e]

KEYWORDS

- Melanoma • Sentinel lymph node biopsy • Lymph node dissection • Lymphedema

KEY POINTS

- Tumor thickness and ulceration are the strongest predictors of nodal spread.
- American Joint Committee on Cancer guidelines from 2018 recommend sentinel lymph node biopsy (SLNB) for any melanoma ≥0.8 mm or any ulcerated melanoma.
- Multicenter Selective Lymphadenectomy Trial (MSLT)-I demonstrated a survival benefit for SLNB.
- The role of completion lymph node dissection (CLND) has evolved given recent domestic (MSLT-II) and international (Dermatologic Cooperative Oncology Group-SLT) level I data demonstrating similar survival rates.
- Immediate lymphatic reconstruction can be performed at the time of CLND to reduce the risk of lymphedema. Lymphovenous anastomoses and vascularized lymph node transfer are microsurgical options to treat lymphedema.

INTRODUCTION

The spread of melanoma occurs radially, vertically, and in-transit through satellite lesions from the primary site. Malignant transformed cells are picked up primarily through the lymphatic system, which can disseminate throughout the body. According to this incubator hypothesis of metastatic spread, sampling the sentinel draining lymph node for any region of the body determines stage and prognosis of the disease. The 8th edition of the American Joint Committee on Cancer (AJCC) guidelines recently updated staging for melanoma in January of 2018 and recommends sentinel lymph node biopsy (SLNB) for most melanomas classified as T1b or greater.[1] This includes cutaneous melanoma with a tumor thickness (Breslow depth) of at least 1 mm or ulcerated lesions, which is similar to the 7th edition recommendations from 2010.[2] Most notably, changes were made to the T category which includes criteria for tumor thickness and presence or absence of ulceration, as these two factors continue to represent important

[a] Brachial Plexus and Tetraplegia Clinic, Institute for Plastic Surgery, Southern Illinois University School of Medicine, 747 N. Rutledge Street, PO Box 19653, Springfield, IL 62794, USA; [b] University of Missouri Columbia, School of Medicine, 1 Hospital Dr, Columbia, MO 65212, USA; [c] Southern Illinois University, School of Medicine, 747 N. Rutledge Street, PO Box 19653, Springfield, IL 62794, USA; [d] Division of Surgical Oncology, Department of Surgery, University of California, Irvine, 333 City Blvd West, Suite 1600, Orange, CA 92868, USA; [e] Division of Plastic Surgery, Indiana University School of Medicine, 545 Barnhill Dr, Suite 232, Indianapolis, IN 46202, USA
* Corresponding author.
E-mail address: bmailey48@siumed.edu

Clin Plastic Surg 48 (2021) 607–616
https://doi.org/10.1016/j.cps.2021.05.005
0094-1298/21/© 2021 Elsevier Inc. All rights reserved.

prognostic factors for survival and influence these recommendations for lymph node sampling.[3,4] Mitoses were removed in the 8th edition as a variable for determining T category in melanoma staging. National Comprehensive Cancer Network (NCCN) guidelines recommend consideration for SLNB for patients based on likelihood of having a positive sentinel node. Patients with a stage Ib or II melanoma (>1.0 mm tumor thickness) and clinically node negative should all be considered for nodal sampling; exceptions are considered in patients with significant comorbidities or very advanced age.

Controversy for SLNB remains for patients with thin melanomas (≤1.0 mm) as the risk of a positive node is low. Among patients with thin melanoma, tumor thickness and ulceration remain strong predictors of nodal spread. In tumor thicknesses less than 0.75 mm, sentinel lymph node (SLN) positivity can be quoted at less than 5%.[5] In contrast, for patients with tumor depths of 0.75 to 1.0 mm, SLN positivity reaches 12.8% in some studies.[5] Based on recent AJCC staging, the NCCN recommends consideration for SLNB for patients with tumor thicknesses 0.8 to 1.0 mm regardless of ulceration and less than 0.8 mm with ulceration or other adverse features, including lymphovascular invasion. This change occurred as a reflection of worse melanoma-specific survival and increased risk of SLN metastasis in this group (T1b, 5% - 12% vs T1a, <5%).[6–9] Importantly, tumor thickness recommendations have been updated and should be rounded to the nearest 0.1 mm (not 0.01 mm, as in prior editions). Thus, treatment recommendations for tumors measuring from 0.95 to 1.04 mm should be identical to those of 1.0 mm[7] To exemplify further, a tumor thickness of 0.95 should warrant an SLNB, and similarly, a tumor of Breslow depth 1.04 (without other prognostic factors) would still be considered to be T1, not T2.

Risks of SLNB are low but include a risk for development of lymphedema. This risk is higher in the lower extremity than in the upper one.[10] Other reported complications include damage to sensory nerves, lymphatic leak requiring prolonged drains, hematoma, and wound infections delaying adjuvant treatments.[10] The role for completion lymph node dissection (CLND) has changed in light of two randomized controlled trials published in 2016 and 2017 comparing CLND to observation,[11,12] with further analysis reporting 5-year outcomes in 2019.[13] This comes as new surgical techniques in lymphatic surgery and treatment options have evolved for the prevention and operative management of lymphedema. This article will review technique and indications for

SLNB in melanoma, the role for CLND, and describe evolving plastic surgery options for prevention (lymphatic microsurgical preventative healing approach [LYMPHA]) and management of lymphedema (lymphovenous anastomosis [LVA] and vascularized lymph node transfer [VLNT]).

SENTINEL LYMPH NODE BIOPSY

The technique for SLNB evolved out of methods described by Holmes and colleagues at the University of California, Los Angeles, and published in 1977.[14] The method they termed cutaneous lymphoscintigraphy was used to predict direction of lymphatic drainage in ambiguous truncal melanoma.[14] Radioactive colloidal gold scanning outlined direction of lymphatic flow to the primary draining regional lymph node group from the melanoma site and reduced the necessity of multiple regional lymphadenectomies. In 1992, Morton and colleagues described the technical details of intraoperative lymphatic mapping for early-stage melanoma.[15] In this study, SLNs were mapped, removed, and then a CLND performed. They demonstrated metastases in 21% of SLNs and 1% of non-SLNs.[15,16] This evolved into SLN intraoperative identification using radiolymphoscintigraphy with 99mTc-labeled albumin. By 2001, the prognostic significance of SLNB had been clearly demonstrated by several studies, and the AJCC incorporated the tumor status of SLNs into its staging system.[17] The modern technique for identifying the first draining lymph node in cutaneous melanoma bore out of this work. SLNB has less complications than CLND and currently is the accepted standard of care for staging patients with clinically node-negative cutaneous melanoma. This technique also provides the strongest predictor of survival and determination for subsequent adjuvant therapies. The prognostic value of micrometastases was formally recognized by the AJCC staging system in 2009.[18] Five-year survival rates range from 70% for micrometastatic disease in one SLN to 39% for patients with 4 or more involved nodes or nodes extensively involved.[6,18]

The first Multicenter Selective Lymphadenectomy Trial (MSLT-I) determined SLNB could reliably be used to identify patients with clinically occult nodal metastases.[19] This trial evaluated two-thousand and one patient between 1994 and 2002 with intermediate thickness melanomas (ITM = 1.2–3.5-mm cutaneous melanomas). Patients were randomized to wide local excision (WLE) with SLNB or WLE with observation. Of the SLN patients, nodal metastases were detected in 16% and another 5% demonstrating nodal disease in non-SLN. This established an overall 20% relative risk of LN metastasis in patients with ITM. The observation group had an incidence of nodal metastases at 10 years of 22%, with 17% of those in the first 1.5 years. Most importantly, however, the 10-year disease-free survival rates were higher in the SLNB group at 71% versus those in the observation group at 65% (*P* = .001).[19]

The current practice of SLNB consists of injection of a radioactive tracer (usually technetium-sulfur-labeled radiocolloid) at 4 sites on each side of the melanoma (**Fig. 1**), preoperative lymphoscintigraphy (**Fig. 2**) with the possibility of using the single photon emission computed tomography/computed tomography (SPECT/CT) hybrid imaging (**Fig. 3**), and intraoperative SLN localization using a handheld gamma probe. This procedure could be supplemented by preoperative injection of blue dye by the surgeon to visually confirm the sentinel lymph node. Tc-labeled injections are identified using gamma-detection imaging performed after injection to localize the primary draining lymph node (**Fig. 4**).

The radioactive tracer (eg, technetium-99 sulfur colloid, technetium Tc 99m tilmanocept) and nonradioactive dyes (eg, methylene blue, isosulfan blue) localize regional lymph nodes. The intraoperative gamma probe quantifies tracer uptake. Based on the tracer concentration and visualization of the blue dye, the surgeon excises the lymph node and places it in formalin. The presence or absence of metastasis in the SLN will stage the disease and determine further treatment recommendations, including potentially removal of the lymph node basin. The tissue is prepared for pathologic analysis by creating 1- to 2-mm serial sections, followed by hematoxylin and eosin staining. This step looks for macrometastasis, variations in LN architecture, melanoma nodules, or other gross signs of metastatic disease. If absent, immunohistochemistry (IHC) is performed with 1 to 3 stains (ie, SOX10, Melan A, S100, PRAME) per section, depending on the institution. Frozen sections are generally not performed, as a true negative diagnosis can only be given after IHC confirmation. Lymphadenectomy can take place should metastasis be present in the sentinel lymph node, generally in a subsequent procedure.

In cases where the radiotracer is encountered in ≥1 lymph node, the presence of multiple sentinel lymph nodes is implied, and each should be sampled. If drainage from the tumor site involves two lymphatic basins, an SLN should be sampled from each site. Such is the case not uncommonly in head and neck melanomas, where cervical SLNs are observed bilaterally. New tracers, SPECT, and new intraoperative devices have advanced progress in melanoma of the head and neck region and in areas of complex anatomy or difficult-to-localize SLNs.[20]

COMPLETION LYMPH NODE DISSECTION

A CLND has been traditionally recommended for all patients with a positive SLN[18]; however, this recommendation has evolved from recent level I domestic and international randomized controlled trials demonstrating similar melanoma-specific survival and limited benefit conferred from clearing out a lymph node basin.[13,19] MSLT I established the clear value of SLNB but also evaluated the ability of lymphadenectomy to yield better patient survival.[19] This study compared patients with immediate CLND to LND when nodal recurrence was identified by ultrasound during scheduled observations. They concluded patients undergoing LND when nodal recurrence was palpable had a lower 10-year melanoma-specific survival rate than those in the SLNB group with a positive SLN and immediate CLND (41.5% vs 62.1%, *P* = .006).[16] These results indicated timing of intervention for nodal disease was an important factor for reducing risk of melanoma-related distant metastases, nodal recurrence, and death in patients with ITM.[19,21]

The second MSLT phase 3 trial began in 2004 and was published in *The New England Journal of Medicine* in 2017.[12] The trial included 63 centers investigating the value of early completion nodal evaluation in patients with SLN metastasis. The goal of this trial, along with the Dermatologic Cooperative Oncology Group (DeCOG-SLT)[11,13] out of Germany, was to examine the survival benefit of complete node dissection after removal of a metastatic SLN, which has been the standard of care. Both studies concluded there was no

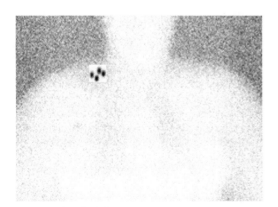

Fig. 1. Radiolabeled tracer is injected at 4 sites surrounding the melanoma. This patient had a malignant melanoma on her right upper back.

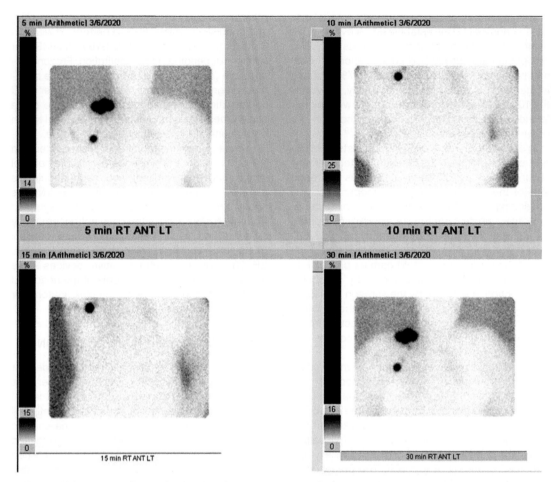

Fig. 2. Serial images are obtained to localize the tracer into specific lymph node basins. This patient's tracer localized to her right axillary lymph node basin.

clinically significant difference in melanoma-specific survival between groups. For the MSLT II, the specific survival between the dissection group and observation group was 86 ± 1.3% and 86 ± 1.2%, respectively, $P = .42$, with the result that there is no significant difference in the mean rate of melanoma-specific survival between the dissection and observation groups.

The DeCOG-SLT was a multicenter, randomized, phase 3 trial published before MSLT II that had a primary endpoint of distant metastasis-free survival. After 3 years, the distant metastasis-free survival was 77% and 75% in the CLND and the observation groups, respectively ($P = .87$). Although the study was underpowered because it did not achieve the required number of events, the analysis showed no difference in survival between the groups. In 2019, they published their final analysis with 72-month follow-up data, demonstrating no significant treatment difference in distant metastasis-free survival between the observation and LND groups (67.6% vs 64.9%, $P = .87$).

Fig. 3. SPECT-CT combines nuclear medicine imaging with CAT scan radiographs to localize sentinel lymph nodes. This patient had a primary melanoma on his temple with primary draining lymph nodes in his parotid and in his cervical lymphatic chain.

LYMPHEDEMA

Lymphedema is chronic limb swelling from inadequate lymphatic function and can occur after

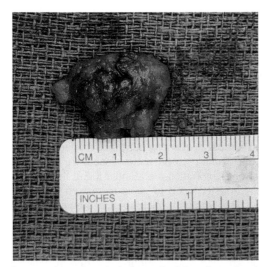

Fig. 4. Enlarged and dark sentinel lymph node obtained from the axillary lymph nodes in a melanoma patient.

lymphadenectomy in the treatment of melanoma. Lymphedema affects 250 million people worldwide.[22] The morbidity associated from this condition includes recurrent cellulitis, pain, and impaired function.[23,24] Symptoms decrease quality of life, have a high health cost burden, and in extreme cases, can lead to amputation.[25,26] There is currently no cure for this progressive disease.[23,24,27]

Lymphatic vessels bud from veins during embryologic development.[28] Lymphatic capillaries transport extracellular fluid from peripheral tissues. The proteinaceous lymph flows though lymphatic collecting vessels which pass through lymph nodes to filter lymph and contribute to immunologic function. Lymph is ultimately returned to the circulatory system via the thoracic duct into the subclavian vein.

Dysfunction in the lymphatic system results in lymphedema, which is categorized as primary (errors in lymphatic development) or secondary (injury to lymphatics). In the United States, the most common cause of the 5 million cases of lymphedema is secondary to treatment of solid tumors, such as melanoma and breast cancer.[29] As many as 30%-50% of patients treated with lymph node dissection develop lymphedema,[30–32] with an average time to onset at 1 year after lymph node removal.[33] Nearly 75% of patients develop lymphedema within 3 years after lymphatic injury.[34] The affected extremity swells distal to the injured regional lymph nodes from unreturned fluid accumulating in adipose tissue and leading to chronic inflammation and fibrosis resulting in progressive limb enlargement.[35]

Pitting edema is initially present because of interstitial lymphatic fluid retention. Progressive subcutaneous fibroadipose deposition over time results in nonpitting edema and is a sign of longer standing disease.[36] The Stemmer sign, the examiner's inability to pinch the dorsal soft tissues between the second and third toe, has a 97% sensitivity and 57% specificity.[37] Obesity remains an independent risk factor for development of lymphedema after lymphadenectomy. Patients are over 3 times more likely to develop lymphedema after axillary lymph node dissection (ALND) if their preoperative body mass index is >30 kg/m².[38] Obese patients that acquire lymphedema exhibit greater morbidity, increased infections, hospitalizations, and larger extremities than nonobese individuals with lymphedema.[39]

Diagnosis of lymphedema is confirmed with lymphoscintigraphy which has 96% sensitivity and 100% specificity.[40] Technetium 99-labeled sulfur colloid is injected intradermally proximal to the 2nd and 4th tarsometatarsal or metacarpophalangeal joints bilaterally for lower and upper extremities, respectively. A positive study exhibits absent or delayed transit of the radioactive tracer to the regional nodes (>45 minutes) or dermal backflow.[41–43] Lymphedema can progress through four stages. Stage 0 is subclinical with a normal examination and imaging showing abnormal lymphatic function. Stage 1 is early edema that improves with extremity elevation. Stage 2 exhibits pitting edema without resolution with limb elevation. Stage 3 is demonstrated by fibroadipose deposition.[44] The increase in limb volume characterizes lymphedema as mild (<20%), moderate (20%–40%), or severe (>40%).[44] Quantification of extremity volume is not standardized. Circumference tape measurement is most commonly used.[45] Although simple to perform, it is inconsistent and the least accurate method. The limb volume must be calculated with the circumference values using the truncated cone equation.[46] Water displacement is time-consuming and contraindicated by the presence of wounds.[47] A perometer using infrared scanning and Vectra 3D camera (Canfield Scientific, Fairfield, NJ) has been used to calculate limb volume.[48,49] Lymphedema can also be quantified by bioimpedance spectroscopy using electrical current resistance in the tissues affected by interstitial fluid.[48,50]

Treatment of lymphedema is challenging, and there is no cure. The mainstay of treatment, compression, decreases limb volume and slows adipose deposition that occurs with high protein fluid in the interstitium.[51] Static compression garments/sleeves can be customized and should be worn frequently. Pneumatic compression devices provide intermittent compression. They are typically worn daily for 2 hours.[52] Complete decongestive therapy is performed by certified therapists and includes manual lymph drainage and applying compressive wraps. Compressive therapies should be optimized before any surgical management. Patient expectations should be set to anticipate the requirement of compression postsurgically.

Operative management of lymphedema is divided into excisional and physiologic procedures. The goal of excisional procedures is to remove tissue to decrease limb volume. Physiologic procedures aim at improving lymph clearance in the extremity. Excisional procedures include the Charles procedure, skin/subcutaneous excision, and suction-assisted lipectomy.[53–55] The Charles procedure involves radical resection of the skin and subcutaneous tissues to the deep fascia with skin grafting.[56] It is seldom performed because of the associated morbidity and potential for causing large open wounds. Skin and subcutaneous excision debulks the extremity with removal of the subcutaneous fibroadipose tissue followed by primary closure. Similarly, suction-assisted lipectomy uses liposuction techniques to remove the abnormally deposited superficial fatty tissue.[57,58] Physiologic procedures include VLNT and lymphovenous bypass (LVB). Right gastroepiploic arteries (**Fig. 5**), deep inferior epigastric artery, superficial circumflex iliac, jejunal, supraclavicular, and axillary/lateral thoracic arteries have been described as donor sites for lymph node free flap transfer.[59–64] LVB involves anastomosing lymphatic vessels to venules in the

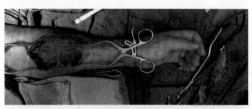
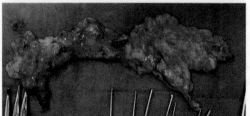

Fig. 5. Free omental vascularized lymph node transfer to the left upper extremity in a patient with lymphedema. The lymphangiogenesis stimulated by the vascularized tissue transfer reduced the patients' arm circumference.

lymphedematous limb.[65–67] The lymphatic channels are typically mapped with indocyanine green (ICG) laser lymphangiography and supermicrosurgery techniques used to shunt lymph into the circulatory system bypassing the injured regional lymph node basin. Systematic review of physiologic procedures has demonstrated an approximately 30% limb volume reduction.[53]

A preventative microsurgical strategy also exists and is most relevant for surgeons managing melanoma. During lymph node dissection, disrupted afferent lymphatics are identified and microsurgically anastomosed to veins to restore lymphatic flow. This lymphatic microsurgical preventing healing approach is now more often termed immediate lymphatic reconstruction (ILR).[32] The technique was first described by Boccardo and colleagues, who showed a 4% lymphedema rate in patients who underwent ALND for breast cancer with immediate LVA compared with the 30% rate in controls.[68] Other groups have also reported success, with lymphedema rates ranging from 0% to 12.5% after ALND.[30,31,33,69–73] A systematic review demonstrated those undergoing ALND and radiation were found to have a 33.4% risk of lymphedema compared with a 10.3% risk with ALND, ILR, and radiation.[33] The feasibility of ILR during axillary or ilioinguinal was shown for the treatment melanoma.[74] The average number of lymphovenous anastomoses was 1.8 in the series.[74]

ILR is performed immediately after axillary or ilioinguinal lymph node dissection. It is facilitated by identification of disrupted critical lymphatics for limb drainage. Localizing the afferent lymphatics involves the use of a dye or fluorescent substance (**Fig. 6**). Isosulfan blue, ICG, and fluorescein have been described.[32,71,74] If isosulfan blue is used, 3 to 5 cc (1% concentration) can be injected in the brachial fascia of the arm, and the injection site is massaged. After completion of the lymphadenectomy and WLE, the lymph node basin is inspected using the operating microscope. Transected lymphatics from the lymph node dissection are identified. The disrupted lymphatics will appear blue with the surgical microscope if isosulfan blue was used. Alternatively, near-infrared laser lymphangiography is used with ICG or a 560-nm filter for the microscope with fluorescein. A venous branch (eg, from axillary vein or thoracodorsal) near the cut lymphatics is selected and mobilized for length as needed for a tension-free LVA. Lymphatic vessels are repaired to the vein using 11 to 0 nylon. A standard end-to-end or end-to-side anastomosis can be performed if there is adequate size match between the lymphatic and the vein. However, more commonly, the injured lymphatic vessels are

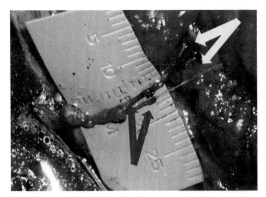

Fig. 6. Immediate lymphatic reconstruction (ILR) to microsurgically prevent lymphedema. Disrupted afferent lymphatics (*yellow arrows*) are anastomosed into vein branches in the axilla (*blue arrows*) to decrease the risk of lymphedema at the time of axillary or ilioinguinal lymph node dissection. The top lymphovenous anastomosis was performed using the sleeve technique with intussusception of the lymphatics into the vein. The lower lymphovenous anastomosis was performed in an end-to-end fashion because of adequate size match.

significantly smaller than the vein branches. Intussusception, also termed the "sleeve technique," can be used. Smaller lymphatics are telescoped within the vein lumen (**Fig. 6**). The sleeve technique can also be performed to anastomose multiple lymphatic vessels. A "U-stich" using 11 to 0 is placed from the adventitia through the lumen of the of the vein, into the lymphatic lumen, and then back through the vein lumen and adventitia. When this suture is tied, the lymphatics are dunked into the vein lumen. Sutures can then be placed between the vein and the perilymphatic adipose. The U-stitch is then removed. Patency is confirmed with ICG or fluorescein. Fibrin glue can further stabilize the anastomosis.

Lymphedema is a difficult problem that can occur after melanoma management. ILR is a promising method to decrease the risk of postsurgical lymphedema, which has been recently adapted for melanoma. Encouraging results in the literature have been reported in retrospective case series. Multiple confounding variables exist such as altered lymph node dissection techniques and selection bias. Lymphedema can occur several years after the operation. Randomized studies and long-term follow-up are necessary to determine the efficacy of ILR.

SUMMARY

The lymphatic system is the primary means for propagation of cancer cells and allowing metastasis to occur. The recommendation for patients

with a malignant melanoma ≥1 mm in depth was to undergo a CLND. In 1992, this was replaced by less invasive SLN sampling, where only the primary drainage lymph nodes were examined for metastasis. MSLT-I confirmed the benefit of SLNB for improving 10-year disease-free survival. Patients undergoing lymph node dissection with positive SLN also demonstrated a disease free survival (DFS) benefit. SLN data have been further refined using location and number of metastases in positive SLNs to guide indications for additional surgery, sparing patients with disease confined to the subcapsular areas of CLND. Recent international (DeCOG-SLT) and US (MSLT-II) randomized control trials added additional level 1 evidence to guide management of stage 3 disease in patients with ITM and clarify the therapeutic role of CLND. They both confirmed a prognostic benefit to SLN sampling and similar melanoma-specific survival in patients with positive SLN undergoing CLND or observation. MSLT-II differed from DeCOG in that DFS was 5% higher for patients who underwent immediate CLND, as opposed to observation by ultrasound for nodal recurrence. It should also be noted in interpreting these results that although melanoma-specific survival rates were similar between groups, they were only measured at 3 and 4 years for DeCOG and MSLT-II, respectively.

In conclusion, information obtained from SLNB remains invaluable for determining prognosis and adjuvant therapies. The role of CLND has changed and can be avoided in many patients; however, a DFS benefit may still remain in some patients. The most feared complication from unnecessary lymph node surgery remains lymphedema. New microsurgical techniques have evolved that can prevent the interruption in lymphatic flow (LYMPHA, ILR) or address symptomatic lymphedema after it occurs (LVA and VLNT). Together, along with advances in adjuvant therapies, the prognosis and treatment options for melanoma have significantly evolved in recent times.

CLINICS CARE POINTS

- Sentinel lymph node biopsy is recommended for melanomas classified at T1b or greater.

- Exceptions for nodal sampling can be made for patients with significant comorbidities, older age, or clinically positive nodal disease.

- Intermediate thickness melanomas (1.2- to 3.5-mm depth) have an overall 20% relative risk of lymph node metastasis.

- Multicenter Selective Lymphadenectomy Trial (MSLT) I demonstrated an improvement in 10-year disease-free survival of 71% versus 65% in the observation group. For patients with a positive SLN, this trial demonstrated a survival benefit for undergoing a lymph node dissection (41% vs 62%).

- MSLT II and De-COG SLT both concluded there was no clinically significant difference in melanoma-specific survival conferred by LND and recommended against routine completion dissection.

- SLNs require permanent sectioning for pathologists to perform immunohistochemistry.

- Immediate lymphatic reconstruction can prevent lymphedema, and lymphovenous anastomosis or vascularized lymph node transfer can treat lymphedema after it has occurred.

DISCLOSURE

The authors have nothing to disclose.

REFERENCES

1. Gershenwald JE, Scolyer RA. Melanoma staging: American joint Committee on cancer (AJCC) 8th edition and beyond. Ann Surg Oncol 2018;25(8): 2105–10.

2. Barreiro-Capurro A, Andres-Lencina JJ, Podlipnik S, et al. Differences in cutaneous melanoma survival between the 7th and 8th edition of the American Joint Committee on Cancer (AJCC). A multicentric population-based study. Eur J Cancer 2021;145: 29–37.

3. Breslow A. Tumor thickness, level of invasion and node dissection in stage I cutaneous melanoma. Ann Surg 1975;182(5):572–5.

4. In 't. Prognostic importance of the extent of ulceration in patients with clinically localized cutaneous melanoma. In: Hout FE, Haydu LE, Murali R, et al, editors. Ann Surg 2012;255(6):1165–70.

5. Vermeeren L, Van der Ent F, Sastrowijoto P, et al. Sentinel lymph node biopsy in patients with thin melanoma: occurrence of nodal metastases and its prognostic value. Eur J Dermatol 2010;20(1):30–4.

6. Gershenwald JE, Scolyer RA, Hess KR, et al. Melanoma staging: evidence-based changes in the American Joint Committee on Cancer eighth edition cancer staging manual. CA Cancer J Clin 2017; 67(6):472–92.

7. Keung EZ, Gershenwald JE. The eighth edition American Joint Committee on Cancer (AJCC) melanoma staging system: implications for melanoma treatment and care. Expert Rev Anticancer Ther 2018;18(8):775–84.

8. Cordeiro E, Gervais MK, Shah PS, et al. Sentinel lymph node biopsy in thin cutaneous melanoma: a systematic review and meta-analysis. Ann Surg Oncol 2016;23(13):4178–88.

9. Murali R, Haydu LE, Quinn MJ, et al. Sentinel lymph node biopsy in patients with thin primary cutaneous melanoma. Ann Surg 2012;255(1):128–33.

10. Hyngstrom JR, Chiang YJ, Cromwell KD, et al. Prospective assessment of lymphedema incidence and lymphedema-associated symptoms following lymph node surgery for melanoma. Melanoma Res 2013;23(4):290–7.

11. Leiter U, Stadler R, Mauch C, et al. Complete lymph node dissection versus no dissection in patients with sentinel lymph node biopsy positive melanoma (De-COG-SLT): a multicentre, randomised, phase 3 trial. Lancet Oncol 2016;17(6):757–67.

12. Faries MB, Thompson JF, Cochran AJ, et al. Completion dissection or observation for sentinel-node metastasis in melanoma. N Engl J Med 2017; 376(23):2211–22.

13. Leiter U, Stadler R, Mauch C, et al. Final analysis of DeCOG-SLT trial: no survival benefit for complete lymph node dissection in patients with melanoma with positive sentinel node. J Clin Oncol 2019; 37(32):3000–8.

14. Holmes EC, Moseley HS, Morton DL, et al. A rational approach to the surgical management of melanoma. Ann Surg 1977;186(4):481–90.

15. Morton DL, Wen DR, Wong JH, et al. Technical details of intraoperative lymphatic mapping for early stage melanoma. Arch Surg 1992;127(4):392–9.

16. Dummer R, Brase JC, Garrett J, et al. Adjuvant dabrafenib plus trametinib versus placebo in patients with resected, BRAF(V600)-mutant, stage III melanoma (COMBI-AD): exploratory biomarker analyses from a randomised, phase 3 trial. Lancet Oncol 2020;21(3):358–72.

17. Balch CM, Gershenwald JE, Soong SJ, et al. Final version of 2009 AJCC melanoma staging and classification. J Clin Oncol 2009;27(36):6199–206.

18. Wong SL, Faries MB, Kennedy EB, et al. Sentinel lymph node biopsy and management of regional lymph nodes in melanoma: american society of clinical oncology and society of surgical oncology clinical practice guideline update. J Clin Oncol 2018; 36(4):399–413.

19. Morton DL, Thompson JF, Cochran AJ, et al. Final trial report of sentinel-node biopsy versus nodal observation in melanoma. N Engl J Med 2014; 370(7):599–609.

20. Wallace AM, Hoh CK, Ellner SJ, et al. Lymphoseek: a molecular imaging agent for melanoma sentinel lymph node mapping. Ann Surg Oncol 2007;14(2): 913–21.

21. Gonzalez A. Sentinel lymph node biopsy: past and present implications for the management of cutaneous melanoma with nodal metastasis. Am J Clin Dermatol 2018;19(Suppl 1):24–30.

22. Schulze H, Nacke M, Gutenbrunner C, et al. Worldwide assessment of healthcare personnel dealing with lymphoedema. Health Econ Rev 2018;8(1):10.

23. Beaulac SM, McNair LA, Scott TE, et al. Lymphedema and quality of life in survivors of early-stage breast cancer. Arch Surg 2002;137(11):1253–7.

24. Norman SA, Localio AR, Kallan MJ, et al. Risk factors for lymphedema after breast cancer treatment. Cancer Epidemiol Biomarkers Prev 2010;19(11):2734–46.

25. Chang SB, Askew RL, Xing Y, et al. Prospective assessment of postoperative complications and associated costs following inguinal lymph node dissection (ILND) in melanoma patients. Ann Surg Oncol 2010;17(10):2764–72.

26. Bundred N, Foden P, Todd C, et al. Increases in arm volume predict lymphoedema and quality of life deficits after axillary surgery: a prospective cohort study. Br J Cancer 2020;123(1):17–25.

27. Shaitelman SF, Cromwell KD, Rasmussen JC, et al. Recent progress in the treatment and prevention of cancer-related lymphedema. CA Cancer J Clin 2015;65(1):55–81.

28. Yang Y, Oliver G. Development of the mammalian lymphatic vasculature. J Clin Invest 2014;124(3):888–97.

29. Rockson SG, Rivera KK. Estimating the population burden of lymphedema. Ann N Y Acad Sci 2008;1131:147–54.

30. Feldman S, Bansil H, Ascherman J, et al. Single institution experience with lymphatic microsurgical preventive healing approach (LYMPHA) for the primary prevention of lymphedema. Ann Surg Oncol 2015;22(10):3296–301.

31. Boccardo F, Casabona F, DeCian F, et al. Lymphatic microsurgical preventing healing approach (LYMPHA) for primary surgical prevention of breast cancer-related lymphedema: over 4 years follow-up. Microsurgery 2014;34(6):421–4.

32. Johnson AR, Singhal D. Immediate lymphatic reconstruction. J Surg Oncol 2018;118(5):750–7.

33. Johnson AR, Kimball S, Epstein S, et al. Lymphedema incidence after axillary lymph node dissection: quantifying the impact of radiation and the lymphatic microsurgical preventive healing approach. Ann Plast Surg 2019;82(4S Suppl 3):S234–41.

34. Petrek JA, Senie RT, Peters M, et al. Lymphedema in a cohort of breast carcinoma survivors 20 years after diagnosis. Cancer 2001;92(6):1368–77.

35. Azhar SH, Lim HY, Tan BK, et al. The unresolved pathophysiology of lymphedema. Front Physiol 2020;11:137.

36. Brorson H, Ohlin K, Olsson G, et al. Breast cancer-related chronic arm lymphedema is associated with excess adipose and muscle tissue. Lymphat Res Biol 2009;7(1):3–10.

37. Goss JA, Greene AK. Sensitivity and specificity of the stemmer sign for lymphedema: a clinical lymphoscintigraphic study. Plast Reconstr Surg Glob Open 2019;7(6):e2295.

38. Ridner SH, Dietrich MS, Stewart BR, et al. Body mass index and breast cancer treatment-related lymphedema. Support Care Cancer 2011;19(6):853–7.

39. Greene AK, Zurakowski D, Goss JA. Body mass index and lymphedema morbidity: comparison of obese versus normal-weight patients. Plast Reconstr Surg 2020;146(2):402–7.

40. Hassanein AH, Maclellan RA, Grant FD, et al. Diagnostic accuracy of lymphoscintigraphy for lymphedema and analysis of false-negative tests. Plast Reconstr Surg Glob Open 2017;5(7):e1396.

41. Gloviczki P, Calcagno D, Schirger A, et al. Noninvasive evaluation of the swollen extremity: experiences with 190 lymphoscintigraphic examinations. J Vasc Surg 1989;9(5):683–9 [discussion: 690].

42. Szuba A, Shin WS, Strauss HW, et al. The third circulation: radionuclide lymphoscintigraphy in the evaluation of lymphedema. J Nucl Med 2003;44(1):43–57.

43. Maclellan RA, Zurakowski D, Voss S, et al. Correlation between lymphedema disease severity and lymphoscintigraphic findings: a clinical-radiologic study. J Am Coll Surg 2017;225(3):366–70.

44. International Society of Lymphology. Lymphology. The diagnosis and treatment of peripheral lymphedema: 2013 Consensus document of the international society of lymphology. Lymphology 2013;46(1):1–11.

45. Sander AP, Hajer NM, Hemenway K, et al. Upper-extremity volume measurements in women with lymphedema: a comparison of measurements obtained via water displacement with geometrically determined volume. Phys Ther 2002;82(12):1201–12.

46. Sitzia J. Volume measurement in lymphoedema treatment: examination of formulae. Eur J Cancer Care (Engl) 1995;4(1):11–6.

47. Ridner SH, Montgomery LD, Hepworth JT, et al. Comparison of upper limb volume measurement techniques and arm symptoms between healthy volunteers and individuals with known lymphedema. Lymphology 2007;40(1):35–46.

48. Keeley V. The early detection of breast cancer treatment-related lymphedema of the arm. Lymphat Res Biol 2020;19(1):51–5.

49. Landau MJ, Kim JS, Gould DJ, et al. Vectra 3D imaging for quantitative volumetric analysis of the upper limb: a feasibility study for tracking outcomes

of lymphedema treatment. Plast Reconstr Surg 2018;141(1):80e–4e.

50. Warren AG, Janz BA, Slavin SA, et al. The use of bio-impedance analysis to evaluate lymphedema. Ann Plast Surg 2007;58(5):541–3.

51. Maclellan RA, Greene AK. Lymphedema. Semin Pediatr Surg 2014;23(4):191–7.

52. Johansson K, Lie E, Ekdahl C, et al. A randomized study comparing manual lymph drainage with sequential pneumatic compression for treatment of postoperative arm lymphedema. Lymphology 1998;31(2):56–64.

53. Carl HMWG, Bello R, Clarke-Pearson, et al. Systematic review of the surgical treatment of extremity lymphedema. J Reconstr Microsurg 2017;33(6):412–25.

54. Chang DW, Masia J, Garza R 3rd, et al. Lymphedema: surgical and medical therapy. Plast Reconstr Surg 2016;138(3 Suppl):209S–18S.

55. Greene AK, Sudduth CL, Taghinia A. Lymphedema (Seminars in pediatric surgery). Semin Pediatr Surg 2020;29(5):150972.

56. Dumanian GA, Futrell JW. The Charles procedure: misquoted and misunderstood since 1950. Plast Reconstr Surg 1996;98(7):1258–63.

57. Hoffner M, Ohlin K, Svensson B, et al. Liposuction gives complete reduction of arm lymphedema following breast cancer treatment-a 5-year prospective study in 105 patients without recurrence. Plast Reconstr Surg Glob Open 2018;6(8):e1912.

58. Schaverien MV, Munnoch DA, Brorson H. Liposuction treatment of lymphedema. Semin Plast Surg 2018;32(1):42–7.

59. Cheng MH, Chen SC, Henry SL, et al. Vascularized groin lymph node flap transfer for postmastectomy upper limb lymphedema: flap anatomy, recipient sites, and outcomes. Plast Reconstr Surg 2013; 131(6):1286–98.

60. Maldonado AA, Chen R, Chang DW. The use of supraclavicular free flap with vascularized lymph node transfer for treatment of lymphedema: a prospective study of 100 consecutive cases. J Surg Oncol 2017;115(1):68–71.

61. Kenworthy EO, Nelson JA, Verma R, et al. Double vascularized omentum lymphatic transplant (VOLT) for the treatment of lymphedema. J Surg Oncol 2018;117(7):1413–9.

62. Hassanein AH, Danforth R, DeBrock W, et al. Deep inferior epigastric artery vascularized lymph node transfer: a simple and safe option for lymphedema.

J Plast Reconstr Aesthet Surg 2020;73(10): 1897–916.

63. Coriddi M, Wee C, Meyerson J, et al. Vascularized jejunal mesenteric lymph node transfer: a novel surgical treatment for extremity lymphedema. J Am Coll Surg 2017;225(5):650–7.

64. Gould DJ, Mehrara BJ, Neligan P, et al. Lymph node transplantation for the treatment of lymphedema. J Surg Oncol 2018;118(5):736–42.

65. Hassanein AH, Sacks JM, Cooney DS. Optimizing perioperative lymphatic-venous anastomosis localization using transcutaneous vein illumination, isosulfan blue, and indocyanine green lymphangiography. Microsurgery 2017;37(8):956–7.

66. Chang DW, Suami H, Skoracki R. A prospective analysis of 100 consecutive lymphovenous bypass cases for treatment of extremity lymphedema. Plast Reconstr Surg 2013;132(5):1305–14.

67. Koshima I, Inagawa K, Urushibara K, et al. Supermicrosurgical lymphaticovenular anastomosis for the treatment of lymphedema in the upper extremities. J Reconstr Microsurg 2000;16(6):437–42.

68. Boccardo FM, Casabona F, Friedman D, et al. Surgical prevention of arm lymphedema after breast cancer treatment. Ann Surg Oncol 2011;18(9):2500–5.

69. Boccardo F, Casabona F, De Cian F, et al. Lymphedema microsurgical preventive healing approach: a new technique for primary prevention of arm lymphedema after mastectomy. Ann Surg Oncol 2009;16(3):703.

70. Casabona F, Bogliolo S, Menada MV, et al. Feasibility of axillary reverse mapping during sentinel lymph node biopsy in breast cancer patients. Ann Surg Oncol 2009;16(9):2459.

71. Cook JASS, Loewenstein SN, DeBrock W, et al. Immediate lymphatic reconstruction: a single institution early experience. Ann Surg Oncol 2021;28(3): 1381–7.

72. HahamoffM GN, MunozD. A lymphedema surveillance programfor breast cancer patients reveals the promise of surgical prevention. J Surg Res 2018;17:30662–5.

73. Schwarz GS, Grobmyer SR, Djohan RS, et al. Axillary reverse mapping and lymphaticovenous bypass: lymphedema prevention through enhanced lymphatic visualization and restoration of flow. J Surg Oncol 2019;120(2):160–7.

74. Cakmakoglu C, Kwiecien GJ, Schwarz GS, et al. Lymphaticovenous bypass for immediate lymphatic reconstruction in locoregional advanced melanoma patients. J Reconstr Microsurg 2020;36(4):247–52.

Dermatologic Follow-up and Assessment of Suspicious Lesions

Julie Iacullo, MD[a], Paola Barriera-Silvestrini, MD[a],
Thomas J. Knackstedt, MD[a,b],*

KEYWORDS

• Guidelines • Monitoring • Melanoma • Surveillance imaging

KEY POINTS

• Follow-up care for melanoma patients varies worldwide, but generally more aggressive surveillance is required for high-stage disease.
• Surveillance methods includes physical examination, laboratory data with S-100 and LDH, and imaging modalities, such as ultrasound (US), chest x-ray (CXR), computer tomography (CT), positron emission tomography-computed tomography (PET-CT), or magnetic resonance imaging (MRI).
• The standard of follow-up care focuses on clinician-led surveillance, but there is increased awareness and incentive for patient-led surveillance for lower stage disease patients.
• Future directions for the assessment of suspicious lesions includes the use of gene-expression profiling, noninvasive imaging technologies, and artificial intelligence.

INTRODUCTION

Cutaneous melanoma incidence has increased significantly over the past decades. Mortality rates increased in parallel during the 1970s and 1980s but have since plateaued, likely due to earlier detection of thinner melanomas.[1,2] Survival rates depend on the stage of the disease as determined by the tumor, node, and metastasis (TMN) system developed by the American Joint Committee on Cancer (AJCC). Survival declines as tumor thickness and disease stage increase. Follow-up recommendations are based on survival and recurrence rates for melanoma set forth by the AJCC. Here, we review melanoma follow-up including national and international guidelines, the use of laboratory data and imaging modalities, future melanoma risk, and the assessment of suspicious lesions.

BACKGROUND

After the diagnosis and appropriate treatment of melanoma, follow-up and early detection of melanoma recurrence becomes a major clinical priority. The main objective of follow-up care is to identify potentially curable locoregional recurrences, second primary melanomas, and low tumor burden distant recurrences, as these are more responsive to systemic therapies.[3–5] The 2-year disease-free survival ranges from 95% for T1b melanoma to 67% for T4b melanomas. The risk of local recurrence is greatest in the first 2–5 years after initial diagnosis and in tumors that are thicker, ulcerated and located on the head, neck, and distal legs. A prospective study of 700 high-risk primary melanoma patients found a 13.4% recurrence rate within 2 years. Of these, 70% were locoregional recurrences and 30% were distant recurrences.

Funding sources: None.
Conflicts of interest: none declared.
This work has not been previously presented or published.
[a] Department of Dermatology, MetroHealth System, 2500 Metrohealth Drive, Cleveland, OH 44109, USA;
[b] Case Western Reserve University, School of Medicine, 2500 Metrohealth Drive, Cleveland, OH 44109, USA
* Corresponding author. 2500 Metrohealth Drive, Cleveland, OH 44109.
E-mail address: thomas.j.knackstedt@gmail.com

Clin Plastic Surg 48 (2021) 617–629
https://doi.org/10.1016/j.cps.2021.05.006

Ultra-late recurrences (>15 years) may occur in an unpredictable manner.[6]

Short-term and long-term monitoring after a melanoma diagnosis have remained an area of debate and controversy as there are few established guidelines and a lack of consensus worldwide. Variation between dermatologic and oncologic organizations exists. Surveillance is mainly focused on history and physical examination, utilization of imaging and laboratory studies for detection of recurrence or metastasis, and duration and frequency of clinical evaluation. Clinical monitoring should include a total-body skin examination, palpation of the primary site and surrounding area for local recurrences, satellitosis, intransit metastases, and a thorough evaluation of lymph nodes. All patients should be asked a review of symptoms, focusing on any new or changing lesions, fatigue, weight loss, headache, vision changes, back pain, and any new and unusual symptoms. Patients should be counseled on regular, monthly skin self-examinations and vigilant sun protection measures.[7]

The degree of follow-up is predicated on the initial melanoma stage and patient characteristics. Generally, more frequent visits and more extensive testing are appropriate for patients with more significant disease or at higher risk for multiple primary lesions. Patients with stages I–II cutaneous melanomas most often present with locoregional recurrences, while those with stages III–IV melanomas will present with progressive systemic metastases (**Fig. 1**).

Major risk factors for developing both primary and subsequent melanoma include genetic, phenotypic and environmental reasons. Some of these factors include: familial cases of melanoma, atypical or dysplastic nevi, number of nevi, sun-sensitive or "red hair phenotype," history of significant ultraviolet exposure, race, and socioeconomic status.

Approximately 10% of all melanomas are familial.[8,9] Patients with multiple cases of invasive melanoma on the same side of the family, multiple primary invasive cutaneous melanomas, early age of onset of cutaneous melanoma, and pancreatic cancer in the family should be considered for genetic screening.[9–11] CDKN2A mutation is the most commonly identified gene mutation, although there is significant genetic heterogeneity among different families suggesting involvement of multiple genes.[9,10] For individuals with multiple primary melanomas, 20.8% are familial cases and 21.0% of those familial cases have mutations in CDKN2A.[12] One study assessed the risk of an additional melanoma in patients with two or more melanomas in both familial and sporadic cases.

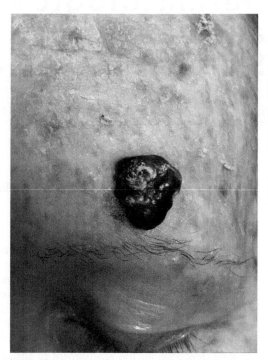

Fig. 1. This patient presented with a large tumor on the right forehead. Further work-up determined this melanoma to be stage IV.

Across both familial and sporadic cases, a two- to three-fold elevated risk for future melanoma was noted.[13] The authors determined that overall risk of second melanoma was higher in individuals with familial melanoma who received a diagnosis before 40 years of age (SIR, 4.7 [95% CI, 3.9–5.6]), especially during the first 5 years of follow-up.[13]

Nevi count and the presence of atypical nevi (also known as Clark's nevi or dysplastic nevi) have been shown to be important independent risk factors for the occurrence of melanoma.[12,14–16] Numerous nevi may indicate a greater genetic tendency to form melanoma or can be indicative of environmental exposures and chronic ultraviolet exposure, depending on the anatomic site.[17,18] There is variability in the literature regarding the threshold nevi count associated with increased melanoma risk. Indeed, some cite greater than 100, others 50–100, and one meta-analysis 25 or more nevi, as increasing melanoma risk.[14,19–21]

Individuals with extensive or repeat high exposure to ultraviolet radiation have higher rates of melanoma.[22–25] An Australian study with 1621 participants randomly assigned participants to an intervention group (directed, daily sunscreen use) and a control group (discretionary sunscreen use) for 4 years. Ten years after the 4-year intervention, participants in the intervention group had 50% fewer primary melanomas compared to the control group (11 vs 22 melanomas, hazard ration [HR] 0.50, 95% CI 0.24–1.02).[26] Vigilant sun protection practices have been the focus of numerous educational campaigns in order to reduce the incidence of melanoma and other non-melanoma skin cancers. However, it is also important to educate melanoma patients on the importance of sun protection measures after a diagnosis of melanoma also. One study assessed sun protection measures after a melanoma diagnosis in relation to the development of future primary melanomas. The authors determined that patients with a history of melanoma doubled their risk of another primary melanoma in the next 2 years if sunscreen use during that time period was inadequate (HR, 2.45; 95% CI, 1.00–6.06).[27–29] For the patients who developed another primary melanoma, 63% were male and 66% were older than 65 years (P<.05).[27] The characteristics associated with risky sun protection behaviors included: male gender, lower education level, having some tanning ability, being a current smoker, not routinely performing skin self-examinations, and having a thinner melanoma at diagnosis.[27] This study showed that the majority of the behavioral modifications were maintained over the 2 years after diagnosis of the initial melanoma. A cancer diagnosis can be a teachable moment. It is important to educate all melanoma patients regarding sun protection measures and being aware as to which populations may be particularly at risk.

CURRENT GUIDELINES FOR MELANOMA SURVEILLANCE

Surveillance follow-up schedules vary significantly depending on country, physician specialty, and stage of disease. These are summarized in **Table 1**.

Special Considerations

In order to complete an effective total-body skin evaluation, both clinicians and patients should maintain a systematic approach and know what clues and signs to look for when examining. Melanomas can appear anywhere on the skin surface, so it is critical to include the scalp, genitals, interdigital skin, and soles of feet in routine examination. These areas, and the back, are particularly challenging for patients to routinely view and are best visualized by clinicians, partners, family members, or friends. The "ugly duckling" sign (melanocytic lesions unlike the patient's classical signature nevus) and the ABCDE rule of melanoma

are tools that can help clinicians and patients identify suspicious lesions that require further evaluation with a biopsy[30] (**Figs. 2** and **3**).

Surveillance imaging is reserved for high-risk disease (stage IIB or higher) in order to detect clinically occult metastasis amenable to surgical or systemic therapy. The overutilization of imaging techniques in early melanoma (AJCC 7 0-IIC) is a cause of concern to Medicare and serves as a quality outcome in performance measure reporting. Detection of occult metastasis has been correlated with increased primary tumor thickness, ulceration of primary tumor, and/or large tumor burden in sentinel lymph nodes.[6] Ultimately, it has not been determined whether presymptomatic detection of distant metastases improves patient outcomes.[31–33] However, with emerging systemic therapies for advanced melanoma, this remains an area of further evaluation as systemic treatments may be more effective in patients with lower tumor burden metastases. Imaging techniques available include ultrasound (US), chest x-ray (CXR), computer tomography (CT), positron emission tomography-computed tomography (PET-CT), or magnetic resonance imaging (MRI). The value of CT, PET-CT, and MRI is directly correlated to the stage of disease. Chest x-ray does not reliably identify pulmonary metastases or lead to the earlier detection of pulmonary metastases.[34] Most studies indicate that if pulmonary metastases are identified by CXR, they are usually unresectable. In addition, they can cause unnecessary patient anxiety, lead to high false-positive rates, and provide additional medical care costs.[34,35] CT is the modality of choice for routine investigations and for staging purposes.[36–39] In addition, CT is the most sensitive for detection of lung metastases, whereas intra-abdominal and soft tissue metastases are better detected by MRI.[36,40,41] MRI can also more readily identify brain metastases compared to CT and PET-CT.[36] In a large meta-analysis evaluating the imaging modalities in surveillance of melanoma patients, PET-CT revealed a higher sensitivity and specificity than CT alone.[42] However, PET-CT is an expensive examination technique, and therefore should not be used indiscriminately. US has been debated in its ability for early detection of locoregional lymph node metastases. The scar of the primary cutaneous melanoma, the lymphatic drainage areas, and the regional lymph node basin should be examined. In one-third of patients, US can detect metastases before they become palpable. Regional nodal US or recurrence detection is a simple and effective examination technique, but is highly user-dependent and requires specific expertise and understanding of

Table 1
Global melanoma surveillance follow-up guidelines proposed by various organizations

Guideline	AJCC Stage	Clinical Examination	Imaging	Imaging Modalities	Laboratory Data	Other
NCCN[8]	Stages IA–IIA	Every 6–12 mo for 5 y, then annually as needed	Not recommended		None	
	Stages IIB–IV	Every 3–6 mo for 2 y; Every 3–12 mo for 3 y; Annually as needed	3–12 mo considered for first 3–5 y	CXR, CT, MRI, PET/CT	None	Imaging between years 3 and 5 not recommended if asymptomatic
ESMO[9]	Stage IA	Every 6 mo for 3 y, then annually	Not recommended		None	
	Stages IB–IIB	Every 3–6 mo for 3 y; Every 6 mo for years 4–10, then annually	Every 6 mo for the first 3 y	Lymph node sonography		
	Stages IIC–IV	Every 3 mo for the first 3 y, every 6 mo for years 4–10, then annually	Sonography every 3–6 mo for first 3 y; Other imaging: Stages IIC–IIIC every 6 mo, IIID every 3–6 mo, IV every 3 mo	Lymph node sonography Other imaging: CXR, CT, MRI, PET/CT	LDH and S-100-beta every 3–6 mo for the first 3 y	Other imaging should be considered for the first 3 y
AAD[10]	Stage 0 MIS	Every 6–12 mo for the first 2 y, then annually	Not recommended		Not recommended	
	Stages IA–IIA	Every 6–12 mo for 2–5 y, then annually	Not recommended		Not recommended	
	Stages IIB–IV	Every 3–6 mo for the first 2 y, every 6 mo for years 3–5, then annually	Can be considered during the first 3–5 y	CXR, CT, MRI, PET/CT	Not recommended	
BAD[11]	Stage 0 MIS	Emphasizes skin self-examination	Not recommended		Not recommended	
	Stage IA	Every 3–6 mo for 1 y; Every 3 mo for 3 y, then every 6 mo for 2 y	Not recommended		Not recommended	
	Stages IB–IIIA		Not recommended		Not recommended	
	Stages IIIB–IV	Every 3 mo for 3 y, then every 6 mo for 2 y, then annually	Can be considered if clinically indicated	Lymph node sonography CXR, CT, MRI, PET/CT		

German Cancer Society and German Dermatologic Society[12]	Stage I < 1 mm	Every 6 mo for the first 5 y, then every 6–12 mo from years 5–10	Not recommended		Not recommended	Abdominal US and CXR on individual basis
	Stage I and II > 1 mm	Every 3 mo for the first 5 y, then every 6 mo for years 5–10	Every 6 mo for the first 5 y	Lymph node sonography	Not recommended	
	Stage III	Every 3 mo for the first 5 y, then every 6 mo for years 5–10	Every 3–6 mo for the first 5 y	Lymph node sonography	S100-beta every 3–6 mo for the first 5 y	
	Stage IV	Not mentioned	Every 6 mo for the first 5 y	Abdominal US, CXR, CT, PET/CT, MRI		
Guidelines for Management of Melanoma in Australia and New Zealand[13]	Stage I	Annually for 10 y	Not recommended		Not recommended	
	Stage IIA	Every 6 mo for 2 y, then annually for 8 y	Not recommended		Not recommended	
	Stages IIB–IIC	Every 3–4 mo for 2 y, then every 6 mo during year 3, then annually for years 5–10	Can be considered every 3–12 mo for the first 3 y for stage IIC		Not recommended	
	Stages IIIA–IIIC	Every 3 mo for 2 y, every 6 mo during year 3, then annually	Can be considered every 3–6 mo for the first 3 y		Not recommended	

Abbreviations: AAD, American Academy of Dermatology; CT, computed tomography; CXR, chest x-ray; ESMO, European Society for Melanoma Oncology; LDH, lactate dehydrogenase; MRI, magnetic resonance imaging; NCCN, National Comprehensive Cancer Network; PET, positron emission tomography; US, ultrasound.

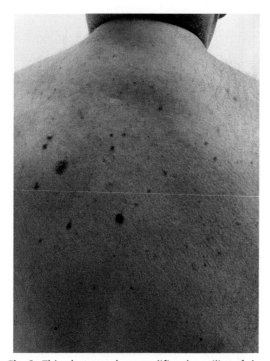

Fig. 2. This photograph exemplifies the utility of the clinical tools of the "ugly duckling" sign and the ABCDE rule of melanoma. The lesion in the central back is unlike the patient's other nevi, given its larger size, darker color, and evolution over time, which would warrant a biopsy to exclude malignancy.

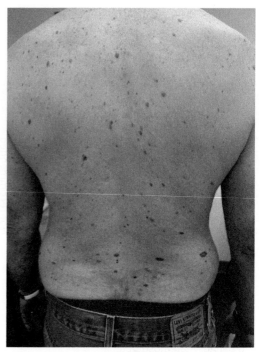

Fig. 3. This photograph illustrates the challenges that can occur during total-body skin examination when patients present with numerous nevi.

established lymph node criteria. Nodal ultrasound is less expensive, noninvasive, and safer than other alternative imaging techniques.[43–47]

There are two potential tumor markers for melanoma, lactate dehydrogenase (LDH) and S100-beta. LDH is found on a multitude of malignant and nonmalignant cells throughout the body. Persistent or recurrent elevation of LDH after treatment of melanoma may indicate recurrence. In the eighth edition of AJCC staging, LDH is incorporated across all M categories, as levels are associated with worse survival and may predict response to therapy in stage IV patients. Its utility for lower stages is negligible.[7,36] S100-beta is an acidic calcium-binding protein that is present within cells of neuroendocrine origin. Its value in the immunohistochemical diagnosis of melanocytic tumors is well established. The use of serum S100-beta has been evaluated in multiple European studies as a possible prognostic biomarker, however, it is not routinely used in the United States. A multivariate analysis of a series of 1007 patients with stages I–III cutaneous melanoma found that elevated serum S-100 was an independent predictor of survival[48–50] One retrospective study analyzing levels of LDH and S100 as predictors

of survival in patients treated with immunotherapy (pembrolizumab alone vs ipilimumab and nivolimumab) found mixed results depending on biomarker and treatment regimen. In the pembrolizumab group, patients with elevated baseline S100B or LDH exhibited significantly impaired overall survival compared with patients with normal S100-beta (1-year OS: 51.1% vs 83.1%, $P<.0001$) and normal LDH (1-year OS: 44.4% vs 80.8%, $P = .00022$), respectively. In patients treated with ipilimumab and nivolumab, baseline S100-beta and increasing S100-beta levels of greater than 145% as well as baseline LDH were associated with impaired OS ($P<.0001$, $P = .00060$, and $P = .0050$, respectively), whereas increasing LDH of greater than 25% was not ($P = .64$).[51]

Localized and metastatic tumors can generate circulating tumor cells, circulating cell-free DNA (cfDNA), and microRNA, which can be detected and quantified from peripheral blood samples, otherwise known as liquid biopsies. One prospective study determined cfDNA can serve as a surrogate marker for tumor burden in metastatic melanoma patients and can be prognostic of overall survival. Baseline cfDNA levels correlated significantly with hazard of death (HR = 2.22 for high cfDNA, $P = .004$). Patients with high cfDNA had shorter overall survival (10.0 vs 22.7 months,

$P = .009$) both in patients with oncogenic mutations (HR 2.12, $P = .0008$) and in wild-type melanoma patients (HR 5.55, $P<.0001$). High baseline cfDNA concentrations were associated with the presence of metastases and higher AJCC stage ($P<.05$).[52,53] Liquid biopsies can serve as novel predictive biomarkers for prognostic purposes and to monitor treatment response, genetic tumor evolution, and acquired drug resistance without performing repeat tissue biopsies.[54,55]

DISCUSSION

The standard model of melanoma follow-up is focused primarily on clinician detection of recurrent or new primary cutaneous melanoma, called clinician-led surveillance. An alternative model is to increase reliance on patient-led surveillance with fewer scheduled office visits and more patient-directed monitoring. This can be accomplished by expanding patient education on skin self-examination.[56] However, observational studies have indicated that clinician-detected melanomas are thinner than those detected by patients during skin self-examination.[57-63] One cumulative review found a 0.55 mm mean tumor thickness difference when comparing lesions initially detected by clinicians versus by patients or patients' significant others.[58] It is known that thinner melanomas carry a better prognosis, indicating a benefit of clinician-led surveillance. Another study in patients with melanoma indicated that routine clinician skin examination was associated with four times the odds of a thinner melanoma at detection, specifically for men greater than 60 years old.[56]

Even still, data on the impact of clinician screening on melanoma-associated mortality do not show a clear benefit. Yet, the importance of skin self-examination for routine detection of suspicious lesions is obvious. Many recurrent melanomas and newly diagnosed primary melanomas are often first detected by the patient or the patient's partner during the intervals between office visits.[64,65] Therefore patient-led surveillance can be considered as the main surveillance tool for low-risk melanoma patients, but should be emphasized for all melanoma patients regardless of risk. Several studies have associated patient skin self-examination with the identification of thinner tumors, reduced risk of advanced melanoma and decreased mortality compared to individuals who do not routinely examine their skin.[64-67] A survey study of 566 newly diagnosed melanoma patients found that routine skin self-examination of some or all of the body was associated with nearly twice the likelihood of a thin melanoma at diagnosis compared with those

who did not examine any part of their body routinely. The greatest benefit was observed in males older than 60 years and in men who used a melanoma picture to aid in self-examination.[56] The MelFo Study UK, an international phase III randomized trial, analyzed the effects of a reduced-frequency, stage-adjusted follow-up schedule for AJCC stages 1B–IIC patients after 3 years. The authors determined that the reduced follow-up strategy was shown to be safe with significant resource usage benefits for national cancer services. In addition, patient acceptance was high and anxiety levels were not increased by a less-intensive follow-up regimen.[68]

Although there are significant data supporting the benefit of clinician-led and patient-led screening, many individuals do not perform regular skin self-examinations. Electronic devices can deliver skills training comparable to other training methods and can be accommodated during the customary outpatient office visit with the physician.[69] One study assessed whether increased performance of skin self-examination can be accomplished via multiple modalities. Patients in the intervention group participated in a computer-assisted learning tutorial, took part in a hands-on skin self-examination tutorial, received monthly telecommunication reminders to perform skin examinations, and received a brochure on melanoma detection. The control group received just the melanoma brochure. After 3 months, the intervention group was more likely to perform skin self-examinations (OR, 2.36; $P<.05$) and was more confident in their ability to identify melanoma (OR, 2.72; $P<.05$).[70] Another randomized control trial revealed that melanoma patients and their partners could reliably perform skin self-examination after participating in a structured skills training program which lasted about 30 minutes with reinforcement every 4 months compared to patients and their partners who received standard care.[71] Studies have also revealed the importance of physician involvement in educating and supporting patients in skin self-examination. Physician influence was positively associated with skin self-examination performance. Melanoma patients may benefit from reminders to check hard-to-see and sensitive areas, develop a plan for conducting skin self-examinations and education on how to use mirrors to see hard-to-reach areas.[72]

Future Directions

In addition to visual screening, research is ongoing to find technologies to help detect melanoma at an earlier stage when a cure is feasible. Some of these tools include gene expression profiling, dermoscopy, computer-assisted diagnosis tools, and artificial intelligence. The 31-gene expression profile test uses tumor biology to categorize melanoma risk as low or high with intermediate subcategories. Multiple studies have highlighted its prognostic utility.[73] A recent meta-analysis showed that the 31 gene-expression profile test accurately identifies patients at increased risk of metastasis, is independent of other clinicopathologic covariates, and augments current risk stratification by reassigning patients to heightened surveillance who were previously categorized as low risk.[74] Noninvasive technologies can facilitate melanoma diagnosis and may reduce the number of skin biopsies obtained from benign skin lesions.[75]

Dermoscopy of suspicious lesions is a noninvasive technique employing polarized light and magnification (**Fig. 4**). Dermoscopy is widely used in dermatologic settings, but not often in primary care settings as it requires training to recognize melanoma-specific features. Characteristic features of melanoma include an atypical pigment network, irregular or brown-black dots or globules, streaks, multiple colors asymmetrically distributed, a blue-whitish veil, and atypical vascular pattern.[76] For those experienced in dermoscopy, sensitivity and specificity of the clinical diagnosis of melanoma increases when used in conjunction with

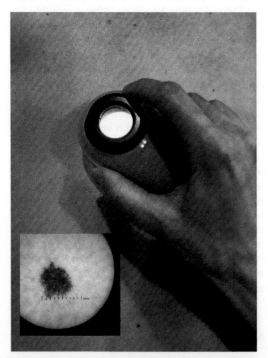

Fig. 4. Dermoscopy requires clinical training in order to reliably identify atypical features that would warrant further investigation with a biopsy

visual inspection rather than when used alone.[77,78] Devices such as MoleMax II (Derma Medical, San Diego, CA) can be used for serial dermoscopic photographs to observe individual lesions over time and monitor for any suspicious changes.[75,78–82] There are several systems that use handheld or video dermatoscopes that communicate with computer software analyzing digital images of skin lesions. A large meta-analysis of these devices that included nearly 9000 lesions and 1063 melanomas found a sensitivity of 90.1% (95% CI 84–94) and 74.3% (95% CI 63.6–82.7).[83] However, limitations of this meta-analysis include considerable variability across the 22 studies in the type of technology used and the algorithm performance, which may contribute to alterations in diagnostic accuracy in certain studies.

Spectrophotometric intracutaneous analysis (SIAscopy) uses handheld scanners with varying light wavelengths to evaluate chromophore imaging and determine microscopic architecture.[75,84] It is a noninvasive multispectral imaging technique intended for pigmented skin lesion assessment and melanoma detection. Calibrated images are analyzed by a series of algorithms that extract information about the distribution, position, and quantity of different chromophores. Multiple studies have assessed the sensitivity and specificity of SIAscopy for melanoma detection alone and in comparison with dermoscopy. SIAscopy does not seem to be superior to dermoscopy in detecting suspicious lesions. It may be useful for primary care settings or other nondermatologists as it does not require specific training or expertise. However, its biggest limitation in primary care settings is its low performance when used for seborrheic keratoses, which are highly prevalent.[75,85–88] MoleMate (MedX, Ontario, Canada) is a multispectral imaging device that uses the SIAscope technology paired with algorithms to improve diagnostic accuracy. It was found to have equivalent sensitivity but reduced specificity, however, it has been approved for use in the European Union, United States, and Canada.[75] MelaFind (MELA Sciences, Irvington, NY) is another multispectral imaging technology that uses a handheld device at varying wavelengths on suspicious skin lesions to create automatic image analysis and uses pattern recognition to determine morphologic disorganization. The utility of MelaFind for melanoma detection has been debated. Some studies suggest that when used as an adjunct for providers, it increases sensitivity but decreases specificity.[75,89]

Convolutional neural networks-based systems (artificial intelligence) use deep learning technologies to efficiently differentiate skin lesions based on image analysis. Studies have shown that these technologies consistently perform equivalent to or better than expert clinicians in diagnosis of melanoma.[90–93] Although such technologies are created to have higher sensitivity, they cannot integrate information from a range of sources like clinicians can to make clinical decisions. In addition, they lack the full spectrum of skin phenotypes and lesions in existing databases.

The use of mobile (smartphone) applications (apps) has grown in parallel with increased access to smartphones worldwide. More than 80% of households in the United States have a smartphone. Health-related apps are becoming more prominent across all health fields, with particular attention to dermatology. A total of 526 dermatology mobile apps have been found, corresponding to an 80% growth in dermatology apps since 2014. The market share of teledermatology increased from 11% to 20% from 2014 to 2017.[94] Some apps function by sending images from smartphone cameras to an experienced professional for review, while others are created to be used for skin self-monitoring. While mobile technology advancements can be beneficial in reducing time to diagnosis, mortality and healthcare costs associated with melanoma, there are concerns about their safety and accuracy. The authors of one systematic review of two large studies examining the utility of five smartphone apps concluded that smartphone apps using artificial intelligence-based analysis have not yet demonstrated sufficient accuracy to draw any implications for clinical practice. This review analyzed a total of 332 lesion images, including 86 melanomas, taken by clinicians in clinical settings. The apps used an algorithm that classified lesions as melanomas or high-risk lesions (necessitating review by clinician) with sensitivities ranging from 7% to 73% and specificities from 37% to 94%. This meant that 27% to 93% of invasive melanomas or atypical melanocytic lesions were not identified, indicating a high likelihood of missing a melanoma.[95] The authors of a more recent systematic review examined nine studies assessing the diagnostic accuracy of six smartphone apps for risk stratification of suspicious lesions also determined that the current algorithm-based smartphone apps cannot reliably detect cases of melanoma.[96] In addition, lesion selection and image acquisition were performed by clinicians rather than smartphone users, inhibiting the generalizability of the study.

These new promising technologies have been created to facilitate detection of melanoma and reduce the practice of obtaining unnecessary biopsy specimens. Their sensitivity and specificity for melanoma detection are largely determined by individual threshold settings used for algorithm classifiers. Therefore, they tend to have greater diagnostic sensitivity and lower specificity due to fear of missing a melanoma. In addition, lesions in these studies have usually been preselected by clinicians and require the lesion to be on a flat surface and accessible. None of these technologies is capable of scanning the entire body or assessing more complex body surfaces, such as on the ears or under the nail plate. These trials also excluded special sites, such as acral, mucosal, and genital lesions. Practitioners will have to carefully consider incorporation and compensation for these devices into their practice as they are currently not covered by most insurance healthcare plans.

SUMMARY

The scope of melanoma staging and therapeutics is ever-changing. The recommendations for melanoma follow-up guidelines also mirror this dynamic landscape. There is currently variability among national guidelines regarding the timing and frequency of clinical surveillance, as well as the use of laboratory data and imaging modalities for detection of melanoma recurrence. However, in general more aggressive surveillance is recommended for more advanced melanomas and for individuals at increased risk for future sporadic or familial melanoma. When examining high-risk individuals, a systematic approach should be followed. Patients and their partners should be educated on the importance of and specific techniques of skin self-examinations. Future considerations include the use of noninvasive imaging techniques and artificial intelligence to enhance detection of melanomas. Understanding the limitations of these special technologies is essential prior to routine incorporation into clinical practice.

CLINICS CARE POINTS

- There is a lack of consensus worldwide regarding optimal follow-up and surveillance methods after a diagnosis of melanoma has been made.

- The standard of follow-up care focuses on clinician-led surveillance, but there is increased awareness and incentive for patient-led surveillance for lower stage disease patients.

- Future directions for the assessment of suspicious lesions include the use of gene-expression profiling, noninvasive technologies and artificial intelligence.

REFERENCES

1. Garbe C, Leiter U. Melanoma epidemiology and trends. Clin Dermatol 2009;27(1):3–9.
2. Siegel RL, Miller KD, Jemal A. Cancer statistics, 2017. CA Cancer J Clin 2017;67(1):7–30.
3. Nishino M, Giobbie-Hurder A, Ramaiya NH, et al. Response assessment in metastatic melanoma treated with ipilimumab and bevacizumab: CT tumor size and density as markers for response and outcome. J Immunother Cancer 2014;2(1):40.
4. Ribas A, Hamid O, Daud A, et al. Association of pembrolizumab with tumor response and survival among patients with advanced melanoma. JAMA 2016;315(15):1600–9.
5. Poklepovic AS, Carvajal RD. Prognostic value of low tumor burden in patients with melanoma. Oncology (Williston Park) 2018;32(9):e90–6.
6. von Schuckmann LA, Hughes MCB, Ghiasvand R, et al. Risk of melanoma recurrence after diagnosis of a high-risk primary tumor. JAMA Dermatol 2019; 155(6):688–93.
7. AJCC Cancer Staging manuel: American Joint Committee on Cancer. 8th ed. New York: Springer; 2017. p. 563–85.
8. Rivers JK. Melanoma. Lancet 1996;347(9004): 803–6.
9. Leachman SA, Carucci J, Kohlmann W, et al. Selection criteria for genetic assessment of patients with familial melanoma. J Am Acad Dermatol 2009;61(4). 677.e1-14.
10. Gabree M, Patel D, Rodgers L. Clinical applications of melanoma genetics. Curr Treat Options Oncol 2014;15(2):336–50.
11. Cust AE, Badcock C, Smith J, et al. A risk prediction model for the development of subsequent primary melanoma in a population-based cohort. Br J Dermatol 2020;182(5):1148–57.
12. Helsing P, Nymoen DA, Ariansen S, et al. Population-based prevalence of CDKN2A and CDK4 mutations in patients with multiple primary melanomas. Genes Chromosomes Cancer 2008;47(2):175–84.
13. Chen T, Fallah M, Försti A, et al. Risk of next melanoma in patients with familial and sporadic melanoma by number of previous melanomas. JAMA Dermatol 2015;151(6):607–15.
14. Gandini S, Sera F, Cattaruzza MS, et al. Meta-analysis of risk factors for cutaneous melanoma: II. Sun exposure. Eur J Cancer 2005;41(1):45–60.
15. Arumi-Uria M, McNutt NS, Finnerty B. Grading of atypia in nevi: correlation with melanoma risk. Mod Pathol 2003;16(8):764–71.
16. Kim CC, Berry EG, Marchetti MA, et al, Pigmented Lesion Subcommittee, Melanoma Prevention Working Group. Risk of subsequent cutaneous melanoma in moderately dysplastic nevi excisionally biopsied but with positive histologic margins. JAMA Dermatol 2018;154(12):1401–8.

17. Olsen CM, Zens MS, Stukel TA, et al. Nevus density and melanoma risk in women: a pooled analysis to test the divergent pathway hypothesis. Int J Cancer 2009;124(4):937–44.
18. Cho E, Rosner BA, Colditz GA. Risk factors for melanoma by body site. Cancer Epidemiol Biomarkers Prev 2005;14(5):1241–4.
19. Bataille V, Bishop JA, Sasieni P, et al. Risk of cutaneous melanoma in relation to the numbers, types and sites of naevi: a case-control study. Br J Cancer 1996;73(12):1605–11.
20. Olsen CM, Carroll HJ, Whiteman DC. Estimating the attributable fraction for cancer: a meta-analysis of nevi and melanoma. Cancer Prev Res (Phila) 2010; 3(2):233–45.
21. Kanzler MH, Mraz-Gernhard S. Primary cutaneous malignant melanoma and its precursor lesions: diagnostic and therapeutic overview. J Am Acad Dermatol 2001;45(2):260–76.
22. US Department of Health and Human Services. The Surgeon General's Call to Action to Prevent Skin Cancer. Washington, DC: US Department of Health and Human Services, Office of the Surgeon General; 2014.
23. Elwood JM, Jopson J. Melanoma and sun exposure: an overview of published studies. Int J Cancer 1997; 73(2):198–203.
24. Gallagher RP, Spinelli JJ, Lee TK. Tanning beds, sunlamps, and risk of cutaneous malignant melanoma. Cancer Epidemiol Biomarkers Prev 2005; 14(3):562–6.
25. International Agency for Research on Cancer Working Group on artificial ultraviolet (UV) light and skin cancer. The association of use of sunbeds with cutaneous malignant melanoma and other skin cancers: a systematic review. Int J Cancer 2007;120(5): 1116–22. Erratum in: Int J Cancer. 2007 Jun 1; 120(11):2526.
26. Green AC, Williams GM, Logan V, et al. Reduced melanoma after regular sunscreen use: randomized trial follow-up. J Clin Oncol 2011;29(3):257–63.
27. von Schuckmann LA, Wilson LF, Hughes MCB, et al. Sun protection behavior after diagnosis of high-risk primary melanoma and risk of a subsequent primary. J Am Acad Dermatol 2019;80(1):139–48.e4.
28. Coit DG, Thompson JA, Albertini MR, et al. Cutaneous melanoma, version 2.2019, NCCN Clinical Practice Guidelines in Oncology. J Natl Compr Canc Netw 2019;17(4):367–402.
29. Garbe C, Amaral T, Peris K, et al. European consensus-based interdisciplinary guideline for melanoma. Part 2: treatment - Update 2019. Eur J Cancer 2020;126:159–77.
30. Grob JJ, Bonerandi JJ. The 'ugly duckling' sign: identification of the common characteristics of nevi in an individual as a basis for melanoma screening. Arch Dermatol 1998;134:103–4.

31. Bhutiani N, Egger ME, Mcmasters KM. Optimizing follow-up assessment of patients with cutaneous melanoma. Ann Surg Onc 2017;24(4):861–3.

32. Swetter SM. Commentary: improved patient outcomes remain elusive after intensive imaging surveillance for high-risk melanoma. J Am Acad Dermatol 2016;75(3):525–7.

33. Freeman M, Laks S. Surveillance imaging for metastasis in high-risk melanoma: importance in individualized patient care and survivorship. Melanoma Manag 2019;6(1):MMT12.

34. Morton RL, Craig J, Thompson JF. The role of surveillance chest x-rays in the follow-up of high-risk melanoma patients. Ann Surg Oncol 2009;16(3):571–7.

35. Brown RE, Stromberg A, Hagendoorn LJ, et al. Surveillance after surgical treatment of melanoma: futility of routine chest radiography. Surgery 2010;148(4):711–6.

36. Swetter SM, Tsao H, Bichakjian CK, et al. Guidelines of care for the management of primary cutaneous melanoma. J Am Acad Dermatol 2019;80(1):208–50.

37. Marsden JR, Newton-Bishop JA, Burrows L, et al. Revised U.K. guidelines for the management of cutaneous melanoma 2010. Br J Dermatol 2010;163:238–56.

38. Dummer R, Siano M, Hunger RE, et al. The updated Swiss guidelines 2016 for the treatment and follow-up of cutaneous melanoma. Swiss Med Wkly 2016;146:w14279.

39. Sladden MJ, Nieweg OE, Howle J, et al. Updated evidence-based clinical practice guidelines for the diagnosis and management of melanoma: definitive excision margins for primary cutaneous melanoma. Med J Aust 2018;208(3):137–42.

40. Müller-Horvat C, Radny P, Eigentler TK, et al. Prospective comparison of the impact on treatment decisions of whole-body magnetic resonance imaging and computed tomography in patients with metastatic malignant melanoma. Eur J Cancer 2006;42(3):342–50.

41. Bronstein Y, Ng CS, Rohren E, et al. PET/CT in the management of patients with stage IIIC and IV metastatic melanoma considered candidates for surgery: evaluation of the additive value after conventional imaging. AJR Am J Roentgenol 2012;198(4):902–8.

42. Xing Y, Bronstein Y, Ross MI, et al. Contemporary diagnostic imaging modalities for the staging and surveillance of melanoma patients: a meta-analysis. J Natl Cancer Inst 2011;103(2):129–42.

43. Bafounta ML, Beauchet A, Chagnon S, et al. Ultrasonography or palpation for detection of melanoma nodal invasion: a meta-analysis. Lancet Oncol 2004;5(11):673–80.

44. Chai CY, Zager JS, Szabunio MM, et al. Preoperative ultrasound is not useful for identifying nodal metastasis in melanoma patients undergoing sentinel node biopsy: preoperative ultrasound in clinically node-negative melanoma. Ann Surg Oncol 2012;19(4):1100–6.

45. Voit C, Van Akkooi AC, Schafer-Hesterberg G, et al. Ultrasound morphology criteria predict metastatic disease of the sentinel nodes in patients with melanoma. J Clin Oncol 2010;28:847–52, 238.

46. Voit CA, Oude Ophuis CM, Ulrich J, et al. Ultrasound of the sentinel node in melanoma patients: echo-free island is a discriminatory morphologic feature for node positivity. Melanoma Res 2016;26:267–71.

47. Voit CA, van Akkooi AC, Schafer-Hesterberg G, et al. Rotterdam criteria for sentinel node (SN) tumor burden and the accuracy of ultrasound (US)-guided fine-needle aspiration cytology (FNAC): can US-guided FNAC replace SN staging in patients with melanoma? J Clin Oncol 2009;27:4994–5000.

48. Aukema TS, Olmos RA, Korse CM, et al. Utility of FDG PET/CT and brain MRI in melanoma patients with increased serum S-100B level during follow-up. Ann Surg Oncol 2010;17(6):1657–61.

49. Tarhini AA, Stuckert J, Lee S, et al. Prognostic significance of serum S100B protein in high-risk surgically resected melanoma patients participating in Intergroup Trial ECOG 1694 [published correction appears in J Clin Oncol. 2012 Nov 1;30(31):3903]. J Clin Oncol 2009;27(1):38–44.

50. Mårtenson ED, Hansson LO, Nilsson B, et al. Serum S-100b protein as a prognostic marker in malignant cutaneous melanoma. J Clin Oncol 2001;19(3):824–31.

51. Wagner NB, Forschner A, Leiter U, et al. S100B and LDH as early prognostic markers for response and overall survival in melanoma patients treated with anti-PD-1 or combined anti-PD-1 plus anti-CTLA-4 antibodies. Br J Cancer 2018;119(3):339–46.

52. Valpione S, Gremel G, Mundra P, et al. Plasma total cell-free DNA (cfDNA) is a surrogate biomarker for tumour burden and a prognostic biomarker for survival in metastatic melanoma patients. Eur J Cancer 2018;88:1–9.

53. Váraljai R, Elouali S, Lueong SS, et al. The predictive and prognostic significance of cell-free DNA concentration in melanoma [published online ahead of print, 2020 Jun 22]. J Eur Acad Dermatol Venereol 2021;35(2):387–95.

54. Gaiser MR, von Bubnoff N, Gebhardt C, et al. Liquid biopsy to monitor melanoma patients. J Dtsch Dermatol Ges 2018;16(4):405–14.

55. Garbe C, Büttner P, Weiss J, et al. Risk factors for developing cutaneous melanoma and criteria for identifying persons at risk: multicenter case-control study of the Central Malignant Melanoma Registry of the German Dermatological Society. J Invest Dermatol 1994;102(5):695–9.

56. Swetter SM, Pollitt RA, Johnson TM, et al. Behavioral determinants of successful early melanoma detection: role of self and physician skin examination. Cancer 2012;118(15):3725–34.

57. Terushkin V, Halpern AC. Melanoma early detection. Hematol Oncol Clin North Am 2009;23(3):481–500, viii.

58. Kovalyshyn I, Dusza SW, Siamas K, et al. The impact of physician screening on melanoma detection. Arch Dermatol 2011;147(11):1269–75.

59. Carli P, De Giorgi V, Palli D, et al. Dermatologist detection and skin self-examination are associated with thinner melanomas: results from a survey of the Italian Multidisciplinary Group on Melanoma. Arch Dermatol 2003;139(5):607–12.

60. Aitken JF, Elwood M, Baade PD, et al. Clinical whole-body skin examination reduces the incidence of thick melanomas. Int J Cancer 2010;126(2):450–8.

61. Epstein DS, Lange JR, Gruber SB, et al. Is physician detection associated with thinner melanomas? JAMA 1999;281(7):640–3.

62. Geller AC, Johnson TM, Miller DR, et al. Factors associated with physician discovery of early melanoma in middle-aged and older men. Arch Dermatol 2009;145(4):409–14.

63. Pollitt RA, Geller AC, Brooks DR, et al. Efficacy of skin self-examination practices for early melanoma detection. Cancer Epidemiol Biomarkers Prev 2009;18(11):3018–23.

64. Berwick M, Begg CB, Fine JA, et al. Screening for cutaneous melanoma by skin self-examination. J Natl Cancer Inst 1996;88(1):17–23.

65. Pollitt RA, Geller AC, Brooks DR, et al. Efficacy of skin self-examination practices for early melanoma detection. Cancer Epidemiol Biomarkers Prev 2009;18(11):3018–23.

66. Johansson M, Brodersen J, Gøtzsche PC, et al. Screening for reducing morbidity and mortality in malignant melanoma. Cochrane Database Syst Rev 2019;6(6):CD012352.

67. Deschner B, Wayne JD. Follow-up of the melanoma patient. J Surg Oncol 2019;119(2):262–8.

68. Moncrieff MD, Underwood B, Garioch JJ, et al. The MelFo study UK: effects of a reduced-frequency, stage-adjusted follow-up schedule for cutaneous melanoma 1B to 2C patients after 3-years. Ann Surg Oncol 2020;27(11):4109–19.

69. Robinson JK, Gaber R, Hultgren B, et al. Skin self-examination education for early detection of melanoma: a randomized controlled trial of Internet, workbook, and in-person interventions. J Med Internet Res 2014;16(1):e7.

70. Aneja S, Brimhall AK, Kast DR, et al. Improvement in patient performance of skin self-examinations after intervention with Interactive education and telecommunication reminders: a randomized controlled study. Arch Dermatol 2012;148(11):1266–72.

71. Robinson JK, Wayne JD, Martini MC, et al. Early detection of new melanomas by patients with melanoma and their partners using a structured skin self-examination skills training intervention: a randomized clinical trial. JAMA Dermatol 2016;152(9):979–85.

72. Czajkowska Z, Hall NC, Sewitch M, et al. The role of patient education and physician support in self-efficacy for skin self-examination among patients with melanoma. Patient Educ Couns 2017;100(8):1505–10.

73. Scott AM, Dale PS, Conforti A, et al. Integration of a 31-gene expression profile into clinical Decision-Making in the treatment of cutaneous melanoma [published online ahead of print, 2020 Aug 5]. Am Surg 2020;86(11):1561–4.

74. Greenhaw BN, Covington KR, Kurley SJ, et al. Molecular risk prediction in cutaneous melanoma: a meta-analysis of the 31-gene expression profile prognostic test in 1,479 patients. J Am Acad Dermatol 2020;83(3):745–53.

75. March J, Hand M, Grossman D. Practical application of new technologies for melanoma diagnosis: Part I. Noninvasive approaches [published correction appears in J Am Acad Dermatol. 2015 Oct;73(4):720]. J Am Acad Dermatol 2015;72(6):929–42.

76. Dinnes J, Deeks JJ, Chuchu N, et al. Dermoscopy, with and without visual inspection, for diagnosing melanoma in adults. Cochrane Database Syst Rev 2018;12(12):CD011902.

77. Vestergaard ME, Macaskill P, Holt PE, et al. Dermoscopy compared with naked eye examination for the diagnosis of primary melanoma: a meta-analysis of studies performed in a clinical setting. Br J Dermatol 2008;159(3):669–76.

78. Kittler H, Pehamberger H, Wolff K, et al. Follow-up of melanocytic skin lesions with digital epiluminescence microscopy: patterns of modifications observed in early melanoma, atypical nevi, and common nevi. J Am Acad Dermatol 2000;43:467–76.

79. Menzies SW, Gutenev A, Avramidis M, et al. Short-term digital surface microscopic monitoring of atypical or changing melanocytic lesions. Arch Dermatol 2001;137:1583–9.

80. Robinson JK, Nickoloff BJ. Digital epiluminescence microscopy monitoring of high-risk patients. Arch Dermatol 2004;140:49–56.

81. Haenssle HA, Krueger U, Vente C, et al. Results from an observational trial: digital epiluminescence microscopy follow-up of atypical nevi increases the sensitivity and the chance of success of conventional dermoscopy in detecting melanoma. J Invest Dermatol 2006;126:980–5.

82. Fuller SR, Bowen GM, Tanner B, et al. Digital dermoscopic monitoring of atypical nevi in patients at risk for melanoma. Dermatol Surg 2007;33:1198–206.

83. Ferrante di Ruffano L, Takwoingi Y, Dinnes J, et al. Computer-assisted diagnosis techniques (dermoscopy and spectroscopy-based) for diagnosing skin cancer in adults. Cochrane Database Syst Rev 2018;12(12):CD013186.

84. Knackstedt T, Knackstedt RW, Couto R, et al. Malignant melanoma: diagnostic and management update. Plast Reconstr Surg 2018;142(2):202e–16e.

85. Haniffa MA, Lloyd JJ, Lawrence CM. The use of a spectrophotometric intracutaneous analysis device in the real-time diagnosis of melanoma in the setting of a melanoma screening clinic. Br J Dermatol 2007; 156(6):1350–2.

86. Govindan K, Smith J, Knowles L, et al. Assessment of nurse-led screening of pigmented lesions using SIAscope. J Plast Reconstr Aesthet Surg 2007;60: 639–45.

87. Haniffa MA, Lloyd JJ, Lawrence CM. The use of a spectrophotometric intracutaneous analysis device in the real-time diagnosis of melanoma in the setting of a melanoma screening clinic. Br J Dermatol 2007; 156:1350–2.

88. Gutkowicz-Krusin D, Elbaum M, Jacobs A, et al. Precision of automatic measurements of pigmented skin lesion parameters with a MelaFind multispectral digital dermoscope. Melanoma Res 2000;10:563–70.

89. MacLellan AN, Price EL, Publicover-Brouwer P, et al. The use of non-invasive imaging techniques in the diagnosis of melanoma: a prospective diagnostic accuracy study [published online ahead of print, 2020 Apr 11]. J Am Acad Dermatol 2020.

90. Hekler A, Utikal JS, Enk AH, et al. Superior skin cancer classification by the combination of human and artificial intelligence. Eur J Cancer 2019;120: 114–21.

91. Maron RC, Weichenthal M, Utikal JS, et al. Systematic outperformance of 112 dermatologists in multiclass skin cancer image classification by convolutional neural networks. Eur J Cancer 2019;119:57–65.

92. Marchetti MA, Liopyris K, Dusza SW, et al. Computer algorithms show potential for improving dermatologists' accuracy to diagnose cutaneous melanoma: results of the International Skin Imaging Collaboration 2017. J Am Acad Dermatol 2020; 82(3):622–7.

93. Brinker TJ, Hekler A, Enk AH, et al. Deep learning outperformed 136 of 157 dermatologists in a head-to-head dermoscopic melanoma image classification task. Eur J Cancer 2019;113:47–54.

94. Flaten HK, St Claire C, Schlager E, et al. Growth of mobile applications in dermatology - 2017 update. Dermatol Online J 2018;24(2). 13030/qt3hs7n9z6.

95. Chuchu N, Takwoingi Y, Dinnes J, et al. Smartphone applications for triaging adults with skin lesions that are suspicious for melanoma. Cochrane Database Syst Rev 2018;12(12):CD013192.

96. Freeman K, Dinnes J, Chuchu N, et al. Algorithm based smartphone apps to assess risk of skin cancer in adults: systematic review of diagnostic accuracy studies [published correction appears in BMJ. 2020 Feb 25;368:m645]. BMJ 2020;368:m127.

Non-Operative Options for Loco-regional Melanoma

Rebecca Knackstedt, MD, PhD[a], Timothy Smile, MD[b], Jennifer Yu, MD, PhD[b], Brian R. Gastman, MD[c],*

KEYWORDS

- Melanoma • Injectable therapy • Radiation therapy • Immunotherapy • Checkpoint inhibitors

KEY POINTS

- There have been numerous recent advances in the medical management of melanoma in-transit metastases.
- Isolated limb infusion was introduced in 1998 as a less invasive alternative to isolated limb perfusion and has demonstrated durable results for patients with melanoma in-transit metastases.
- In December 2015, TVEC was approved by the Food and Drug Administration as the first oncolytic immunotherapy for adults with stages IIIb, IIIc, and IV M1a melanoma without bone, brain, lung, or visceral disease manifestations. It can be used independently or in concert with other targeted therapy.
- For patients with bulky locoregional disease and in-transit metastasis, the addition of hyperthermia to radiation therapy can be considered and has demonstrated favorable results.

INTRODUCTION

Malignant melanoma is the 5th most common cancer and stage IV melanoma accounts for approximately 4% of new melanoma diagnoses in the United States. The prognosis for advanced disease is poor, with 5-year survival rates for stage IIID melanoma less than 30%.[1] Up to 10% of patients with melanoma may develop recurrent locoregional disease, often presenting as in-transit metastasis.[2,3] The 8th edition of AJCC melanoma staging includes in-transit metastases as a microsatellite lesion (MSI). The presence of MSI leads to a pathologic stage of at least N1c and, thus, overall stage of IIIb. For N2 and N3 lesions, the presence of MSI leads to an upstaging to N2c and N3c, respectively. Various treatment options exist for in-transit metastases, depending on the presentation, which can range from small to bulky lesions. While simple excision can be employed for small, single lesions, this is not an option for bulky disease. The optimal treatment for these lesions would be feasible, have the potential for repeat utilization, if required, and have tolerable local and systemic toxicity.[4] There have been numerous recent advances in the medical management of melanoma in-transit metastases. The goal of this paper is to review currently accepted treatment options for in-transit metastases and introduce emerging therapies.

Limb Perfusion

Isolated limb perfusion (ILP), a treatment option for bulky or multifocal disease, was developed by Creech and colleagues in 1958.[5,6] Melphalan (L-phenylalanine mustard) is considered the standard drug for ILP due to its efficacy[7,8] and toxicity profile.[9] Drugs commonly used in the treatment of melanoma have been tested in ILP, but no drug or drug combination has achieved results superior

The authors have no disclosures.
[a] Department of Plastic Surgery, Cleveland Clinic, 2049 East 100th Street, Desk A60, Cleveland, OH 44195, USA;
[b] Department of Radiation Oncology, Cleveland Clinic, Taussig Cancer Center, 10201 Carnegie Avenue, Cleveland, OH 44195, USA; [c] Department of Plastic Surgery, Cleveland Clinic, Cleveland Clinic Lerner College of Medicine, 2049 East 100th Street, Desk A60, Cleveland, OH 44195, USA
* Corresponding author.
E-mail address: gastmab@ccf.org

Clin Plastic Surg 48 (2021) 631–642
https://doi.org/10.1016/j.cps.2021.05.007
0094-1298/21/© 2021 Elsevier Inc. All rights reserved.

to those of melphalan. The only alternative still in use is the combination of melphalan and actinomycin-D.[10]

A randomized trial published in 2006 compared melphalan with ILP (M-ILP) to combination therapy with melphalan and TNF-alpha (TM-ILP). While this trial demonstrated no beneficial effect to adding TNF-alpha, the response rate was assessed at 3 months as opposed to when the maximum response is reached, which is usually after 3–6 months.[11] Thus, the results of this trial were met with much criticism. A retrospective review comparing M-ILP to TM-ILP demonstrated a significantly improved complete response (CR) rate when TM-ILP was employed.[12] The results of TM-ILP in large series published after 2000 have demonstrated that CR rates are typically greater than 60%.[13–16] A systematic review of over 2000 patients undergoing ILP found a median overall response rate (ORR) of 90% and a CR of 58% with improved responses with the addition of TNF-alpha.[17] A study of 64 patients randomized patients to melphalan, TM-ILP, or the combination of melphalan, TNF-alpha, and IFN-gamma. Compared to melphalan-only historical controls, ORR were 78%, 91%, and 100% for melphalan, melphalan/TNF-alpha, and melphalan/TNF-alpha/IFN-gamma, respectively.[18] These studies are summarized in **Table 1**.

It has been shown that the response to ILP is dependent on the extent of disease. The best responses are observed in patients with in-transit metastases but no nodal disease, followed by in-transit metastases with nodal disease, and lastly by stage IV disease.[19] These differences have been demonstrated in many series and may be due to the aggressiveness of melanoma.[20,21] Long-term results of a Swedish trial confirmed that adjuvant ILP after the excision of high-risk primary melanomas does not improve survival.[22] Reported recurrence rates after ILP are approximately 50%.[17] The management of limb recurrences after ILP is essentially the same as for the initial presentation, with local excision if feasible, and repeated perfusion for extensive disease.[23] Repeat ILPs have produced response rates of 72% to 96% with similar toxicity profiles to initial procedures.[24,25]

Limb Infusion

Isolated limb infusion (ILI) was introduced in 1998 as a less invasive alternative to ILP.[26] A series of 316 ILI procedures for patients with melanoma performed over a 15-year period at five Australian institutions demonstrated an ORR of 75%. Patients with a CR had longer overall survival (OS)

than those with a partial response (PR).[20] In the United States, 148 ILI procedures for melanoma performed over a 10-year period demonstrated an ORR of 59%. Responders had better outcomes, including longer OS. After ILI, 26% of the cohort was resected to no evidence of disease.[27] A prospective study of 61 ILI treatments demonstrated an ORR of 44%.[28] A cohort study of 31 patients demonstrated an ORR of 52% and a CR of 26%.[29] A study of 62 patients, 58 of whom had melanoma, who underwent ILI demonstrated a median response duration of 12 months after CR. The 5-year survival after CR was 91% versus 34% with stable disease or progression.[30] An international, multi-institutional study examined ILI for stages IIIB/C melanoma. Among 687 cases, the ORR was 64.1% and median OS was 38.2 months. Superior outcomes were observed in responders compared with nonresponders, with longer OS (46.5 vs 24.4 months).[31]

After intra-arterial therapy, approximately 20% to 50% of patients recur locoregionally.[25,32,33] Repeat ILIs performed at a median of 11 to 14 months after the index procedure have response rates of 71% to 83% with fewer CR.[33,34] Some series report more grade ≥3 toxicities after repeat ILI.[34] A planned double ILI protocol (4 weeks after the initial infusion) did not improve ORR or response duration (88 vs 82%, 18 vs 17 months), but toxicity was higher after the second ILI (grade ≥3; 76 vs 52%).[33]

There have been no randomized comparisons of ILI and ILP. However, retrospective studies have been performed. At Duke University, 59 ILPs were compared to 61 ILIs. ORRs were better for ILP than ILI (ORR 88 vs 44% and CR 57 vs 30%), but more patients experienced a grade ≥3 toxicity after ILP.[28,35] Updated results included 72 ILPs and 144 ILIs and demonstrated similar ORR (81 vs 43%) and CR (55 vs 30%), but no difference in OS (32 vs 33 months). Grade ≥3 toxicity was reported in 27% after ILP and 22% after ILI.[35] A comparison of 94 ILIs performed at Moffitt Cancer Center and 109 ILPs at Sahlgrenska University Hospital also found higher ORR for ILP than ILI (80 vs 53%) but similar OS (40 vs 46 months).[36]

Radiation Therapy

Melanoma is historically considered relatively radioresistant based on in vitro studies. However, clinical studies support that radiation plays a key role in the management of primary cutaneous melanoma,[37–44] particularly for patients who are medically inoperable or patients for whom surgery would be disfiguring.[45] In the adjuvant setting, multiple studies have demonstrated excellent

Table 1
Summary of studies investigating interventions in limb perfusion for melanoma

Intervention	Outcome	Citation
Limb perfusion		
M-ILP vs TM-ILP	No difference in outcomes	Cornett et al.,[11] 2006
M-ILP vs TM-ILP	Improved complete response with TM-ILP	Rossi et al.,[12] 2010
M-ILP vs TM-ILP	Improved complete response and overall response rate with TM-ILP	Moreno-Ramirez et al.,[17] 2010
M-ILP vs TM-ILP vs TM-ILP and IFN-gamma	Overall response rates were 78%, 91%, and 100% for melphalan, melphalan/TNF-alpha, and melphalan/TNF-alpha/IFN-gamma,	Lienard et al.,[18] 1999

Abbreviations: M-ILP, melphalan isolated limb perfusion, TM-ILP, TNF-alpha and melphalan isolated limb perfusion.

regional control rates for postoperative radiation after lymph node dissection.[46–48] These studies led to the landmark ANZMTG 01.02/TROG 02.01 study that established the role of radiation therapy for improved regional lymph node control. The addition of radiation to lymph node dissection reduced 6-year nodal recurrence rates to 21% compared to 36% without radiation.[49] Not unexpectedly, there was no difference in overall survival. Risk factors on surgical pathology for adjuvant radiation included extracapsular spread, $\geq$ 1 parotid node, $\geq$ 2 cervical or axillary nodes, $\geq$ 3 inguinal nodes, size $\geq$ 3 cm cervical or axillary node, or size $\geq$ 4 cm inguinal node. Adjuvant radiation to the inguinofemoral nodes increased the incidence of lower extremity lymphedema from 7% with nodal dissection alone to 15%, but cervical and axillary radiation did not significantly increase lymphedema rates.

Radiotherapy techniques and fractionation
Radiation can be delivered by many techniques including en-face electron therapy, three-dimensional conformal radiotherapy (3D-CRT), intensity-modulated radiotherapy (IMRT) in standard fractionated and hypofractionated regimens, orthovoltage x-ray therapy, and brachytherapy. For superficial melanoma, en-face electrons, orthovoltage x-rays, and brachytherapy techniques can achieve adequate coverage of the target lesion. For deeper infiltrating tumors or lymph nodes, 3D-CRT and IMRT techniques can penetrate to deeper tissues to achieve adequate radiation dose coverage.

Clinical trials comparing conventionally fractionated radiation to hypofractionated radiation regimens (higher dose per fraction in fewer total fractions) demonstrated no significant difference in outcomes.[50–52] Nevertheless, moderately hypofractionated radiotherapy has been used on many trials and has become a widely accepted treatment. Commonly employed radiation dose and fractionation regimens for nodal relapse or in-transit metastases include 30 Gy in five fractions delivered over 2.5 weeks and 55 Gy in 20 fractions delivered daily over 4 weeks.

Palliative radiotherapy
Radiation can be utilized for patients with nodal recurrence or satellitosis/in-transit metastases that have progressed despite systemic therapy in an effort to achieve local control and durable palliation. The choice of local therapy depends on the burden of metastatic disease and performance status. For consideration in treating patients with less favorable prognosis, a nonrandomized prospective study of standard palliative radiation for patients with metastatic melanoma demonstrated a 65% pain relief rate with a duration of response corresponding to 57% of remaining lifetime when adjusted for survival.[52]

Radiotherapy with hyperthermia
For patients with bulky locoregional disease and in-transit metastasis, the addition of hyperthermia can be considered. Hyperthermia is a well-known radiosensitizer and has been shown to improve tumor control in many cancers including melanoma, head and neck, and breast cancer.[53–56] In many treatment-resistant cancers, such as soft-tissue sarcomas, ovarian, gastric, pancreatic cancers, and glioblastoma, hyperthermia also confers an overall survival benefit when added to chemotherapy and/or radiation.[57–61] Two phase III clinical trials support the benefit of hyperthermia to radiation for patients with melanoma.

Overgaard and colleagues randomized 70 patients with 134 recurrent metastatic melanoma lesions to receive radiation with or without hyperthermia.[55] Hyperthermia was prescribed to 43° C for 60 minutes given shortly after each radiation fraction. Patients received 24 to 27 Gy in three fractions. The 2-year local control (LC) rates were significantly improved with hyperthermia (46% vs 28%, $P = .008$). As expected, the higher dose of radiation led to better local control (56% vs 25%, $P = .02$). Notably, patients for whom all known disease was controlled with local therapy had 38% overall survival at 5 years. The addition of hyperthermia did not significantly increase acute or late radiation toxicity.

Jones and colleagues randomized 109 patients with superficial tumors (≤ 3 cm depth) to radiation with or without hyperthermia to examine the primary endpoints of complete response and duration of local control.[56] About 10% of patients had melanoma. The addition of hyperthermia to radiation resulted in a complete response rate of 66.1% compared to 42.3% without hyperthermia, and the odds ratio for complete response was 2.7 (95% CI, 1.2–5.8; $P = .02$). The authors reported the greatest complete response benefit among previously irradiated patients with CR rates of 68.2% versus 24.5% with and without hyperthermia, respectively. There was no overall survival benefit with the addition of hyperthermia.

There are several mechanisms by which therapeutic hyperthermia increases the efficacy of radiotherapy. First, hyperthermia fosters radiosensitivity in hypoxic tumor environments by increasing blood flow and therefore the degree of oxygen-mediated DNA damage fixation.[62] Hyperthermia also facilitates degradation of the DNA damage response protein BRCA2,[63] leading to accumulation of DNA damage and consequently cell death. Additionally, hyperthermia increases the susceptibility of tumor cells in the radioresistant S-phase of the cell cycle to the effects of ionizing radiation.[62] Hyperthermia can also increase the cytotoxicity in radioresistant clones and the radioresistant cancer stem cell population.[64,65] Melanoma is a robustly immunogenic histology, and hyperthermia can also potentiate the immunogenic potential of melanoma.[66–68] Hyperthermia augments the antigen presentation and improves immune cell infiltration into the tumor, enabling a robust antitumor response.[69,70] These data suggest that hyperthermia may complement immune checkpoint inhibitors.

Injectables

Talimogene laherparepvec (TVEC)

Talimogene laherparepvec (TVEC) is perhaps the most widely recognized injectable utilized for in-transit melanoma metastases. In December 2015, TVEC was approved by the Food and Drug Administration (FDA) as the first oncolytic immunotherapy for adults with stages IIIb, IIIc, and IV M1a melanoma without bone, brain, lung, or visceral

disease manifestations. TVEC is derived from the herpes simplex virus type 1 with the neurovirulence factor, the ICP34.5 loci, removed.[71,72] The virus has been modified such that upon lysis, it releases tumor-associated antigens and provides cytokine stimulation by expressing granulocyte macrophage colony-stimulating factor (GM-CSF).[71–73] The combination of tumor destruction, release of tumor antigens, and GM-CSF expression enhances tumor antigen presentation to T cells and stimulates a targeted immune response.[74] TVEC has also shown to increase the levels of circulating and tumor-infiltrating T cells.[75–77] Numerous studies have investigated the safety and efficacy of TVEC.

In 2010, a phase II clinical trial demonstrated a 28% ORR in patients injected with TVEC. A direct oncolytic effect in injected tumors and a secondary immune-mediated antitumor effect on noninjected tumors was observed. This study was the nidus for a prospective, randomized phase III clinical trial in patients with unresectable stages IIIb, IIIc, or IV melanoma,[78] the OPTiM trial. In OPTiM, 436 melanoma patients with stages IIIb, IIIc, or IV were treated with TVEC or GM-CSF alone. In this study, the ORR was higher in the TVEC cohort (26.4% compared to 5.7%). The median OS for the TVEC cohort was improved at 23.3 months compared to 18.9 months, even though this did not reach statistical significance. TVEC was most effective in patients with stages IIIB, IIIC, or IVM1a disease and in patients with treatment-naive disease. The most common adverse events observed with TVEC were fatigue, chills, and pyrexia, and there were no fatal adverse events (AEs).[77] A subgroup analysis focused on the patterns and time course of response to TVEC. Analysis demonstrated that TVEC resulted in a decrease in size by greater than 50% in 64% of injected lesions, 34% of noninjected nonvisceral lesions, and 15% of visceral lesions. There was a complete resolution in 47% of injected lesions, 22% of noninjected nonvisceral lesions, and 9% of visceral lesions.[79] A second subgroup analysis focused on patients with IIIB–IVM1a melanoma. This analysis of 249 patients (57.1% of the original population) derived greater benefit in ORR from TVEC as compared to GM-CSF.[80] In the final planned analysis of OPTiM, the median OS was 23.3 and 18.9 months in the TVEC and GM-CSF cohorts, respectively. The ORR was 31.5% and 6.4%, respectively. Fifty (16.9%) patients and one (0.7%) patient in the TVEC and GM-CSF arms, respectively, achieved a CR. For TVEC patients, the median time to CR was 8.6 months and among patients with a CR, 88.5% were estimated to survive at a 5-year landmark analysis.[81]

Other retrospective studies and small case reports of patients with metastatic melanoma treated with TVEC have supported these positive findings.[82–84]

Talimogene laherparepvec combination therapy

The mechanism of action for TVEC can be complementary to that of checkpoint inhibitor-based tumor immunotherapies. Checkpoint inhibitors include blockade of cytotoxic T-lymphocyte antigen 4 (CTLA-4) or programmed death protein and its ligand (PD-1/PD-L1). Ipilimumab, a human monoclonal antibody against CTLA-4, was approved by the FDA in March 2011 for the treatment of unresectable or metastatic melanoma after a survival benefit was demonstrated in two phase III clinical trials (MDX010-20 and CA184-042).[85,86] CTLA-4 is expressed on the surface of T cells and binding to its ligand on antigen-presenting calls inhibits T-cell activation. Ipilimumab prevents this interaction to augment T-cell responses.[87,88] Pembrolizumab and nivolumab, both of which are human monoclonal antibodies targeting PD-1, were FDA approved in September and December 2014, respectively.[89] PD-1 is a checkpoint inhibitor, that, when engaged by its ligands, dampens T-effector functions by inhibiting downstream signaling.[90] Thus, inhibiting this interaction augments the T-cell response.

TVEC can be complementary to checkpoint inhibitor-based tumor immunotherapies by helping effector T cells overcome negative regulation during priming and in the effector stage. This may be especially pertinent in the control of systemic disease.[75] TVEC contributes to anti-PD-1 immunotherapy by augmenting the inflammatory state of the tumor microenvironment, which allows for increased homing and activation of tumor-reactive T cells whose activity is prolonged by PD-1 blockade.[91,92] Promoting the influx of T cells into the tumor is especially important for patients with low intratumoral T cells that cannot respond adequately to PD-1 blockade.[75] Interestingly, it has been found that after combination treatment with TVEC and PD-1 blockade, there are elevated levels of PD-1-expressing, circulating T cells among complete responders as compared to partial-responders.[93]

In 2016, the results of a multicenter, phase Ib trial of TVEC in combination with ipilimumab were published. The medial duration of TVEC treatment was 13.3 weeks and median follow-up time for survival analysis was 20.0 months. Nineteen patients were included in the safety analysis. Grades 3/4 treatment-related AEs were seen in 26.3% of patients; 15.8% had AEs attributed to TVEC, and 21.1% had AEs attributed to ipilimumab. There were no dose-limiting toxicities. The ORR was 50%, and 18-month OS was 67%. Thus, the combination of TVEC and ipilimumab was found to have a tolerable safety profile and a greater efficacy than TVEC or ipilimumab monotherapy.[94]

In 2018, a phase II clinical trial investigated the combination of TVEC plus ipilimumab compared to ipilimumab monotherapy in patients with unresectable stages IIIB to IV melanoma. Patients were eligible if they had no more than one prior therapy if BRAF wild-type, no more than two prior therapies if BRAF mutant, measurable/injectable disease, and were without symptomatic autoimmunity or clinically significant immunosuppression. Thirty-eight patients (39%) in the combination arm and 18 patients (18%) in the ipilimumab arm had an objective response. Responses were not limited to injected lesions and decreases in visceral lesion were observed in 52% of patients in the combination arm and 23% of patients in the ipilimumab arm. Adverse events included fatigue (combination, 59%; ipilimumab, 42%), chills (combination, 53%; ipilimumab alone, 3%) and diarrhea (combination, 42%; ipilimumab alone, 35%). The incidence of grade 3 or higher AEs was 45% and 35% in the combination and ipilimumab monotherapy cohorts, respectively. Thus, combination therapy was found to have improved antitumor activity without additional safety concerns versus ipilimumab monotherapy.[95]

In 2017, a phase 1b trial, Masterkey-265, analyzed the combination of TVEC with pembrolizumab in 21 patients with advanced melanoma with dermal, subcutaneous, or nodal lesions amenable to intratumoral injection. For these patients, the ORR was 61.9%. In 82% of injected, 43% of noninjected nonvisceral, and 33% of noninjected visceral lesions, the melanoma burden decreased by greater than 50%. Interestingly, TVEC responses were independent of baseline CD8+ infiltration, PD-L1 status, or IFN-gamma signature, but were associated with increased intratumoral inflammation with enhanced CD8+ T-cell infiltration and elevated IFN-gamma gene expression. This suggested that TVEC can alter the tumor microenvironment to encourage T-cell activity in response to PD-1 blockade.[76]

A case series from our institution, published in 2018, of 10 patients with stages IIIC to IVM1b melanoma treated with TVEC plus checkpoint inhibitors (pembrolizumab, ipilimumab/nivolumab, or nivolumab) demonstrated an ORR for on-target lesions of 90%, with six patients experiencing a CR in injected lesions. Two patients had off-target lesions that completely resolved after treatment. Blood samples were tested for the three complete responders and two partial responders. CD4:CD8 ratio and frequencies of circulating PD1+ CD4 and CD8 T cells were elevated in complete responders as compared to partial responders. It was proposed that the higher response rates in this cohort might have been attributable to the patients who received nivolumab or nivolumab plus ipilimumab. In addition, when comparing the results of this study to MASTERKEY-265, the majority of patients in this cohort were started on checkpoint inhibition either before or simultaneously with TVEC injection, whereas MASTERKEY-265 administered pembrolizumab 5 weeks after initiation of TVEC.[96] Studies summarizing investigating Talimogene laherparepvec (TVEC) and combination therapy for melanoma can be found in **Table 2**.

Other injectables

Several other injectables have been investigated for utilization in patients with in-transit melanoma lesions.

PV-10, a sterile, nonpyrogenic 10% solution of rose bengal, causes direct tumor lysis, promotes selective lymphocyte-mediated tumor destruction, and results in a local and systemic antitumor response.[97–100] Research on PV-10 is rather limited to small trials and case series; however, early results are promising. A case series of 19 patients injected with PV-10 demonstrated an ORR of 52% and a CR of 26%.[101] A phase I trial of 11 patients injected with PV-10 demonstrated an ORR of 48%.[102] A study of 45 patients demonstrated a CR of 42%, ORR 87%, and OS of 25 months from first PV-10 treatment.[103] A phase II trial of 80 patients demonstrated an ORR of 51% and a 26% CR. Uninjected lesions demonstrated a 33% ORR. Adverse effects associated with PV-10 were most commonly related to injection site pain, erythema, swelling, and photosensitivity.[104]

Toll-like receptors (TLRs) are a family of pattern recognition receptors that are components of the innate immunity and have the ability to activate the innate and adaptive immune responses.[105] TLRs play a role in cancer development and their agonists have been investigated as a cancer therapy.[106] SD-101 (Dynavax Technologies, Berkeley, CA) is a synthetic TLR9 agonist. In a phase Ib study, patients with unresectable or metastatic melanoma were treated with intratumoral SD-101 and intravenous pembrolizumab.[23] Combination therapy resulted in an ORR of 78% among nine patients who were naive to anti-PD-1 and PD-L1 therapy and an ORR of 15% among 13 patients who had received prior anti-PD-1 and PD-L1 therapy. In patients naive to anti-PD-1/PD-L1 therapy, the 12-month PFS was 88%, and the OS was

89%. The most common AEs were injection-site reactions and transient flu-like symptoms.[107] Tilsotolimod (IMO-2125; Idera Pharmaceuticals, Cambridge, MA) and CMP-001 (Checkmate Pharmaceuticals, Cambridge, MA) are other TLR9 agonists that have been investigated in concert with checkpoint inhibitors in the treatment of melanoma. In a phase I/II study, the combination of tilsotolimod and ipilimumab led to an ORR of 38% in patients with metastatic melanoma refractory to anti-PD-1 therapy.[25]

Coxsackievirus A21 (CAVATAK, Merck & Co., Inc. Kenilworth, NJ) is a naturally occurring, genetically unaltered oncolytic virus which selectively infects tumor cells to result in cell lysis.[108] A phase Ib study evaluated the safety and efficacy of CAVATAK and ipilimumab in patients with treated or untreated unresectable stages IIIC–IVM1c melanoma. Of the 18 patients evaluable for response assessment, the ORR was 50%. The ORR was 60% in patients who were naive to checkpoint inhibitors and 38% in those who had prior checkpoint inhibitor therapy. Responses were observed in both injected and uninjected lesions.[50]

A summary of intralesional therapies under clinical trial can be round in reference.[109] Future studies are needed to further delineate the role that these emerging injectables could play with other systemic or local therapies for in-transit lesions.

Topical Therapy

There has also been investigation into topical options for melanoma in-transit disease. Imiquimod, through activation of immune cells via the toll-like receptor 7 (TLR7)-MyD88-dependent signaling pathway, induces the production of antitumor cytokines including IFN-α, TNF, and IL-12.[110–115] Several neoplasms have been successfully treated with imiquimod including basal cell carcinoma, squamous cell carcinoma, extramammary Paget's disease, lymphoma, and melanoma[113,114,116–124] However, it has been shown that subcutaneous and dermal melanomas are often resistant to imiquimod, likely due to developed resistance to apoptotic pathways, poor drug penetration, or another yet to be identified mechanism.[116,125–130] While it is not recommended as monotherapy, systematic reviews have concluded that imiquimod can lead to locoregional control and may be beneficial for patients in whom conventional therapies have failed.[124,131] Imiquimod was utilized with IL-2 and retinoid therapy in a retrospective case series of 11 patients with cutaneous metastatic melanoma and resulted in a 100% complete local

Table 2
Summary of studies investigating talimogene laherparepvec (TVEC) and combination therapy for melanoma

Intervention	Outcome	Citation
TVEC		
Phase II trial; TVEC only	28% ORR	Christie and Tiver,[44] 1996
Phase III trial; TVEC vs GM-CSF	TVEC improved ORR, OS	Lee et al.,[43] 2011
Phase III trial; TVEC vs GM-CSF; subgroup analysis	TVEC resulted in a decrease in size by ≥ 50% in 64% of injected lesions, 34% of noninjected nonvisceral lesions, and 15% of visceral lesions.	National Comprehensive Cancer Network,[45] 2020
Phase III trial; TVEC vs GM-CSF; subgroup analysis; IIIB–IVM1a melanoma	249 patients (57.1% of the original population) derived greater benefit in ORR from TVEC as compared to GM-CSF	Ang et al.,[46] 1994
TVEC plus ipilimumab		
Phase Ib trial; TVEC plus ipilimumab	ORR was 50% and 18-month OS was 67%	van der Horst et al.,[60] 2018
Phase II trial; TVEC plus ipilimumab vs ipilimumab	Combination therapy improved objective response. Responses not limited to injected lesions	Sneed et al.,[61] 1998
TVEC plus pembrolizumab		
Phase Ib trial; TVEC plus pembrolizumab	61.9% ORR	Tsang et al.,[42] 1994
TVEC plus checkpoint inhibitor		
Case series	90% ORR	Hall,[62] 2019

Abbreviations: ORR, overall response rate; OS, overall survival.

response at an average of 24 months.[132] Another topical therapy option, diphencyprone (DPCP), a contact sensitizer which induces contact hypersensitivity, was used in a case series of 50 patients with in-transit melanoma for at least 1 month and led to complete clearance of cutaneous disease in 46% and a partial response in a further 38%.[133–135] Thus, while research on topical therapies is somewhat limited, consideration to topical treatment could be given for patients who have failed conventional therapies.

SUMMARY

The treatment paradigm for in-transit melanoma metastases continues to evolve with the development of newer injectables and combination therapies. While the ideal treatment protocol has yet to be determined, advances continue to improve response rates and survival. Further research must be performed to determine the most efficacious therapy that offers an acceptable toxicity profile. Multicenter trials will be required to answer the numerous questions that remain in the treatment of in-transit metastases.

CLINICS CARE POINTS

- There have been numerous recent advances in the medical management of melanoma in-transit metastases and the treatment paradigm continues to evolve.

- Numerous clinical trials are currently ongoing investigating new therapeutic options and combination therapy for patients with in-transit metastases

- Patients with in-transit metastases should be treated in a multidisciplinary setting in order to consider appropriately all surgical and medical options.

REFERENCES

1. Gershenwald JE, Scolyer RA, Hess KR, et al. Melanoma staging: evidence-based changes in the American Joint Committee on Cancer eighth edition cancer staging manual. CA Cancer J Clin 2017;67(6):472–92.
2. Borgstein PJ, Meijer S, van Diest PJ. Are locoregional cutaneous metastases in melanoma predictable? Ann Surg Oncol 1999;6(3):315–21.
3. Pawlik TM, Ross MI, Johnson MM, et al. Predictors and natural history of in-transit melanoma after sentinel lymphadenectomy. Ann Surg Oncol 2005; 12(8):587–96.
4. Gabriel E, Skitzki J. The role of regional therapies for in-transit melanoma in the era of improved systemic options. Cancers (Basel) 2015;7(3):1154–77.
5. Creech O Jr, Krementz ET, Ryan RF, et al. Chemotherapy of cancer: regional perfusion utilizing an extracorporeal circuit. Ann Surg 1958;148(4): 616–32.
6. Madu MF, Deken MM, van der Hage JA, et al. Isolated limb perfusion for melanoma is safe and effective in elderly patients. Ann Surg Oncol 2017;24(7):1997–2005.
7. Nieweg OE, Kroon BB. Isolated limb perfusion with melphalan for melanoma. J Surg Oncol 2014; 109(4):332–7.
8. Grunhagen DJ, Kroon HM, Verhoef C. Perfusion and infusion for melanoma in-transit metastases in the era of effective systemic therapy. Am Soc Clin Oncol Educ Book 2015;e528–34.
9. Thompson JF, Gianoutsos MP. Isolated limb perfusion for melanoma: effectiveness and toxicity of cisplatin compared with that of melphalan and other drugs. World J Surg 1992;16(2):227–33.
10. Sanki A, Kam PC, Thompson JF. Long-term results of hyperthermic, isolated limb perfusion for melanoma: a reflection of tumor biology. Ann Surg 2007;245(4):591–6.
11. Cornett WR, McCall LM, Petersen RP, et al. Randomized multicenter trial of hyperthermic isolated limb perfusion with melphalan alone compared with melphalan plus tumor necrosis factor: American College of Surgeons Oncology Group Trial Z0020. J Clin Oncol 2006;24(25):4196–201.
12. Rossi CR, Pasquali S, Mocellin S, et al. Long-term results of melphalan-based isolated limb perfusion with or without low-dose TNF for in-transit melanoma metastases. Ann Surg Oncol 2010;17(11): 3000–7.
13. Hoekstra HJ, Veerman K, van Ginkel RJ. Isolated limb perfusion for in-transit melanoma metastases: melphalan or TNF-melphalan perfusion? J Surg Oncol 2014;109(4):338–47.
14. Di Filippo F, Giacomini P, Rossi CR, et al. Prognostic factors influencing tumor response, locoregional control and survival, in melanoma patients with multiple limb in-transit metastases treated with TNFalpha-based isolated limb perfusion. In Vivo 2009;23(2):347–52.
15. Deroose JP, Grunhagen DJ, van Geel AN, et al. Long-term outcome of isolated limb perfusion with tumour necrosis factor-alpha for patients with melanoma in-transit metastases. Br J Surg 2011; 98(11):1573–80.
16. Olofsson R, Mattsson J, Lindner P. Long-term follow-up of 163 consecutive patients treated with isolated limb perfusion for in-transit metastases of malignant melanoma. Int J Hyperthermia 2013; 29(6):551–7.
17. Moreno-Ramirez D, de la Cruz-Merino L, Ferrandiz L, et al. Isolated limb perfusion for malignant melanoma: systematic review on effectiveness and safety. Oncologist 2010;15(4):416–27.
18. Lienard D, Eggermont AM, Koops HS, et al. Isolated limb perfusion with tumour necrosis factor-alpha and melphalan with or without interferon-gamma for the treatment of in-transit melanoma metastases: a multicentre randomized phase II study. Melanoma Res 1999;9(5):491–502.
19. Deroose JP, Eggermont AM, van Geel AN, et al. 20 years experience of TNF-based isolated limb perfusion for in-transit melanoma metastases: TNF dose matters. Ann Surg Oncol 2012;19(2): 627–35.
20. Kroon HM, Coventry BJ, Giles MH, et al. Australian multicenter study of isolated limb infusion for melanoma. Ann Surg Oncol 2016;23(4):1096–103.
21. Noorda EM, Vrouenraets BC, Nieweg OE, et al. Isolated limb perfusion for unresectable melanoma of the extremities. Arch Surg 2004;139(11):1237–42.
22. Olofsson Bagge R, Mattsson J, Hafstrom L. Regional hyperthermic perfusion with melphalan after surgery for recurrent malignant melanoma of the extremities–long-term follow-up of a randomised trial. Int J Hyperthermia 2014;30(5):295–8.
23. Deroose JP, Grunhagen DJ, Eggermont AM, et al. Repeated isolated limb perfusion in melanoma patients with recurrent in-transit metastases. Melanoma Res 2015;25(5):427–31.
24. Noorda EM, Vrouenraets BC, Nieweg OE, et al. Repeat isolated limb perfusion with TNFalpha and melphalan for recurrent limb melanoma after failure of previous perfusion. Eur J Surg Oncol 2006;32(3): 318–24.
25. Grunhagen DJ, van Etten B, Brunstein F, et al. Efficacy of repeat isolated limb perfusions with tumor necrosis factor alpha and melphalan for multiple in-transit metastases in patients with prior isolated limb perfusion failure. Ann Surg Oncol 2005; 12(8):609–15.
26. Thompson JF, Kam PC, Waugh RC, et al. Isolated limb infusion with cytotoxic agents: a simple

alternative to isolated limb perfusion. Semin Surg Oncol 1998;14(3):238–47.

27. O'Donoghue C, Perez MC, Mullinax JE, et al. Isolated limb infusion: a single-center experience with over 200 infusions. Ann Surg Oncol 2017; 24(13):3842–9.

28. Beasley GM, Petersen RP, Yoo J, et al. Isolated limb infusion for in-transit malignant melanoma of the extremity: a well-tolerated but less effective alternative to hyperthermic isolated limb perfusion. Ann Surg Oncol 2008;15(8):2195–205.

29. Brady MS, Brown K, Patel A, et al. Isolated limb infusion with melphalan and dactinomycin for regional melanoma and soft-tissue sarcoma of the extremity: final report of a phase II clinical trial. Melanoma Res 2009;19(2):106–11.

30. Steinman J, Ariyan C, Rafferty B, et al. Factors associated with response, survival, and limb salvage in patients undergoing isolated limb infusion. J Surg Oncol 2014;109(5):405–9.

31. Miura JT, Kroon HM, Beasley GM, et al. Long-term oncologic outcomes after isolated limb infusion for locoregionally metastatic melanoma: an international multicenter analysis. Ann Surg Oncol 2019; 26(8):2486–94.

32. Grunhagen DJ, Brunstein F, Graveland WJ, et al. One hundred consecutive isolated limb perfusions with TNF-alpha and melphalan in melanoma patients with multiple in-transit metastases. Ann Surg 2004;240(6):939–47 [discussion: 947–8].

33. Lindner P, Thompson JF, De Wilt JH, et al. Double isolated limb infusion with cytotoxic agents for recurrent and metastatic limb melanoma. Eur J Surg Oncol 2004;30(4):433–9.

34. Kroon HM, Lin DY, Kam PC, et al. Efficacy of repeat isolated limb infusion with melphalan and actinomycin D for recurrent melanoma. Cancer 2009; 115(9):1932–40.

35. Raymond AK, Beasley GM, Broadwater G, et al. Current trends in regional therapy for melanoma: lessons learned from 225 regional chemotherapy treatments between 1995 and 2010 at a single institution. J Am Coll Surg 2011;213(2):306–16.

36. Dossett LA, Ben-Shabat I, Olofsson Bagge R, et al. Clinical response and regional toxicity following isolated limb infusion compared with isolated limb perfusion for in-transit melanoma. Ann Surg Oncol 2016;23(7):2330–5.

37. Harwood AR. Conventional fractionated radiotherapy for 51 patients with lentigo maligna and lentigo maligna melanoma. Int J Radiat Oncol Biol Phys 1983;9(7):1019–21.

38. Farshad A, Burg G, Panizzon R, et al. A retrospective study of 150 patients with lentigo maligna and lentigo maligna melanoma and the efficacy of radiotherapy using Grenz or soft X-rays. Br J Dermatol 2002;146(6):1042–6.

39. Hedblad MA, Mallbris L. Grenz ray treatment of lentigo maligna and early lentigo maligna melanoma. J Am Acad Dermatol 2012;67(1):60–8.

40. Fogarty GB, Hong A, Scolyer RA, et al. Radiotherapy for lentigo maligna: a literature review and recommendations for treatment. Br J Dermatol 2014;170(1):52–8.

41. Schmid-Wendtner MH, Brunner B, Konz B, et al. Fractionated radiotherapy of lentigo maligna and lentigo maligna melanoma in 64 patients. J Am Acad Dermatol 2000;43(3):477–82.

42. Tsang RW, Liu FF, Wells W, et al. Lentigo maligna of the head and neck. Results of treatment by radiotherapy. Arch Dermatol 1994;130(8):1008–12.

43. Lee H, Sowerby LJ, Temple CL, et al. Carbon dioxide laser treatment for lentigo maligna: a retrospective review comparing 3 different treatment modalities. Arch Facial Plast Surg 2011;13(6): 398–403.

44. Christie DR, Tiver KW. Radiotherapy for melanotic freckles. Australas Radiol 1996;40(3):331–3.

45. National Comprehensive Cancer Network. Cutaneous Melanoma (Version 3.2020). 2020. 8/21/2020. Available at: https://www.nccn.org/professionals/physician_gls/pdf/cutaneous_melanoma.pdf.

46. Ang KK, Peters LJ, Weber RS, et al. Postoperative radiotherapy for cutaneous melanoma of the head and neck region. Int J Radiat Oncol Biol Phys 1994;30(4):795–8.

47. Ballo MT, Bonnen MD, Garden AS, et al. Adjuvant irradiation for cervical lymph node metastases from melanoma. Cancer 2003;97(7):1789–96.

48. Burmeister BH, Mark Smithers B, Burmeister E, et al. A prospective phase II study of adjuvant postoperative radiation therapy following nodal surgery in malignant melanoma-Trans Tasman Radiation Oncology Group (TROG) Study 96.06. Radiother Oncol 2006;81(2):136–42.

49. Henderson MA, Burmeister BH, Ainslie J, et al. Adjuvant lymph-node field radiotherapy versus observation only in patients with melanoma at high risk of further lymph-node field relapse after lymphadenectomy (ANZMTG 01.02/TROG 02.01): 6-year follow-up of a phase 3, randomised controlled trial. Lancet Oncol 2015;16(9):1049–60.

50. Konefal JB, Emami B, Pilepich MV. Analysis of dose fractionation in the palliation of metastases from malignant melanoma. Cancer 1988;61(2):243–6.

51. Chang DT, Amdur RJ, Morris CG, et al. Adjuvant radiotherapy for cutaneous melanoma: comparing hypofractionation to conventional fractionation. Int J Radiat Oncol Biol Phys 2006;66(4):1051–5.

52. Huguenin PU, Kieser S, Glanzmann C, et al. Radiotherapy for metastatic carcinomas of the kidney or melanomas: an analysis using palliative end points. Int J Radiat Oncol Biol Phys 1998;41(2):401–5.

53. Datta NR, Puric E, Klingbiel D, et al. Hyperthermia and radiation therapy in locoregional recurrent breast cancers: a systematic review and meta-analysis. Int J Radiat Oncol Biol Phys 2016;94(5): 1073–87.

54. Datta NR, Rogers S, Ordóñez SG, et al. Hyperthermia and radiotherapy in the management of head and neck cancers: a systematic review and meta-analysis. Int J Hyperthermia 2016;32(1):31–40.

55. Overgaard J, Gonzalez Gonzalez D, Hulshof MC, et al. Randomised trial of hyperthermia as adjuvant to radiotherapy for recurrent or metastatic malignant melanoma. European Society for Hyperthermic Oncology. Lancet 1995;345(8949):540–3.

56. Jones EL, Oleson JR, Prosnitz LR, et al. Randomized trial of hyperthermia and radiation for superficial tumors. J Clin Oncol 2005;23(13):3079–85.

57. Issels RD, Lindner LH, Verweij J, et al. Effect of neoadjuvant chemotherapy plus regional hyperthermia on long-term outcomes among patients with localized high-risk soft tissue sarcoma: the EORTC 62961-ESHO 95 randomized clinical trial. JAMA Oncol 2018;4(4):483–92.

58. van Driel WJ, Koole SN, Sikorska K, et al. Hyperthermic intraperitoneal chemotherapy in ovarian cancer. N Engl J Med 2018;378(3):230–40.

59. Yang XJ, Huang CQ, Suo T, et al. Cytoreductive surgery and hyperthermic intraperitoneal chemotherapy improves survival of patients with peritoneal carcinomatosis from gastric cancer: final results of a phase III randomized clinical trial. Ann Surg Oncol 2011;18(6):1575–81.

60. van der Horst A, Versteijne E, Besselink MGH, et al. The clinical benefit of hyperthermia in pancreatic cancer: a systematic review. Int J Hyperthermia 2018;34(7):969–79.

61. Sneed PK, Stauffer PR, McDermott MW, et al. Survival benefit of hyperthermia in a prospective randomized trial of brachytherapy boost +/- hyperthermia for glioblastoma multiforme. Int J Radiat Oncol Biol Phys 1998;40(2):287–95.

62. Hall EJ, GA. Radiobiology for the radiologist. 8th edition. Philadelphia: Wolters Kluwer; 2019.

63. Krawczyk PM, Eppink B, Essers J, et al. Mild hyperthermia inhibits homologous recombination, induces BRCA2 degradation, and sensitizes cancer cells to poly (ADP-ribose) polymerase-1 inhibition. Proc Natl Acad Sci U S A 2011;108(24):9851–6.

64. Man J, Shoemake JD, Ma T, et al. Hyperthermia sensitizes glioma stem-like cells to radiation by inhibiting AKT signaling. Cancer Res 2015;75(8): 1760–9.

65. Atkinson RL, Zhang M, Diagaradjane P, et al. Thermal enhancement with optically activated gold nanoshells sensitizes breast cancer stem cells to radiation therapy. Sci Transl Med 2010;2(55): 55ra79.

66. Werthmöller N, Frey B, Rückert M, et al. Combination of ionising radiation with hyperthermia increases the immunogenic potential of B16-F10 melanoma cells in vitro and in vivo. Int J Hyperthermia 2016;32(1):23–30.

67. Vatner RE, Cooper BT, Vanpouille-Box C, et al. Combinations of immunotherapy and radiation in cancer therapy. Front Oncol 2014;4:325.

68. Schildkopf P, Frey B, Ott OJ, et al. Radiation combined with hyperthermia induces HSP70-dependent maturation of dendritic cells and release of pro-inflammatory cytokines by dendritic cells and macrophages. Radiother Oncol 2011;101(1): 109–15.

69. Repasky EA, Evans SS, Dewhirst MW. Temperature matters! And why it should matter to tumor immunologists. Cancer Immunol Res 2013;1(4):210–6.

70. Chu KF, Dupuy DE. Thermal ablation of tumours: biological mechanisms and advances in therapy. Nat Rev Cancer 2014;14(3):199–208.

71. Kohlhapp FJ, Kaufman HL. Molecular pathways: mechanism of action for talimogene laherparepvec, a new oncolytic virus immunotherapy. Clin Cancer Res 2016;22(5):1048–54.

72. Hercus TR, Thomas D, Guthridge MA, et al. The granulocyte-macrophage colony-stimulating factor receptor: linking its structure to cell signaling and its role in disease. Blood 2009;114(7):1289–98.

73. Agarwala SS. Intralesional therapy for advanced melanoma: promise and limitation. Curr Opin Oncol 2015;27(2):151–6.

74. Hoeller C, Michielin O, Ascierto PA, et al. Systematic review of the use of granulocyte-macrophage colony-stimulating factor in patients with advanced melanoma. Cancer Immunol Immunother 2016; 65(9):1015–34.

75. Dummer R, Hoeller C, Gruter IP, et al. Combining talimogene laherparepvec with immunotherapies in melanoma and other solid tumors. Cancer Immunol Immunother 2017;66(6):683–95.

76. Ribas A, Dummer R, Puzanov I, et al. Oncolytic virotherapy promotes intratumoral T cell infiltration and improves anti-PD-1 immunotherapy. Cell 2017;170(6):1109–19.e10.

77. Andtbacka RH, Kaufman HL, Collichio F, et al. Talimogene laherparepvec improves durable response rate in patients with advanced melanoma. J Clin Oncol 2015;33(25):2780–8.

78. Kaufman HL, Bines SD. OPTIM trial: a Phase III trial of an oncolytic herpes virus encoding GM-CSF for unresectable stage III or IV melanoma. Future Oncol 2010;6(6):941–9.

79. Andtbacka RH, Ross M, Puzanov I, et al. Patterns of clinical response with talimogene laherparepvec (T-VEC) in patients with melanoma treated in the OPTiM phase III clinical trial. Ann Surg Oncol 2016;23(13):4169–77.

80. Harrington KJ, Andtbacka RH, Collichio F, et al. Efficacy and safety of talimogene laherparepvec versus granulocyte-macrophage colony-stimulating factor in patients with stage IIIB/C and IVM1a melanoma: subanalysis of the Phase III OPTiM trial. Onco Targets Ther 2016;9:7081–93.

81. Andtbacka RHI, Collichio F, Harrington KJ, et al. Final analyses of OPTiM: a randomized phase III trial of talimogene laherparepvec versus granulocyte-macrophage colony-stimulating factor in unresectable stage III-IV melanoma. J Immunother Cancer 2019;7(1):145.

82. Zhou AY, Wang DY, McKee S, et al. Correlates of response and outcomes with talimogene laherperpvec. J Surg Oncol 2019;120(3):558–64.

83. Blackmon JT, Stratton MS, Kwak Y, et al. Inflammatory melanoma in transit metastases with complete response to talimogene laherparepvec. JAAD Case Rep 2017;3(4):280–3.

84. Perez MC, Miura JT, Naqvi SMH, et al. Talimogene Laherparepvec (TVEC) for the treatment of advanced melanoma: a single-institution experience. Ann Surg Oncol 2018;25(13):3960–5.

85. Wolchok JD, Neyns B, Linette G, et al. Ipilimumab monotherapy in patients with pretreated advanced melanoma: a randomised, double-blind, multicentre, phase 2, dose-ranging study. Lancet Oncol 2010;11(2):155–64.

86. Hodi FS, O'Day SJ, McDermott DF, et al. Improved survival with ipilimumab in patients with metastatic melanoma. N Engl J Med 2010;363(8):711–23.

87. Callahan MK, Wolchok JD. At the bedside: CTLA-4- and PD-1-blocking antibodies in cancer immunotherapy. J Leukoc Biol 2013;94(1):41–53.

88. Walker LS, Sansom DM. The emerging role of CTLA4 as a cell-extrinsic regulator of T cell responses. Nat Rev Immunol 2011;11(12):852–63.

89. Ribas A, Hamid O, Daud A, et al. Association of pembrolizumab with tumor response and survival among patients with advanced melanoma. JAMA 2016;315(15):1600–9.

90. Topalian SL, Drake CG, Pardoll DM. Targeting the PD-1/B7-H1(PD-L1) pathway to activate anti-tumor immunity. Curr Opin Immunol 2012;24(2):207–12.

91. Orloff M. Spotlight on talimogene laherparepvec for the treatment of melanoma lesions in the skin and lymph nodes. Oncolytic Virother 2016;5:91–8.

92. Liu Z, Ravindranathan R, Kalinski P, et al. Rational combination of oncolytic vaccinia virus and PD-L1 blockade works synergistically to enhance therapeutic efficacy. Nat Commun 2017;8:14754.

93. Gros A, Parkhurst MR, Tran E, et al. Prospective identification of neoantigen-specific lymphocytes in the peripheral blood of melanoma patients. Nat Med 2016;22(4):433–8.

94. Puzanov I, Milhem MM, Minor D, et al. Talimogene laherparepvec in combination with ipilimumab in previously untreated, unresectable stage IIIB-IV melanoma. J Clin Oncol 2016;34(22):2619–26.

95. Chesney J, Puzanov I, Collichio F, et al. Randomized, open-label phase II study evaluating the efficacy and safety of talimogene laherparepvec in combination with ipilimumab versus ipilimumab alone in patients with advanced, unresectable melanoma. J Clin Oncol 2018;36(17):1658–67.

96. Sun L, Funchain P, Song JM, et al. Talimogene Laherparepvec combined with anti-PD-1 based immunotherapy for unresectable stage III-IV melanoma: a case series. J Immunother Cancer 2018; 6(1):36.

97. Toomey P, Kodumudi K, Weber A, et al. Intralesional injection of rose bengal induces a systemic tumor-specific immune response in murine models of melanoma and breast cancer. PLoS One 2013; 8(7):e68561.

98. Maker AV, Prabhakar B, Pardiwala K. The potential of intralesional rose bengal to stimulate T-cell mediated anti-tumor responses. J Clin Cell Immunol 2015;6(4).

99. Liu H, Innamarato PP, Kodumudi K, et al. Intralesional rose bengal in melanoma elicits tumor immunity via activation of dendritic cells by the release of high mobility group box 1. Oncotarget 2016;7(25): 37893–905.

100. Qin J, Kunda N, Qiao G, et al. Colon cancer cell treatment with rose bengal generates a protective immune response via immunogenic cell death. Cell Death Dis 2017;8(2):e2584.

101. Lippey J, Bousounis R, Behrenbruch C, et al. Intralesional PV-10 for in-transit melanoma-A single-center experience. J Surg Oncol 2016;114(3): 380–4.

102. Thompson JF, Hersey P, Wachter E. Chemoablation of metastatic melanoma using intralesional Rose Bengal. Melanoma Res 2008;18(6):405–11.

103. Read TA, Smith A, Thomas J, et al. Intralesional PV-10 for the treatment of in-transit melanoma metastases-Results of a prospective, non-randomized, single center study. J Surg Oncol 2018;117(4): 579–87.

104. Thompson JF, Agarwala SS, Smithers BM, et al. Phase 2 study of intralesional PV-10 in refractory metastatic melanoma. Ann Surg Oncol 2015; 22(7):2135–42.

105. Takeda K, Kaisho T, Akira S. Toll-like receptors. Annu Rev Immunol 2003;21:335–76.

106. Shi M, Chen X, Ye K, et al. Application potential of toll-like receptors in cancer immunotherapy: systematic review. Medicine (Baltimore) 2016;95(25): e3951.

107. Ribas A, Medina T, Kummar S, et al. SD-101 in combination with pembrolizumab in advanced melanoma: results of a phase Ib, multicenter study. Cancer Discov 2018;8(10):1250–7.

108. Xiao C, Bator-Kelly CM, Rieder E, et al. The crystal structure of coxsackievirus A21 and its interaction with ICAM-1. Structure 2005;13(7):1019–33.

109. Hamid O, Ismail R, Puzanov I. Intratumoral immunotherapy-update 2019. Oncologist 2020;25(3): e423–38.

110. Hemmi H, Kaisho T, Takeuchi O, et al. Small antiviral compounds activate immune cells via the TLR7 MyD88-dependent signaling pathway. Nat Immunol 2002;3(2):196–200.

111. Gorden KB, Gorski KS, Gibson SJ, et al. Synthetic TLR agonists reveal functional differences between human TLR7 and TLR8. J Immunol 2005;174(3): 1259–68.

112. O'Neill LA, Golenbock D, Bowie AG. The history of Toll-like receptors - redefining innate immunity. Nat Rev Immunol 2013;13(6):453–60.

113. Beutner KR, Geisse JK, Helman D, et al. Therapeutic response of basal cell carcinoma to the immune response modifier imiquimod 5% cream. J Am Acad Dermatol 1999;41(6):1002–7.

114. Mackenzie-Wood A, Kossard S, de Launey J, et al. Imiquimod 5% cream in the treatment of Bowen's disease. J Am Acad Dermatol 2001;44(3):462–70.

115. Edwards L, Ferenczy A, Eron L, et al. Self-administered topical 5% imiquimod cream for external anogenital warts. HPV Study Group. Human PapillomaVirus. Arch Dermatol 1998;134(1):25–30.

116. Green DS, Bodman-Smith MD, Dalgleish AG, et al. Phase I/II study of topical imiquimod and intralesional interleukin-2 in the treatment of accessible metastases in malignant melanoma. Br J Dermatol 2007;156(2):337–45.

117. Suchin KR, Junkins-Hopkins JM, Rook AH. Treatment of stage IA cutaneous T-Cell lymphoma with topical application of the immune response modifier imiquimod. Arch Dermatol 2002;138(9):1137–9.

118. Deeths MJ, Chapman JT, Dellavalle RP, et al. Treatment of patch and plaque stage mycosis fungoides with imiquimod 5% cream. J Am Acad Dermatol 2005;52(2):275–80.

119. Zampogna JC, Flowers FP, Roth WI, et al. Treatment of primary limited cutaneous extramammary Paget's disease with topical imiquimod monotherapy: two case reports. J Am Acad Dermatol 2002;47(4 Suppl):S229–35.

120. Ahmed I, Berth-Jones J. Imiquimod: a novel treatment for lentigo maligna. Br J Dermatol 2000; 143(4):843–5.

121. Steinmann A, Funk JO, Schuler G, et al. Topical imiquimod treatment of a cutaneous melanoma metastasis. J Am Acad Dermatol 2000;43(3): 555–6.

122. Naylor MF, Crowson N, Kuwahara R, et al. Treatment of lentigo maligna with topical imiquimod. Br J Dermatol 2003;149(Suppl 66):66–70.

123. Bong AB, Bonnekoh B, Franke I, et al. Imiquimod, a topical immune response modifier, in the treatment of cutaneous metastases of malignant melanoma. Dermatology 2002;205(2):135–8.

124. Scarfi F, Patrizi A, Veronesi G, et al. The role of topical imiquimod in melanoma cutaneous metastases: a critical review of the literature. Dermatol Ther 2020;e14165.

125. Turza K, Dengel LT, Harris RC, et al. Effectiveness of imiquimod limited to dermal melanoma metastases, with simultaneous resistance of subcutaneous metastasis. J Cutan Pathol 2010;37(1):94–8.

126. Schon MP, Wienrich BG, Drewniok C, et al. Death receptor-independent apoptosis in malignant melanoma induced by the small-molecule immune response modifier imiquimod. J Invest Dermatol 2004;122(5):1266–76.

127. Suzuki H, Wang B, Shivji GM, et al. Imiquimod, a topical immune response modifier, induces migration of Langerhans cells. J Invest Dermatol 2000; 114(1):135–41.

128. Burns RP Jr, Ferbel B, Tomai M, et al. The imidazoquinolines, imiquimod and R-848, induce functional, but not phenotypic, maturation of human epidermal Langerhans' cells. Clin Immunol 2000; 94(1):13–23.

129. Gibson SJ, Lindh JM, Riter TR, et al. Plasmacytoid dendritic cells produce cytokines and mature in response to the TLR7 agonists, imiquimod and resiquimod. Cell Immunol 2002;218(1-2):74–86.

130. Dusza SW, Delgado R, Busam KJ, et al. Treatment of dysplastic nevi with 5% imiquimod cream, a pilot study. J Drugs Dermatol 2006;5(1):56–62.

131. Sisti A, Sisti G, Oranges CM. Topical treatment of melanoma skin metastases with imiquimod: a review. Dermatol Online J 2014;21(2).

132. Shi VY, Tran K, Patel F, et al. 100% Complete response rate in patients with cutaneous metastatic melanoma treated with intralesional interleukin (IL)-2, imiquimod, and topical retinoid combination therapy: results of a case series. J Am Acad Dermatol 2015;73(4):645–54.

133. Damian DL, Saw RP, Thompson JF. Topical immunotherapy with diphencyprone for in transit and cutaneously metastatic melanoma. J Surg Oncol 2014;109(4):308–13.

134. van der Steen PH, Happle R. Topical immunotherapy of alopecia areata. Dermatol Clin 1993; 11(3):619–22.

135. Buckley DA, Du Vivier AW. The therapeutic use of topical contact sensitizers in benign dermatoses. Br J Dermatol 2001;145(3):385–405.

Radiation Therapy for Local Cutaneous Melanoma

Parinaz J. Dabestani, BS[a], Amanda J. Dawson, MD[b],*,
Michael W. Neumeister, MD[c], C. Matthew Bradbury, MD, PhD[d]

KEYWORDS

- Cutaneous melanoma • Radiation • Lentigo maligna • Adjuvant radiotherapy
- Definitive radiotherapy

KEY POINTS

- Definitive radiotherapy can be used in cases of primary melanoma in situ and lentigo maligna type when surgical resection is not feasible.
- Adjuvant radiation therapy has a role in improving locoregional control for high-risk tumor recurrence.
- Radiation is generally well tolerated; however, long-term effects of radiation, particularly cutaneous manifestation and lymphedema, remain a concern for this treatment modality.

INTRODUCTION

Radiation therapy is a commonly used modality for treatment of cancer. Distinct from other local (ie, surgical) treatments or systemic (ie, biological or chemotherapy) treatments, radiation therapy is directed toward a specific body site that harbors gross or microscopic disease, and exerts its effects through ionization events in tumor cells, which results in the production of free radicals, DNA damage, and preferential tumor cell killing.[1] To achieve this tumoricidal effect, radiation therapy is delivered in a fractionated schema, where serial treatments are delivered over multiple sessions to complete a prescribed course.

A clear role of radiation therapy in the treatment of primary melanoma has not been well defined. This is due, in part, to preclinical studies in human cell lines that suggested melanoma was intrinsically radioresistant, or needed a higher dose per fraction radiotherapy to produce a response.[2–5] In more modern clinical situations, the paucity of phase III clinical studies characterizing the use of radiation therapy for primary melanoma represents a challenge for oncologists seeking to form treatment plans.

Among the treatment intents associated with radiation therapy are definitive, adjuvant, and palliative. The goal of this chapter is to elucidate an evidence basis for the use of radiation therapy in the treatment of primary cutaneous melanoma. Due to this chapter's focus on primary cutaneous melanoma, emphasis will be place on definitive and adjuvant radiotherapy approaches to local disease. Mucosal and uveal melanoma, elective regional lymph node therapy, and palliative treatment for metastasis, are beyond the scope of this chapter.

Radiation Delivery, Dose, and Fractionation

As opposed to normal somatic tissues, cancer cells lack much of the cellular machinery to repair certain types of damage induced by ionizing radiation. Delivery of radiation therapy in fractionated doses allows normal human cells to repair

[a] Creighton University School of Medicine, 2500 California Plaza, Omaha, NE 68178, USA; [b] 717 N. 190th Plaza, Suite 2200, Omaha, NE 68022, USA; [c] Southern Illinois University School of Medicine, Institute for Plastic Surgery, 747 N. Rutledge St #3, Springfield, IL 62702, USA; [d] Springfield Clinic Cancer Center and Southern Illinois University School of Medicine, 900 N. 1st Street, Springfield, IL 62702, USA
* Corresponding author.
E-mail address: Amanda.Dawson@nmhs.org

Clin Plastic Surg 48 (2021) 643–649
https://doi.org/10.1016/j.cps.2021.05.008

themselves, while tumor cells do not.[1] Fundamentally, it is the exploitation of these radiobiological differences between normal cells and tumor cells that permits radiation therapy to be delivered safely and effectively.

In the past, radiation therapy in the form of low energy x-rays (eg, Grenz rays) and higher energy orthovoltage x-rays was used in the management of primary cutaneous melanoma. In such circumstances, considerations for the penetration of radiation therapy into the dermis are important, as low-voltage, superficial radiotherapy may not penetrate sufficiently deep. In order to effectively treat below hair follicles, which have been shown to extend a median of 1.5 mm below the skin surface, it has been suggested that radiation therapy must penetrate 5 mm below the skin surface.[6] At present, national treatment guidelines conclude that there are insufficient data to support routine use of electronic surface brachytherapy in the management of cutaneous melanoma.[7]

Following broader availability of linear accelerators, electron beam therapy approaches were used. More recently, intensity-modulated radiation therapy using megavoltage photons and image guidance allows sculpting of radiation delivery to complex treatment volumes.[8] Each of these techniques has distinct roles defined by the evolution of technology and understanding of melanoma biology.

In the middle of the last century, Miescher and colleagues[9] were among the pioneers researching radiation therapy for melanoma. Radiobiological studies showed wide initial shoulders on cell survival curves, which suggest benefit with treatment using higher fractionation.[3] Subsequent in vitro studies have shown that multiple melanoma subtypes are susceptible to radiation through exploitation of radiobiological features.[10–12]

Because of the previous biological data showing the radioresistance of melanoma, it was thought that decreasing the number of fractions and using a higher dose per fraction, a concept known as hypofractionation, may result in greater tumor response in patients. A retrospective review in 114 patients with 204 malignant melanoma lesions showed that a higher dose per fraction (ie, > 4 Gy vs < 4 Gy) showed a 57% complete response compared to a 24% complete response with a lower dose per fraction. Though higher doses per fraction showed better response in this study, total cumulative dose and treatment time did not show any correlation with tumor response.[13]

Another study of melanoma among a series of 121 patients with 239 recurrent or metastatic malignant melanomas found that the cells exhibited characteristics of late-responding normal tissue.

Through radiobiological modeling, the authors suggested that about 6 Gy per fraction - based on their multifraction linear-quadratic model - would be effective for malignant melanoma.[14]

Additionally, a multi-institutional phase III randomized clinical trial by the Radiation Therapy Oncology Group (RTOG) for patients with metastatic melanoma[15] demonstrated that radiation therapy in higher dose per fraction radiotherapy (ie, 8 Gy/fraction × 4 weekly fractions) did not produce superior outcomes when compared to lower fraction radiation treatment (ie, 2.5 Gy/fraction × 20 daily fractions). The study did show, however, that complete or partial remission was seen in approximately 24% and 35% of patients, respectively, supporting the use of radiation therapy for melanoma.

Recent clinical data appear to support the notion of hypofractionated radiation therapy in the management of cutaneous melanoma. Ang and colleagues[16] described their experience of 174 patients who received postoperative radiation therapy following wide local excision or regional nodal dissection, and were assessed to have a 50% risk of locoregional recurrence based on historical experience. Radiation therapy was 6 Gy/fraction × 5 fractions over 2.5 weeks; actuarial 5-year locoregional control was 88% and survival was 47%. Furthermore, acute and late side effects were relatively rare. These data represent an improvement over expected historical outcomes and support the use of hypofractionated radiation therapy as adjuvant management of melanoma.

Definitive Radiotherapy

Patients with melanoma may experience local recurrence, in-transit metastasis, regional nodal involvement, and distant spread.[8] Due in part to the perception of melanoma's resistance to radiation therapy as well as the combined diagnostic and therapeutic capability of surgery, surgical wide local excision is the primary definitive treatment for localized melanoma. Current national treatment guidelines limit consideration for definitive radiotherapy for primary melanoma in situ and lentigo maligna type in patients who are not surgical candidates or in cases where surgical morbidity would be prohibitive.[7]

Surgical resection affords excellent disease control at the primary site when adequate margins are achieved, rendering little additional benefit for radiation therapy in such circumstances.[17] Primary radiation has been shown to be effective in some cases, but does not show overall benefit when compared to surgical excision.[18–20] For example, one study compared surgical excision and radiotherapy for melanoma in situ, and found a lower 5-year recurrence rate of 6.8% (n = 1041) with surgical excision versus 13.2% (n = 15) for radiotherapy alone.[21] This may be due, in part, to the small sample size of patients receiving radiation therapy for melanoma. The study did find, however, that patients chosen for definitive radiotherapy were of older age and had tumors localized to the face and neck region.

Most studies suggesting a role for definitive radiotherapy for primary melanoma focus on lentigo maligna type, which has a characteristically slower rate of growth and is less likely to progress to invasive disease. Although surgery remains the preferred treatment, there are roles for definitive radiation therapy over surgery in situations where margin-negative excision is not feasible, as in expansive lesions over the head and neck.

Experiences with radiation therapy for lentigo maligna type were initially heterogeneous in their conclusions. An older study from the 1970s exploring the use of radiation therapy in 16 patients with lentigo maligna found five (31%) local recurrences or persistent lesions, with three progressing to metastatic melanoma.[22] These conclusions are in contrast to a more recent study which showed a 97% cure rate with primary radiation therapy for lentigo maligna melanoma at 10 years.[23] Furthermore, a recent literature review incorporating data from nine clinical studies (n = 537) investigating the use of radiation therapy for lentigo maligna type melanoma showed a 5% local recurrence rate, and a 1.4% progression to invasive disease.[24] Some retrospective studies (n = 807) have shown clinical efficacy for primary radiation treatment of lentigo maligna with recurrence rates ranging from 0% to 17%.[25-28] Thus, while surgical resection is preferred, some clinical situations would support the use of radiation therapy for definitive melanoma management.

Taken together, while surgery is the therapeutic mainstay for definitive melanoma management, there is a defined role for radiation therapy in cases of lentigo maligna that do not otherwise lend themselves well to a primary surgical approach. In these situations, radiation therapy can be delivered with the expectation for durable and safe local control.

Adjuvant Radiotherapy

In the presence of certain patient and/or tumor factors, the locoregional recurrence of melanoma following surgical excision alone is high.[29] However, following adjuvant radiation therapy delivery using a variety of fractionation schema has shown clinical benefit in multiple settings, with 5-year local control rates of 87% to 95%.[16,30-35] As such, radiation therapy following surgical excision of local tumors has been shown to be effective for locoregional control of melanoma.

Prior investigations have delineated high-risk factors for melanoma recurrence following surgical resection. In a study among 629 patients with melanoma treated over a 30-year period at the Sydney Melanoma Unit, rates of local recurrence increased incrementally with tumor thickness, culminating with a 20% risk for ≥4 mm thickness.[36] Additionally, among other investigations, the presence of positive regional lymph nodes has been associated with a 24% risk of relapse at the primary site.[37]

Among melanoma subtypes, multiple studies - including a phase II trial and retrospective reviews - have shown a benefit of adjuvant radiation therapy for local control of desmoplastic melanoma; these studies do not show benefit in overall survival when compared to surgical excision alone.[35,38-41] A 2019 retrospective study looked at 2390 patients with desmoplastic melanoma in the National Cancer Database and compared treatment outcomes between wide local excision and wide local excision with adjuvant radiotherapy. This study found that overall survival was significantly improved for patients with adjuvant radiotherapy compared to surgical excision alone only if tumor size was factored into the equation. While adjuvant radiotherapy has been shown in some cases to reduce local tumor recurrence, this study is the first study suggesting a survival benefit with the use of adjuvant radiotherapy for primary melanoma.[42] Other studies evaluating a role for adjuvant radiation therapy to nodal basins have not demonstrated improvement in either relapse-free survival or overall survival.[43]

In a trial conducted by the Trans-Tasman Radiation Oncology Group (TROG), Burmeister and colleagues (2006) reviewed 234 node-positive melanoma patients managed with lymph node dissection and adjuvant radiation therapy.[44] Sites of disease include head and neck, axilla, and inguinal nodal basins, with the majority having two or more involved lymph nodes and extracapsular extension. Patients were treated using a 48 Gy/fraction × 20 fraction schema (which is slightly hypofractionated) with 5-year results demonstrating 91% regional control and 36% overall survival and lymphedema being the primary late effect of treatment. In that regard, radiation therapy improves outcomes not only at the primary site of melanoma involvement, but also in association with the treatment of high-risk nodal basins.

For these reasons, guidelines based on retrospective reports have advocated for the use of adjuvant radiation therapy for desmoplastic cutaneous melanoma with high-risk features, including Breslow thickness greater than 4 mm, anatomic location of the head and neck, and narrow deep-margin resection.[6,35,45] However, advances in other treatment modalities have improved outcomes in such patients and radiation therapy is not routinely offered to patients with thick tumor, lymphovascular invasion, or perineural invasion in the absence of other pathologic features.

Current National Comprehensive Cancer Network (NCCN) guidelines suggest consideration for adjuvant radiation therapy for primary disease in select cases of high-risk desmoplastic melanoma with risk factors including head and neck location, extensive neurotropism, and situations where clear surgical margins are not able to be attained and/or the surgeon is not able to resect greater margins for cosmetic and/or anatomic reasons, or where locally recurrent disease exists.[7] As per these guidelines, adjuvant radiation therapy may be delivered following resected melanoma nodal involvement, in the presence of adverse pathologic features including nodal extracapsular extension, involvement of nodes (any nodes in parotid, $\geq$ 2 cervical/axillary, and $\geq$ 3 inguinofemoral), or large nodal deposits (ie, $\geq$3 cm cervical or axillary or $\geq$4 cm inguinofemoral node) by tumor.[7] Such treatment may be delivered in conventional or hypofractionated schema. Which treatment decision is chosen is in part determined by the expediency for delivery of adjuvant systemic therapy and the volume and location of the radiation target.

In sum, adjuvant radiation therapy likely has a role in improving locoregional control in patients with melanoma at high risk for tumor recurrence, but its effect on survival has not been demonstrated in a prospective fashion. Additionally, such treatments appear safe and effective.

Toxicity

Radiation delivery itself is painless and not perceptible by the patient. However, it conveys expected tumoricidal effects as well as effects upon normal surrounding tissues. Mechanistically, low-dose radiation causes nuclear changes and apoptosis, whereas high-dose radiation causes cytoplasmic swelling and disruption of other organelles resulting in cellular necrosis.[46] This depends in part on radiation dose and fractionation, size and location of target, radiosensitivity of the native tissue, and genetics of the individual as related to the DNA repair mechanisms.[47]

Radiation-induced skin reactions have been studied through the treatment of other cancer types and result from the inflammatory and oxidative properties of radiation therapy.[47] These reactions can be classified in terms of short-term and long-term toxicity; short-term toxicity being less than 90 days posttreatment whereas long-term toxicity is after 90 days following treatment.[48] The National Cancer Institute's Common Terminology Criteria for Adverse Events provides grading schema following radiation. Based on progressive severity, it ranges from the absence of skin findings, to erythema, desquamation, edema, and skin necrosis.[49]

In the short term, preventing dryness of skin, through the use of topical skin products with hydrophilic/colloidal preparations and products to prevent itching, may be used to treat the dermatitis. Erythema begins to occur 3 weeks into treatment and desquamation can present after 4 weeks of treatment.[50] Subjective discomfort of the treated skin region occasionally occurs, and must also be managed.

In the longer term, fibrosis of the skin and subcutaneous tissue, pain, and nerve damage are other potential effects,[51] as are cosmetic changes such as persistent hyperpigmentation in the treated field and lymphedema. With regard to lymphedema, rates may vary between 10% to 30% following radiation therapy, noting that the risk of lymphedema following surgery alone may also approach 20%.[31,44]

Current national treatment guidelines advise that hypofractionated radiation therapy regimens may increase the risk of long-term side effects and complications,[7] particularly where a large volume of tissue must be treated or cosmesis is a concern. Hypofractionated radiation therapy delivered to cervical lymph nodes after surgical excision of involved lymph nodes is associated with a complication rate of less than 10% and nodal field control rate greater than 90% at 5 years.[52] Thus, with the use of sentinel node lymphadenectomy and nodal basin dissection evolving for melanoma treatment, the role of radiation therapy in terms of risk and benefit is also likely to evolve.

Future Directions

There are limited data available regarding the use of radiotherapy for primary local cutaneous melanoma. Much of the preclinical and initial translational data are based on studies conducted decades ago. In addition, the paucity of more recent phase III trials limits the selection of radiation therapy for primary melanoma. As such, radiation therapy is unlikely to displace wide surgical resection as the gold standard in definitive management of local cutaneous melanoma.

Nonetheless, exciting developments in radiation therapy delivery and current understanding of melanoma tumor biology impart the promise of meaningful interventions ahead. For example, use of advanced radiation therapy techniques such as stereotactic body radiation therapy (SBRT) allows for increased conformality and fraction size while adhering to a high margin of safety in a relatively short treatment course, resulting in more effective treatment of oligometastatic disease.[53] In addition, delivery of SBRT with biological targets (eg, BRAF/MAPK pathway) and checkpoint inhibitor immunotherapy have been postulated to have a synergistic effect.[54]

SUMMARY

The use of radiation therapy for melanoma continues to be investigated. Surgery remains the preferred treatment modality for definitive treatment of melanoma, but primary radiotherapy can be used in cases of lentigo maligna where surgical excision is not indicated. Adjuvant radiation therapy has been shown to be effective for desmoplastic melanoma lesions. Both conventional and hypofractionated radiation therapy delivery have been used safely and effectively, particularly in the adjuvant setting. Side effects of radiation therapy are dependent on patient, tumor, and treatment factors, but treatment is generally well tolerated. As the field progresses, additional innovations will likely further expand the role for radiation therapy in primary cutaneous melanoma, and multidisciplinary collaboration will be essential to achieve optimal patient outcomes.

CLINICS CARE POINTS

- Primary radiation has been shown to be effective in certain cases for the treatment of melanoma, but this does not show overall benefit when compared to surgical resection. Limit considerations to definitive radiotherapy for melanoma in situ and lentigo maligna type when surgical intervention is not feasible.

- Current NCCN guidelines support the use of adjuvant radiation therapy in high-risk desmoplastic melanoma with factors concerning for head and neck location, extensive neurotropism, scenarios where clear margins are not able to be obtained, and/or the surgeon

is not able to resect greater margins due to anatomy/cosmesis, or where locally recurrent disease exists.

- Toxicity of radiation with cutaneous manifestations, fibrosis, and lymphedema continue to be problematic with the treatment modality. Hypofractionated radiation may increase the risk of long-term side effects and complications.

DISCLOSURE

None.

REFERENCES

1. Maani EV, Maani CV. Radiation Therapy. In: StatPearls. StatPearls Publishing; 2020. http://www.ncbi.nlm.nih.gov/books/NBK537036/. [Accessed 7 September 2020].
2. Doss LL, Memula N. The radioresponsiveness of melanoma. Int J Radiat Oncol Biol Phys 1982;8(7):1131–4.
3. Fertil B, Malaise EP. Intrinsic radiosensitivity of human cell lines is correlated with radioresponsiveness of human tumors: analysis of 101 published survival curves. Int J Radiat Oncol 1985;11(9):1699–707.
4. Barranco SC, Romsdahl MM, Humphrey RM. The radiation response of human malignant melanoma cells grown in vitro. Cancer Res 1971;31(6):830–3.
5. Berk LB. Radiation therapy as primary and adjuvant treatment for local and regional melanoma. Cancer Control J Moffitt Cancer Cent 2008;15(3):233–8.
6. Swetter SM, Tsao H, Bichakjian CK, et al. Guidelines of care for the management of primary cutaneous melanoma. J Am Acad Dermatol 2019;80(1):208–50.
7. Melanoma. Cutaneous in National Comprehensive Cancer Network NCCN clinical practice guidelines in oncology version 1.2021. NCCN.org; 2020.
8. Mendenhall WM. Adjuvant radiotherapy for cutaneous melanoma. In: Radiation therapy for skin cancer. New York: Springer Science+Business Media; 2013. p. 575–605.
9. Miescher G. [Melanotic precancerosis]. Oncologia 1954;7(2):92–4.
10. Rofstad EK. Radiation biology of malignant melanoma. Acta Radiol Oncol 1986;25(1):1–10.
11. Aninditha KP, Weber KJ, Brons S, et al. In vitro sensitivity of malignant melanoma cells lines to photon and heavy ion radiation. Clin Transl Radiat Oncol 2019;17:51–6.
12. Owens JM, Roberts DB, Myers JN. The role of postoperative adjuvant radiation therapy in the treatment of mucosal melanomas of the head and neck region. Arch Otolaryngol Head Neck Surg 2003;129(8):864–8.

13. Overgaard J, Overgaard M, Hansen PV, et al. Some factors of importance in the radiation treatment of malignant melanoma. Radiother Oncol J Eur Soc Ther Radiol Oncol 1986;5(3):183–92.

14. Bentzen SM, Overgaard J, Thames HD, et al. Clinical radiobiology of malignant melanoma. Radiother Oncol J Eur Soc Ther Radiol Oncol 1989;16(3):169–82.

15. Sause WT, Cooper JS, Rush S, et al. Fraction size in external beam radiation therapy in the treatment of melanoma. Int J Radiat Oncol Biol Phys 1991;20(3):429–32.

16. Ang KK, Peters LJ, Weber RS, et al. Postoperative radiotherapy for cutaneous melanoma of the head and neck region. Int J Radiat Oncol Biol Phys 1994;30(4):795–8.

17. Ballo MT, Ang KK. Radiotherapy for cutaneous malignant melanoma: rationale and indications. Oncol Williston Park N 2004;18(1):99–107. discussion 107-110, 113-114.

18. Harwood AR. Radiotherapy of acral lentiginous melanoma of the foot. J La State Med Soc 1999;151(7):373–6.

19. Mortier L, Mirabel X, Modiano P, et al. [Interstitial brachytherapy in management of primary cutaneous melanoma: 4 cases]. Ann Dermatol Venereol 2006;133(2):153–6.

20. Hellriegel W. Radiation therapy of primary and metastatic melanoma. Ann N Y Acad Sci 1963;100:131–41.

21. Zalaudek I, Horn M, Richtig E, et al. Local recurrence in melanoma in situ: influence of sex, age, site of involvement and therapeutic modalities. Br J Dermatol 2003;148(4):703–8.

22. Kopf AW, Bart RS, Gladstein AH. Treatment of melanotic freckle with X-rays. Arch Dermatol 1976;112(6):801–7.

23. Drakensjö IRT, Rosen E, Nilsson MF, et al. Ten-year follow-up study of Grenz ray treatment for lentigo maligna and early lentigo maligna melanoma. Acta Derm Venereol 2020. https://doi.org/10.2340/00015555-3631.

24. Fogarty GB, Hong A, Scolyer RA, et al. Radiotherapy for lentigo maligna: a literature review and recommendations for treatment. Br J Dermatol 2014;170(1):52–8.

25. Farshad A, Burg G, Panizzon R, et al. A retrospective study of 150 patients with lentigo maligna and lentigo maligna melanoma and the efficacy of radiotherapy using Grenz or soft X-rays. Br J Dermatol 2002;146(6):1042–6.

26. Hedblad M-A, Mallbris L. Grenz ray treatment of lentigo maligna and early lentigo maligna melanoma. J Am Acad Dermatol 2012;67(1):60–8.

27. Schmid-Wendtner MH, Brunner B, Konz B, et al. Fractionated radiotherapy of lentigo maligna and lentigo maligna melanoma in 64 patients. J Am Acad Dermatol 2000;43(3):477–82.

28. Tsang RW, Liu FF, Wells W, et al. Lentigo maligna of the head and neck. Results of treatment by radiotherapy. Arch Dermatol 1994;130(8):1008–12.

29. Mendenhall WM, Amdur RJ, Grobmyer SR, et al. Adjuvant radiotherapy for cutaneous melanoma. Cancer 2008;112(6):1189–96.

30. Chang DT, Amdur RJ, Morris CG, et al. Adjuvant radiotherapy for cutaneous melanoma: comparing hypofractionation to conventional fractionation. Int J Radiat Oncol Biol Phys 2006;66(4):1051–5.

31. Ballo MT, Ross MI, Cormier JN, et al. Combined-modality therapy for patients with regional nodal metastases from melanoma. Int J Radiat Oncol Biol Phys 2006;64(1):106–13.

32. Burmeister BH, Smithers BM, Poulsen M, et al. Radiation therapy for nodal disease in malignant melanoma. World J Surg 1995;19(3):369–71.

33. Stevens G, Thompson JF, Firth I, et al. Locally advanced melanoma: results of postoperative hypofractionated radiation therapy. Cancer 2000;88(1):88–94.

34. Corry J, Smith JG, Bishop M, et al. Nodal radiation therapy for metastatic melanoma. Int J Radiat Oncol Biol Phys 1999;44(5):1065–9.

35. Strom EA, Ross MI. Adjuvant radiation therapy after axillary lymphadenectomy for metastatic melanoma: toxicity and local control. Ann Surg Oncol 1995;2(5):445–9.

36. O'Brien CJ, Coates AS, Petersen-Schaefer K, et al. Experience with 998 cutaneous melanomas of the head and neck over 30 years. Am J Surg 1991;162(4):310–4.

37. Shen P, Wanek LA, Morton DL. Is adjuvant radiotherapy necessary after positive lymph node dissection in head and neck melanomas? Ann Surg Oncol 2000;7(8):554–9. discussion 560-561.

38. Foote MC, Burmeister B, Burmeister E, et al. Desmoplastic melanoma: the role of radiotherapy in improving local control. ANZ J Surg 2008;78(4):273–6.

39. Rule WG, Allred JB, Pockaj BA, et al. Results of NCCTG N0275 (Alliance) - a phase II trial evaluating resection followed by adjuvant radiation therapy for patients with desmoplastic melanoma. Cancer Med 2016;5(8):1890–6.

40. Oliver DE, Patel KR, Switchenko J, et al. Roles of adjuvant and salvage radiotherapy for desmoplastic melanoma. Melanoma Res 2016;26(1):35–41.

41. Guadagnolo BA, Prieto V, Weber R, et al. The role of adjuvant radiotherapy in the local management of desmoplastic melanoma. Cancer 2014;120(9):1361–8.

42. Abbott JL, Qureshi MM, Truong MT, et al. Comparing survival outcomes in early stage desmoplastic melanoma with or without adjuvant radiation. Melanoma Res 2019;29(4):413–9.

43. Henderson MA, Burmeister BH, Ainslie J, et al. Adjuvant lymph-node field radiotherapy versus

observation only in patients with melanoma at high risk of further lymph-node field relapse after lymphadenectomy (ANZMTG 01.02/TROG 02.01): 6-year follow-up of a phase 3, randomised controlled trial. Lancet Oncol 2015;16(9):1049–60.

44. Burmeister BH, Mark Smithers B, Burmeister E, et al. A prospective phase II study of adjuvant postoperative radiation therapy following nodal surgery in malignant melanoma-Trans Tasman Radiation Oncology Group (TROG) Study 96.06. Radiother Oncol J Eur Soc Ther Radiol Oncol 2006;81(2): 136–42.

45. Rao NG, Yu H-HM, Trotti A, et al. The role of radiation therapy in the management of cutaneous melanoma. Surg Oncol Clin N Am 2011;20(1):115–31.

46. Mendelsohn FA, Divino CM, Reis ED, et al. Wound care after radiation therapy. Adv Skin Wound Care 2002;15(5):216–24.

47. Wei J, Meng L, Hou X, et al. Radiation-induced skin reactions: mechanism and treatment. Cancer Manag Res 2018;11:167–77.

48. Shuff JH, Siker ML, Daly MD, et al. Role of radiation therapy in cutaneous melanoma. Clin Plast Surg 2010;37(1):147–60.

49. Hymes SR, Strom EA, Fife C. Radiation dermatitis: clinical presentation, pathophysiology, and treatment 2006. J Am Acad Dermatol 2006;54(1):28–46.

50. Dunne-Daly CF. Skin and wound care in radiation oncology. Cancer Nurs 1995;18(2):144–60. quiz 161-162.

51. Wada-Ohno M, Ito T, Furue M. Adjuvant therapy for melanoma. Curr Treat Options Oncol 2019;20(8):63.

52. Ballo MT, Garden AS, Myers JN, et al. Melanoma metastatic to cervical lymph nodes: can radiotherapy replace formal dissection after local excision of nodal disease? Head Neck 2005;27(8): 718–21.

53. Palma DA, Olson R, Harrow S, et al. Stereotactic ablative radiotherapy for the comprehensive treatment of oligometastatic cancers: long-term results of the SABR-COMET Phase II Randomized Trial. J Clin Oncol 2020;38(25):2830–8.

54. Sundahl N, Seremet T, Van Dorpe J, et al. Phase 2 trial of nivolumab combined with stereotactic body radiation therapy in patients with metastatic or locally advanced inoperable melanoma. Int J Radiat Oncol Biol Phys 2019;104(4):828–35.

Adjuvant and Neoadjuvant Therapeutics for the Treatment of Cutaneous Melanoma

William J. Bruce, MD[a], Jessie L. Koljonen, MD[a],
Michael R. Romanelli, MD, MA[a], Aziz U. Khan, MD[b],
Michael W. Neumeister, MD, FRCS[c],*

KEYWORDS

- Adjuvant • Neoadjuvant • Targeted therapy • Immunotherapy • Chemotherapy • Cancer vaccines
- Melanoma

KEY POINTS

- Adjuvant therapy is integral in the treatment of stage III and IV melanoma after surgical resection.
- Trials for neoadjuvant therapeutics are ongoing; these are most beneficial for presurgical treatment of disease that is surgically resectable and carries a high risk of recurrence.
- Immune modulating therapeutics—including interferon-alpha-2b, CTLA-4 inhibitors, and PD-1 inhibitors—act to enhance the response of the immune system against melanoma cells.
- Mutation-specific targeted therapy exploits one of the most common mutations in melanoma (BRAF-V600E/K substitution). These medications inhibit the BRAF/MEK pathway to prevent unregulated cell growth.
- Oncolytic vaccines—including 6-MHP and T-VEC—work to induce a specific, targeted tumor-antigen immune response against melanoma cells.

INTRODUCTION

Adjuvant and neoadjuvant therapies for melanoma have evolved to benefit patients who are at highest risk of disease recurrence after surgical resection.

Neoadjuvant therapy is used for locally and regionally advanced neoplasms (stage IIIB–D and IVA) to reduce tumor burden and activity preoperatively to aid in the surgical and medical management of the patient.[1] Without neoadjuvant treatment, regionally advanced disease with palpable lymph nodes is associated with a 5-year survival of less than 30%, and local recurrence is associated with a less than 10% 5-year survival.[2,3] In addition, pathologic response to neoadjuvant therapy can offer prognostic value, predict response to adjuvant therapy, and identify markers that correlate with outcomes.[1] Combined regimens of neoadjuvant and adjuvant therapies in many cases show superior results in both disease-free survival and eradication of metastasis.[4]

Systemic adjuvant therapy is administered after surgery to increase survival and decrease recurrence by suppressing or eliminating residual malignancy. Adjuvant therapy for melanoma is most beneficial in patients with a high risk of recurrence and death from metastatic disease after excision of the primary tumor, typically in stage III and stage IV melanoma (**Table 1**).[5] Lymph node involvement

[a] Institute for Plastic Surgery, Southern Illinois University School of Medicine, 747 North Rutledge Street #3, Springfield, IL 62702, USA; [b] Division of Hematology/Oncology, Department of Internal Medicine, Southern Illinois University School of Medicine, 315 West Carpenter Street, Springfield, IL 62702, USA; [c] Institute for Plastic Surgery, Southern Illinois University School of Medicine, P.O. Box 19653, Springfield, IL 62794-9653, USA
* Corresponding author.
E-mail address: mneumeister@siumed.edu

Clin Plastic Surg 48 (2021) 651–658
https://doi.org/10.1016/j.cps.2021.06.001

Table 1
Adjuvant treatment algorithm for cutaneous melanoma categorized by American Joint Committee on Cancer guidelines

American Joint Committee on Cancer TNM Staging[†]	Treatment
0 IA IB IIA	Surgical excision, adjuvant therapy not indicated except in the context of a formal clinical trial
IIB IIC	Adjuvant therapy not recommended given favorable prognosis and associated adverse effects of therapeutics
IIIA	Disease recurrence risk is <20%, consider observation
IIIB IIIC IIID	1 y of immunotherapy nivolumab or pembrolizumab; if BRAF V600+, then dabrafenib and trametinib could be an alternative
IV	1 y immunotherapy with 4 doses of induction nivolumab plus ipilimumab, followed by maintenance nivolumab

Data from Cohen JV, Buchbinder EI. The evolution of adjuvant therapy for melanoma. Curr Oncol Rep 2019;21(12):1–7.
  † Gershenwald JE, Scolyer RA, Hess KR, et al. Melanoma of the Skin. In: Amin AB, Edge SB, Greene, FL, et al. (Eds). AJCC Cancer Staging Manual. 8th Ed. New York: Springer; 2017:563-585.

and sentinel node tumor size greater than 1 mm carry increased risk of recurrence and mortality.[6,7] Trials are ongoing to evaluate the use of adjuvant therapy in high-risk, node-negative disease.

In both the adjuvant and neoadjuvant settings, early chemotherapeutic and biochemical antitumor agents are making their way to newer immune therapies, mutation-specific targeted therapies, and oncolytic vaccines that are transforming the treatment of malignant melanoma (**Table 2**). The use of these systemic therapies in addition to surgical resection has been shown to increase overall survival. The side-effect profiles of many of these medications are significant and must be considered along with patient functional status and comorbidities before selection of a treatment course.

IMMUNE THERAPY

Immunotherapeutic agents in the treatment of melanoma focus on inhibition of checkpoint molecules that are bypassed by the typical mutations in melanoma cells. The most promising of these are high-dose interferon-alpha-2b (IFN- alpha-2b; HDI), Cytotoxic T-Lymphocyte Antigen 4 (CTLA-4) inhibitors (ipilimumab), and Programmed Cell Death-1 (PD-1) pathway inhibitors (pembrolizumab, nivolumab).

Interferon-alpha

Interferon-alpha-based drugs are derived from human proteins, which cause nonspecific activation of the adaptive immune system through the JAK-STAT pathway, ultimately leading to stimulation of apoptosis in malignant cell lines.[8]

Immunotherapeutics have shown efficacy as a treatment for a variety of malignant or virally induced conditions.

Interferon-alpha-2b was the only approved drug for patients with high-risk cutaneous melanoma before 2015 and the development of newer immune therapies.[7]

Two separate phase 2 trials have evaluated high-dose neoadjuvant IFN-alpha-2b. Moschos and colleagues[4] trialed 4 weeks of preoperative HDI as a single agent in patients with IIIB/C melanoma. Fifteen percent of patients achieved pathologic complete response (pCR) with 55% of patients overall responding to therapy. Pathologic evaluation also demonstrated an increase in the intratumoral adaptive immune response with increases in mature natural killer cells (CD83+), T-lymphocytes (CD3+), and mononuclear cells (CD11+) in the patients who responded to treatment. Similarly, regimens with neoadjuvant HDI combined with interleukin-2 and standard biochemical therapy demonstrated an increase in relapse-free survival (RFS) and overall radiographic response.[9]

A 2015 trial evaluating the effect of adjuvant IFN-alpha-2b on distant metastasis-free interval and overall survival found no improvement in outcomes for patients with stage III melanomas.[10] A subsequent large meta-analysis of 14 randomized controlled trials showed that adjuvant treatment with IFN-alpha resulted in a statistically significant improvement in disease-free survival and overall survival; however, the clinical benefit was marginal (hazard ratio [HR] for disease recurrence and death 0.82 and 0.89, respectively).[11]

Table 2
Categories of adjuvant and neoadjuvant therapeutics

Category of Therapy	Treatment	Mechanism of Action
Immune therapy	Interferon-α-2b (IFN-α-2b)	Activates JAK-STAT pathway
	Pegylated interferon	Activates JAK-STAT pathway
	Ipilimumab	CTLA-4 inhibitor
	Pembrolizumab	PD-1 inhibitor
	Nivolumab	PD-1 inhibitor
Targeted therapy	Vemurafenib	BRAF inhibitor
	Dabrafenib	BRAF inhibitor
	Encorafenib	BRAF inhibitor
	Trametinib	MEK inhibitor
	Cobimetinib	MEK inhibitor
	Binimetinib	MEK inhibitor
Chemotherapy	Dacarbazine	Alkylating agent
Radiation therapy	Externalized beam therapy	Localized damage to DNA
	Stereotactic therapy	Localized damage to DNA
Cancer vaccines	6-HMP	Immune presentation of melanoma peptides
	T-VEC	Activation/recruitment of antigen-presenting cells

Toxicity is a major concern in patients taking IFN-alpha-2b, with all patients experiencing fevers/chills and constitutional flulike symptoms, in addition to a high rate of myelosuppression, hepatotoxicity, and neurologic and psychological effects.[12] Pegylated interferon-alpha-2b was later approved; however, use of both agents remains limited by frequent and difficult-to-tolerate side effects, which make year-long adjuvant therapy challenging.[5] The reduced time course of neoadjuvant therapies makes HDI more manageable for short-term use. With newer, more efficacious, more tolerable therapies now available, the use of IFN-alpha-2b has fallen out of favor. Interferon therapy remains useful in situations where newer therapies are unavailable. In addition, IFN-alpha-2b specifically benefits patients with ulcerated melanoma, and its continued use is indicated in this subset of patients.[13]

Cytotoxic T-Lymphocyte Antigen-4 Inhibitors: Ipilimumab

Whereas IFN class medications nonspecifically activate the immune system, newer classes of immunotherapeutics target pathways in the activation of adaptive immunity that are specific to neoplastic cell lines. Mutations in checkpoint regulatory molecules PD-1 and CTLA-4 are common to melanoma cells and cause downregulation of the adaptive immune response to the cancer cells. Checkpoint inhibitors that target PD-1 and CTLA-4 have shown improved outcomes in disease-free survival and disease recurrence in patients with advanced melanoma.

Adjuvant use of ipilimumab—a human monoclonal antibody that inhibits CTLA-4—to augment antitumor immune responses was approved by the Food and Drug Administration (FDA) in 2015, based on randomized controlled trials showing survival benefits for patients with unresectable stage III and stage IV disease.[14,15] When comparing ipilimumab to placebo, the 5-year rate of recurrence-free survival in patients with advanced melanoma who were given ipilimumab was 40.8% compared with 30.3% in the placebo group (HR for recurrence, 0.76). The 5-year rate of overall survival was 65.4%, versus 54.4% with placebo (HR for death, 0.72).[16]

Patients taking ipilimumab often experience a high rate of immune-related adverse effects (41.6%). Gastrointestinal (16.1%), hepatic (10.8%), and endocrine (7.9%) effects are the most common, followed by pruritis, rash, fatigue, and death (1.1%).[16,17] These effects, and the development of more efficacious and tolerable therapies, including the anti-PD-1 antibodies, have shifted therapy away from ipilimumab as a first-line option for adjuvant treatment of advanced melanoma.

After initial use in adjuvant therapies, ipilimumab was evaluated for neoadjuvant use but was found to be ineffective and poorly tolerated as a monotherapy.[18,19] Additional studies using ipilimumab in combination with PD-1 inhibitors or HDI have shown some promise. Ipilimumab in combination with HDI demonstrated up to a 32% pCR with a significant increase in the amount of tumor infiltrating lymphocytes.[19]

Programmed Cell Death-1 Inhibitors: Pembrolizumab and Nivolumab

Monoclonal PD-1 inhibitors pembrolizumab and nivolumab are now standard therapy in the adjuvant treatment of advanced stage melanoma and are highly effective as neoadjuvant. Compared with the anti-CTLA-4 antibody ipilimumab, pembrolizumab was found to be associated with longer progression-free survival, higher overall survival, and decreased high-grade adverse events in patients with advanced melanoma.[20–23]

Pembrolizumab and nivolumab have shown promise alone and in combination as neoadjuvant therapy. The trial by Amaria and colleagues[24,25] comparing neoadjuvant nivolumab alone to combination ipilimumab/nivolumab was discontinued early because of the high rate (73%) of serious adverse events in the combination group. Interim data however showed good effectiveness (25% pCR) and tolerability (8% adverse events) in the neoadjuvant nivolumab monotherapy group; surgical pathology of this group also demonstrated an increase in the concentration of tumor infiltrating lymphocytes.

The OpaCIN and OpaCIN-neo trials in the Netherlands compared dosing regimens for both adjuvant and neoadjuvant administration of ipilimumab and nivolumab.[26,27] The neoadjuvant trials demonstrated an increasing adverse event rate concurrent with an increased pCR. The specific combination of low-dose ipilimumab and high-dose nivolumab demonstrated the most successful results, with a 64% pCR and a 20% rate of high-grade adverse events. Overall, use of this combination therapy in high-risk resectable melanoma demonstrated significant improvement in RFS from 60% to 78% when used as neoadjuvant therapy as compared with adjuvant alone.

Pembrolizumab has also shown efficacy as single-dose monotherapy before surgery in high-risk resectable melanoma; this schedule demonstrates up to 19% pCR with minimal toxicity.[28]

A recent phase 3 adjuvant trial evaluating pembrolizumab in patients with resected, high-risk stage III melanoma demonstrated that the use of pembrolizumab resulted in a higher rate of RFS. At 1 year, the risk of recurrence or death was 43% lower in the pembrolizumab group compared with the placebo group.[29]

Although less severe than IFN or CTLA-4 therapies, patients taking pembrolizumab do experience a higher rate of immune-related effects compared with placebo, including endocrine disorders (hypothyroidism, diabetes mellitus), colitis, pruritis, and rash. Many of these adverse effects resolve after cessation of the treatment regimen.[29,30]

Nivolumab has shown similarly promising results as adjuvant therapy in patients with stage III or IV melanoma. Among these patients, those treated with adjuvant nivolumab experienced a significantly longer RFS rate and a lower rate of severe adverse events when compared with ipilimumab.[31]

Interestingly, the response of a tumor to PD-1 blockade can also be somewhat predicted with monitoring of IFN-gamma gene expression. These data have potential in use for targeting PD-1 blockade therapy specifically to the patients who will benefit most.[32,33]

TARGETED THERAPY
BRAF/MEK Inhibitor Combinations: Dabrafenib/Trametinib, Vemurafenib/Cobimetinib, Encorafenib/Binimetinib

Targeted therapies for melanoma are considered first-line therapy in the adjuvant treatment of advanced melanoma. These monoclonal antibodies target mutated proteins in the mitogen-activated protein kinase (MAPK) pathway, specifically resulting from common BRAF (B-Rapidly Accelerated Fibrosarcoma) and MEK (Mitogen Activated Protein Kinase Kinase) gene mutations that lead to unregulated cell growth. Targeted therapy is predicated on tumor oncotyping for specific somatic mutations. Fifty percent of malignant melanomas have a mutation in the BRAF proto-oncogene, with 90% of these BRAF mutations occurring as a Glutamine-to-Lysine substitution at the v600 allele.[34,35] This mutation alters the MAPK signaling pathway responsible for cell differentiation.[36] The first BRAF targeting medication vemurafenib was shown to prolong both progression-free survival and overall survival when used as adjuvant therapy.[37,38] The combination of the BRAF inhibitor dabrafenib and the MEK inhibitor trametinib is also particularly useful in this subset of patients with a BRAF v600E/K mutant melanoma and shows significantly improved overall survival and decreased recurrence when compared with either of the BRAF inhibitors alone.[39,40] Newer combination BRAF/MEK inhibitors, including vemurafenib/cobimetinib, as well as encorafenib/binimetinib, have shown improvement in survival rates when compared with vemurafenib monotherapy,[22] with a much more tolerable side-effect profile.[41] Compared with placebo, adjuvant use of this combination therapy in patients with stage III BRAF-mutant melanoma resulted in a significantly lower risk of recurrence and higher rate of survival. At 3 years, the rate of RFS was 50% in the therapy group versus 39% in placebo (HR for relapse or death, 0.47).[42]

Neoadjuvant therapy with dabrafenib alone was noted to have a very short-lived response; however, combination with trametinib increased the initial response rate up to 68% and prolonged response up to 11.5 months.[34,35,43,44]

The NeoCombi Trial showed similarly promising results with use of combination dabrafenib and trametinib neoadjuvant therapy, demonstrating an overall 49% pCR and 51% partial response.[40] A pCR in this trial was associated with 82% and 63% 1- and 2-year recurrence-free survival, respectively.

When the combination of dabrafenib plus trametinib was given as both neoadjuvant and adjuvant therapy in the MDACC trial for patients with high-risk resectable BRAF v600E/K melanomas, significantly more patients receiving neoadjuvant therapy were alive without progression of their disease, compared with those receiving adjuvant only.[24,25] pCR was shown to predict improved distant metastasis-free survival. Despite marked toxicity with 67% of patients experiencing grade III adverse events, the study was ultimately halted early because of the significant benefit in event-free survival noted with the neoadjuvant combination on interim analysis.

The most common adverse effects for this combination treatment were chills, headache, pyrexia, and diarrhea. Other adverse effects included increased risk of nonmelanoma skin cancer, rash, and ocular toxicity.[5]

ONCOLYTIC VACCINES

Research focused on oncolytic viral therapy (also known as cancer vaccines) for the treatment of advanced-stage melanoma is rapidly advancing. Vaccines can induce a specific, targeted tumor-antigen immune response, with the benefit of low systemic toxicity.

The 6-Melanoma Helper Peptide (6-MHP) vaccine is currently undergoing promising clinical trials. This vaccine combines 6 shared melanoma peptides presented in immune major histocompatibility complex class II (MHC-II) molecules. When the 6-MHP vaccine was given to patients with resected stage IV melanoma, median survival was significantly higher than in unvaccinated case-matched controls.[45]

Viral vectors are promising, as normal cells with intact antiviral defenses can prevent replication of the virus, but the vector can replicate freely in melanoma cells. The talimogene laherparepvec or T-VEC is one such viral therapy derived from an attenuated Herpes Simplex Virus (HSV-1) strain with a granulocyte-macrophage colony-stimulating factor (GM-CSF) gene insertion. The GM-CSF gene product recruits and activates antigen-presenting cells to the tumor microenvironment to process and present tumor antigens; this in turn drives an effector T-cell response against the neoplastic cells. T-VEC currently remains the only oncolytic viral therapy approved by the FDA.

In the neoadjuvant OPTiM trial, T-VEC was shown to be a superior vector to systemic GM-CSF alone in the treatment of high-risk resectable melanomas with a 16.3% durable response compared with 2.1% for systemic GM-CSF alone.[46] In additional neoadjuvant trials performed by Dummer and colleagues,[47,48] the use of neoadjuvant T-VEC sustained a pCR rate of 17%, improved R0 resectability from 41% to 56% and raised the 1-year recurrence-free survival rate in these patients from 22% to 34%. This trial demonstrated generally well-tolerated adverse effects, which included fatigue, chills, injection pain, and cellulitis. Unfortunately, 25% of enrolled patients had disease progression that precluded surgery during the initial neoadjuvant window.

This is a promising field with huge potential in the treatment of melanoma.

SUMMARY

Today, surgical excision remains the sole method of treatment for patients with low-risk, stage I and IIA cutaneous melanoma.

Neoadjuvant therapy carries the most benefit for patients with borderline resectable disease that carries a high risk of recurrence. Immune modulating therapies, targeted therapies, and newly emerging cancer vaccines show great promise in this realm, and patients should be evaluated for inclusion in relevant clinical trials whenever possible.

Adjuvant treatment significantly decreases disease recurrence and death in patients with advanced stage resected melanoma and nodal metastasis. Current standards of care for stage III cutaneous melanoma include the PD-1 antibody therapies (pembrolizumab and nivolumab) as a first-line adjuvant. The combination BRAF/MEK inhibitors (dabrafenib plus trametinib) are used in patients with a BRAF mutation. Use of these therapies decreases the risk of disease recurrence and death after surgical resection. In patients with stage IV cutaneous melanoma, nivolumab with ipilimumab is recommended.[49]

The anti-CTLA-4 antibody (ipilimumab) and IFN-alpha-2b have historically been used but have fallen out of favor because of the emergence of newer, more-effective, and less-toxic therapies. In countries where access may be limited and for specific subtypes of melanoma, these older therapies may still be considered.

Multimodal adjuvant and neoadjuvant therapeutics have made great strides over the last 10 years, which have resulted in the ability to personalize therapy based on a patient's prognosis and tolerance of adverse effects. Long-term use studies, as well as further developments and newer therapies, are currently being investigated.

CLINICS CARE POINTS

- Medications for the systemic adjuvant and neoadjuvant treatment of melanoma can be classified into classic chemotherapeutic and biochemical agents, immune therapies, mutation-specific targeted therapies, and oncolytic vaccines.

- Stage III cutaneous melanoma is treated with immunotherapy using the Programmed Cell Death-1 inhibitor nivolumab or pembrolizumab.

- If tumor oncotyping reveals a BRAF V600 mutation, this can be treated with the combination of targeted medications dabrafenib and trametinib.

- Stage IV cutaneous melanoma should be treated with nivolumab with ipilimumab if tolerated.

DISCLOSURE

The authors have nothing to disclose.

REFERENCES

1. Khunger A, Buchwald ZS, Lowe M, et al. Neoadjuvant therapy of locally/regionally advanced melanoma. Ther Adv Med Oncol 2019;11. 1758835919866959.

2. Karakousis CP, Balch CM, Urist MM, et al. Local recurrence in malignant melanoma: long-term results of the multiinstitutional randomized surgical trial. Ann Surg Oncol 1996;3(5):446–52.

3. Balch CM, Soong S-J, Smith T, et al. Long-term results of a prospective surgical trial comparing 2 cm vs. 4 cm excision margins for 740 patients with 1–4 mm melanomas. Ann Surg Oncol 2001;8(2):101–8.

4. Moschos SJ, Edington HD, Land SR, et al. Neoadjuvant treatment of regional stage IIIB melanoma with high-dose interferon alfa-2b induces objective tumor regression in association with modulation of tumor infiltrating host cellular immune responses. J Clin Oncol 2006;24(19):3164–71.

5. Cohen JV, Buchbinder EI. The evolution of adjuvant therapy for melanoma. Curr Oncol Rep 2019;21(12):1–7.

6. Morton DL, Thompson JF, Cochran AJ, et al. Final trial report of sentinel-node biopsy versus nodal observation in melanoma. N Engl J Med 2014;370(7):599–609.

7. Kwak M, Farrow NE, Salama AK, et al. Updates in adjuvant systemic therapy for melanoma. J Surg Oncol 2019;119(2):222–31.

8. Theofilopoulos AN, Baccala R, Beutler B, et al. Type I interferons (α/β) in immunity and autoimmunity. Annu Rev Immunol 2005;23:307–35.

9. Lewis KD, Robinson WA, McCarter M, et al. Phase II multicenter study of neoadjuvant biochemotherapy for patients with stage III malignant melanoma. J Clin Oncol 2006;24(19):3157–63.

10. Eggermont AM, Suciu S, MacKie R, et al. Post-surgery adjuvant therapy with intermediate doses of interferon alfa 2b versus observation in patients with stage IIb/III melanoma (EORTC 18952): randomised controlled trial. Lancet 2005;366(9492):1189–96.

11. Mocellin S, Pasquali S, Rossi CR, et al. Interferon alpha adjuvant therapy in patients with high-risk melanoma: a systematic review and meta-analysis. J Natl Cancer Inst 2010;102(7):493–501.

12. Hauschild A, Gogas H, Tarhini A, et al. Practical guidelines for the management of interferon-α-2b side effects in patients receiving adjuvant treatment for melanoma: expert opinion. Cancer Interdiscip Int J Am Cancer Soc 2008;112(5):982–94.

13. Ives NJ, Suciu S, Eggermont AM, et al. Adjuvant interferon-α for the treatment of high-risk melanoma: an individual patient data meta-analysis. Eur J Cancer 2017;82:171–83.

14. Hodi FS, O'Day SJ, McDermott DF, et al. Improved survival with ipilimumab in patients with metastatic melanoma. N Engl J Med 2010;363(8):711–23.

15. Robert C, Thomas L, Bondarenko I, et al. Ipilimumab plus dacarbazine for previously untreated metastatic melanoma. N Engl J Med 2011;364(26):2517–26.

16. Eggermont AM, Chiarion-Sileni V, Grob J-J, et al. Prolonged survival in stage III melanoma with ipilimumab adjuvant therapy. N Engl J Med 2016;375(19):1845–55.

17. Berman D, Parker SM, Siegel J, et al. Blockade of cytotoxic T-lymphocyte antigen-4 by ipilimumab results in dysregulation of gastrointestinal immunity in patients with advanced melanoma. Cancer Immun Archive 2010;10(1).

18. Tarhini AA, Edington H, Butterfield LH, et al. Neoadjuvant ipilimumab in locally/regionally advanced melanoma: clinical outcome and biomarker analysis. Am Soc Clin Oncol 2012;76–76.

19. Tarhini AA, Edington H, Butterfield LH, et al. Immune monitoring of the circulation and the tumor microenvironment in patients with regionally advanced melanoma receiving neoadjuvant ipilimumab. PLoS One 2014;9(2):e87705.

20. Robert C, Schachter J, Long GV, et al. Pembrolizumab versus ipilimumab in advanced melanoma. N Engl J Med 2015;372(26):2521–32.

21. Robert C, Ribas A, Schachter J, et al. Pembrolizumab versus ipilimumab in advanced melanoma (KEYNOTE-006): post-hoc 5-year results from an open-label, multicentre, randomised, controlled, phase 3 study. Lancet Oncol 2019;20(9):1239–51.

22. Ascierto PA, Long GV, Robert C, et al. Survival outcomes in patients with previously untreated BRAF wild-type advanced melanoma treated with nivolumab therapy: three-year follow-up of a randomized phase 3 trial. JAMA Oncol 2019;5(2):187–94.

23. Hwang SJE, Fernández-Peñas P. Adverse reactions to biologics: melanoma (ipilimumab, nivolumab, pembrolizumab). Curr Probl Dermatol 2018;53: 82–92.

24. Amaria RN, Prieto PA, Tetzlaff MT, et al. Neoadjuvant plus adjuvant dabrafenib and trametinib versus standard of care in patients with high-risk, surgically resectable melanoma: a single-centre, open-label, randomised, phase 2 trial. Lancet Oncol 2018; 19(2):181–93.

25. Amaria RN, Reddy SM, Tawbi HA, et al. Neoadjuvant immune checkpoint blockade in high-risk resectable melanoma. Nat Med 2018;24(11):1649–54.

26. Blank CU, Rozeman EA, Fanchi LF, et al. Neoadjuvant versus adjuvant ipilimumab plus nivolumab in macroscopic stage III melanoma. Nat Med 2018; 24(11):1655–61.

27. Rozeman EA, Menzies AM, van Akkooi AC, et al. Identification of the optimal combination dosing schedule of neoadjuvant ipilimumab plus nivolumab in macroscopic stage III melanoma (OpACIN-neo): a multicentre, phase 2, randomised, controlled trial. Lancet Oncol 2019;20(7):948–60.

28. Huang AC, Orlowski RJ, Xu X, et al. A single dose of neoadjuvant PD-1 blockade predicts clinical outcomes in resectable melanoma. Nat Med 2019; 25(3):454–61.

29. Eggermont AM, Blank CU, Mandala M, et al. Adjuvant pembrolizumab versus placebo in resected stage III melanoma. N Engl J Med 2018;378(19): 1789–801.

30. Eggermont AM, Robert C, Ribas A. The new era of adjuvant therapies for melanoma. Nat Rev Clin Oncol 2018;15(9):535–6.

31. Weber J, Mandala M, Del Vecchio M, et al. Adjuvant nivolumab versus ipilimumab in resected stage III or IV melanoma. N Engl J Med 2017;377(19):1824–35.

32. Ayers M, Lunceford J, Nebozhyn M, et al. IFN-γ–related mRNA profile predicts clinical response to PD-1 blockade. J Clin Invest 2017;127(8):2930–40.

33. Cristescu R, Mogg R, Ayers M, et al. Pan-tumor genomic biomarkers for PD-1 checkpoint blockade–based immunotherapy. Science 2018; 362(6411).

34. Chapman PB, Hauschild A, Robert C, et al. Improved survival with vemurafenib in melanoma with BRAF V600E mutation. N Engl J Med 2011; 364(26):2507–16.

35. Hauschild A, Grob J-J, Demidov LV, et al. Dabrafenib in BRAF-mutated metastatic melanoma: a multicentre, open-label, phase 3 randomised controlled trial. Lancet 2012;380(9839):358–65.

36. Curtin JA, Fridlyand J, Kageshita T, et al. Distinct sets of genetic alterations in melanoma. N Engl J Med 2005;353(20):2135–47.

37. Maio M, Lewis K, Demidov L, et al. Adjuvant vemurafenib in resected, BRAFV600 mutation-positive melanoma (BRIM8): a randomised, double-blind, placebo-controlled, multicentre, phase 3 trial. Lancet Oncol 2018;19(4):510–20.

38. Anforth R, Fernandez-Peñas P, Long GV. Cutaneous toxicities of RAF inhibitors. Lancet Oncol 2013;14(1): e11–8.

39. Lugowska I, Koseła-Paterczyk H, Kozak K, et al. Trametinib: a MEK inhibitor for management of metastatic melanoma. OncoTargets Ther 2015;8:2251.

40. Long GV, Saw RP, Lo S, et al. Neoadjuvant dabrafenib combined with trametinib for resectable, stage IIIB–C, BRAFV600 mutation-positive melanoma (NeoCombi): a single-arm, open-label, single-centre, phase 2 trial. Lancet Oncol 2019;20(7): 961–71.

41. Gogas HJ, Flaherty KT, Dummer R, et al. Adverse events associated with encorafenib plus binimetinib in the COLUMBUS study: incidence, course and management. Eur J Cancer 2019;119:97–106.

42. Long GV, Hauschild A, Santinami M, et al. Adjuvant dabrafenib plus trametinib in stage III BRAF-mutated melanoma. N Engl J Med 2017;377(19): 1813–23.

43. Long GV, Stroyakovskiy D, Gogas H, et al. Combined BRAF and MEK inhibition versus BRAF inhibition alone in melanoma. N Engl J Med 2014;371(20): 1877–88.

44. Larkin J, Ascierto PA, Dréno B, et al. Combined vemurafenib and cobimetinib in BRAF-mutated melanoma. N Engl J Med 2014;371(20):1867–76.

45. Hu Y, Kim H, Blackwell CM, et al. Long-term outcomes of helper peptide vaccination for metastatic melanoma. Ann Surg 2015;262(3):456.

46. Andtbacka R, Kaufman HL, Collichio F, et al. Talimogene laherparepvec improves durable response rate in patients with advanced melanoma. J Clin Oncol 2015;33(25):2780–8.

47. Andtbacka RHI, Dummer R, Gyorki DE, et al. Interim analysis of a randomized, open-label phase 2 study of talimogene laherparepvec (T-VEC) neoadjuvant treatment (neotx) plus surgery (surgx) vs surgx for resectable stage IIIB-IVM1a melanoma (MEL). Am Soc Clin Oncol 2018;9508–9508.

48. Dummer R, Gyorki DE, Hyngstrom JR, et al. One-year (yr) recurrence-free survival (RFS) from a randomized, open label phase II study of neoadjuvant (neo) talimogene laherparepvec (T-VEC) plus surgery (surgx) versus surgx for resectable stage IIIB-IVM1a melanoma (MEL). Am Soc Clin Oncol 2019;9520–9520.

49. Zimmer L, Livingstone E, Hassel JC, et al. Adjuvant nivolumab plus ipilimumab or nivolumab monotherapy versus placebo in patients with resected stage IV melanoma with no evidence of disease (IMMUNED): a randomised, double-blind, placebo-controlled, phase 2 trial. Lancet 2020;395(10236):1558–68.

Extirpative Considerations of Melanoma of the Head and Neck

Danielle Olla, MD[a],*, Anthony P. Tufaro, DDS, MD[b],
Michael W. Neumeister, MD, FRCSC[c]

KEYWORDS

- Melanoma ● Head and neck melanoma ● Head and neck ● Surgical considerations
- Surgical management ● Sentinel lymph node biopsy

KEY POINTS

- Head and neck melanomas account for 25% of all melanomas, and lentigo maligna and desmoplastic melanomas have higher incidence in the head and neck region.
- The National Comprehensive Cancer Network guideline recommendations for surgical margins and sentinel lymph node biopsy (SLNB) for cutaneous melanoma remain unchanged for head and neck melanoma but may require case-by-case modifications depending on the location of the melanoma and structures involved in and around the suggested margins.
- Lymphatic drainage in the head and neck is variable and complex and single-photon emission computed tomography has been shown to help identify sentinel lymph nodes.
- Recent MSTL-II trial has shown improvement in regional control and slight improvement in disease-free survival in completion lymph-node dissection versus observation after positive SLNB but there was no difference in melanoma-specific survival.
- Regional control in the head and neck may be more important than other anatomic locations given the critical structures within this region.

INTRODUCTION

The incidence of melanoma is continuing to rise in the United States, as other cancer incidences appear to have stabilized.[1] Head and neck melanomas account for 25% of all cutaneous melanomas and require special considerations when performing wide local excision, sentinel lymph node biopsy (SLNB), and reconstruction.[2]

DEMOGRAPHICS

The lifetime risk for a male individual developing melanoma is 1 in 27 and for a female individual 1 in 42.[1] The American Cancer Society estimates that in 2021 there will be approximately 106,110 new melanomas diagnosed, with approximately 62,260 in male and 43,850 in female individuals, but these numbers are likely an underestimate, as many superficial and in situ melanomas treated in the outpatient setting are not reported to tumor registries. There are expected to be 7180 deaths in 2021 attributed to melanoma. Over the past 50 years, the annual percentage change in mortality rate has increased steadily at 1.8% each year.[3] Approximately 25% of all cutaneous melanomas arise in the head and neck region with a male predominance and median age of diagnosis of 59 years.[2] Tumors are most commonly found in the face (48.1%) and scalp/neck (34.2%), with fewer than 20% arising from the lip, ear, or

[a] Institute for Plastic Surgery, Southern Illinois University, 747 North Rutledge Street #3, Springfield, IL 62702, USA; [b] University Hospitals Cleveland Medical Center, 11100 Euclid Aveune, Suite 5206, Cleveland, OH 44106, USA; [c] Department of Surgery, The Elvin G Zook Endowed Chair - Institute for Plastic Surgery, Southern Illinois University, 747 North Rutledge Street #3, Springfield, IL 62702, USA
* Corresponding author.
E-mail address: dolla41@siumed.edu

Clin Plastic Surg 48 (2021) 659–668
https://doi.org/10.1016/j.cps.2021.06.003

eyelid.[4,5] Men have been found to develop primary lesions significantly more frequently than women in the left peripheral regions of the head and neck.[6]

RISK FACTORS

Risk factors for melanoma include Fitzpatrick skin types I-III, blonde or red hair, blue or green eyes, personal history or family history of melanoma, and rare genetic mutations.[3,7] Excess sun exposure and UV tanning contribute to development of melanoma. Tanning booths and sun beds are associated with early-onset melanoma and have been classified as a carcinogen by the World Health Organization. The risk of melanoma from tanning booth exposure is greater than developing lung cancer from smoking.[8]

TYPES OF MELANOMA IN THE HEAD AND NECK

The most common subtypes of melanoma found in the head and neck include superficial spreading, nodular, lentigo maligna, and desmoplastic.[7] Lentigo maligna and desmoplastic subtypes are related to chronic sun exposure, whereas superficial spreading and nodular melanomas are related to acute intermittent sun exposure.[9] Lentigo melanoma is more commonly found in the head and neck compared with other regions.[10] Desmoplastic melanoma is an uncommon form, accounting for only 1% of melanomas, with 51% of all cases found in the head and neck region.[3,7] Rare variants of melanoma are found in **Table 1**.[11,12]

Epidemiologic analysis has led to the proposal of early-onset and late-onset melanoma. The early-onset melanoma category is predominately associated with female sex, superficial spreading, and found in the lower extremities. The late-onset category is predominately associated with male sex, lentigo maligna, and found in the head and neck region.[13]

Presentations[7,14]:

- Superficial spreading melanoma: Presents as an irregular pigmented macule or plaque and often occurs in young patients. There is an initial radial growth phase pattern with eventual development of a vertical growth phase.
- Nodular melanoma: Presents as an ulcerated black or blue nodule and has a vertical growth from its onset.
- Lentigo maligna melanoma: Presents as a slow enlarging, asymmetric, brown to black macule with irregular pigmentation on sun-exposed skin and has a prolonged radial growth phase.

- Desmoplastic melanoma: Presents as an amelanotic and deeply infiltrative lesion or associated with lentigo maligna or other melanocytic lesions. Characterized by infrequent metastasis but a higher local recurrence rate and perineural involvement.

PROGNOSTIC FACTORS AND SURVIVAL

Cutaneous melanoma of the head and neck has been found to have a worse prognosis compared with other sites.[15] At presentation, approximately 85% of patients with head and neck melanoma have localized disease, 10% have regional disease, and 5% have systemic disease.[16] Breslow thickness, ulceration status, and mitotic rate are important characteristics independently predictive of outcome.[17]

Studies have found lower rates of positive sentinel lymph nodes (SLNs) in head and neck melanomas (10.8%) compared with extremity (16.8%) and trunk (19.3%), but had the worst 5-year disease-free survival and 5-year overall survival.[15] Patients with melanoma in the head and neck region when adjusted for other prognostic parameters were 1.84 times more likely to die of the disease when compared with melanomas arising in other sites.[18] Other studies have found a survival difference between scalp/neck melanoma and melanoma of other sites.[4] The 5-year and 10-year Kaplan-Meier survival for scalp/neck melanoma were 83.1% and 76.2% compared with 92.1% and 88.7% for melanomas of other sites, including extremities, face, and ears.[18]

BIOPSY

An excisional biopsy with 1-mm to 3-mm margins should be performed when a suspicious lesion is identified.[19] If an excisional biopsy is not appropriate due to the location, such as a cosmetically sensitive area on the face, a full-thickness incisional biopsy or punch biopsy of the clinically thickest portion may be acceptable. The goal of the biopsy is to provide accurate primary tumor microstaging without interfering with definitive local therapy. Compared with excisional biopsy, punch and shave biopsy had a significantly increased risk for inaccurate microstaging.[20] For larger lesions with indistinct margins, such as seen in lentigo maligna, a number of punch biopsies can be taken from normal-appearing skin 3 to 5 mm from the obvious border of the tumor. The presence of negative findings on the punch biopsies will allow the surgeon to ensure negative radial margins on the excision.

Table 1
Rare variants of malignant melanoma

Verrucous melanoma	Many consider verrucous melanoma a variant of superficial spreading melanoma characterized by an exophytic papilliferous growth pattern.
Animal melanoma	Animal melanoma is a rare dermal-based melanocytic neoplasm with sheets of heavily pigmented epithelioid or spindle cells with many melanophages.
Nevoid melanoma	These lesions resemble ordinary compound or dermal nevi. Clues to the malignant nature of these lesions include pleomorphism, impaired maturation, asymmetry, and mitoses.
Malignant blue nevus	Malignant blue nevus, a misnomer, refers to either de novo melanoma that simulates a cellular blue nevus or melanoma that arises in association with a blue nevus.
Balloon cell melanoma	Characterized by the presence of balloon cells that are epithelioid cells containing abundant eosinophilic or foamy cytoplasm.
Clear cell soft part sarcoma	Rare variant of a soft tissue sarcoma showing melanocytic differentiation. These affect soft tissue in the foot and ankle of young adults.
Spitzoid melanoma	Spitz nevus and melanoma histologically simulate one another. Features that favor melanoma include asymmetry, prominent confluence, high cellular density of melanocytes, failure of maturation, deep invasion, increased mitotic rate, deep mitoses, lack of Kamino bodies, and necrosis en masse.
Sarcomatoid melanoma	Rare melanoma with features that simulate a spindle cell or epithelioid cell sarcoma.
Spindle cell melanoma	Proliferation of spindle-shaped melanocytes arranged in fascicles and sheets. These lesions do not demonstrate diffuse and deep involvement.
Follicular melanoma	Follicular melanoma involves hair follicles. Atypical melanocytes may involve the entire length of the hair follicle including the sebaceous duct with extension into the adjacent papillary dermis.
Signet ring cell melanoma	Seen in <0.5% of melanomas and should prompt consideration of metastatic adenocarcinoma. Ultrastructural examination reveals that the vacuolated appearance is most often imparted by the intracytoplasmic accumulation of vimentin.
Myxoid melanoma	Presents as a metastatic tumor deposit that is associated with a primary neoplasm that does not manifest a myxoid morphology. Primary myxoid melanoma has been described in skin and extracutaneous sites including sino-nasal passages.
Rhabdoid melanoma	Rhabdoid features in melanoma consist of sheets of polygonal cells with abundant cytoplasms containing eosinophilic inclusions and peripherally displaced nuclei.
Small cell melanoma	Most frequently encountered in the setting of a melanoma that has arisen in a giant congenital nevus. May show nuclear molding reminiscent of small cell carcinoma or may mimic lymphoblastic lymphoma.

Data from Refs.[11,12]

WORKUP

A complete dermatologic examination is recommended after a patient is diagnosed with melanoma. A detailed personal and family history should be performed as well as physical examination of the head and neck with special attention to local regional areas and lymph node drainage basins of the known primary.

Clinical staging is determined by the examination, biopsy and nodal pathology, and imaging results. In general, staging for cutaneous melanoma is categorized as localized disease (stage I and II), regional disease (stage III), and distant metastatic disease (stage IV).[21]

For stage I-II, no additional workup is needed, as the yield of blood work and imaging studies for asymptomatic distant metastatic disease is low. The National Comprehensive Cancer Network (NCCN) guidelines recommend additional imaging in the setting of a positive review of systems. Consider nodal basin ultrasound before sentinel lymph node biopsy (SLNB) for patients with melanoma with an equivocal regional lymph node physical examination. Abnormalities or suspicious lesions noted on nodal basin ultrasound should be confirmed histologically.

For clinical stage III, an ultrasound-guided fine needle aspiration can be used to confirm metastatic melanoma within lymph nodes. In stage IIIA, consider cross-sectional imaging for baseline staging. Cross-sectional imaging studies include neck/chest/abdominal/pelvic computed tomography (CT) with intravenous (IV) contrast and/or whole-body PET with fludeoxyglucose (FDG)/CT. For stage IIIB/C/D cross-sectional imaging is recommended with or without brain MRI with IV contrast for baseline staging.

Stage IV patients require workup for systemic metastasis. This includes lactate dehydrogenase levels, cross-sectional imaging, and brain MRI with IV contrast. Early detection and treatment of subclinical central nervous system (CNS) metastases are important. Clinically symptomatic CNS metastases are associated with significant morbidity and poor survival. Outcomes after treatment are markedly better in patients with lower CNS tumor burden and/or asymptomatic metastases.[21,22]

CURRENT STAGING

The eighth edition of the American Joint Committee on Cancer (AJCC) staging system is currently the most widely accepted approach to melanoma staging and classification at initial diagnosis. Tables 2 to 4 show the current staging for cutaneous melanoma (**Tables 2–4**).[17,23]

Table 2
T category (primary tumor) criteria in cutaneous melanoma

T Category	Thickness	Ulceration Status
TX: Primary tumor thickness cannot be assessed	Not applicable	Not applicable
T0: No evidence of primary tumor	Not applicable	Not applicable
Tis (melanoma in situ)	Not applicable	Not applicable
T1	≤1 mm	Unknown or unspecified
T1a	<0.8 mm	Without ulceration
T1b	<0.8 mm 0.8–1.0 mm	With ulceration With or without ulceration
T2	>1.0–2.0 mm	Unknown or unspecified
T2a	>1.0–2.0 mm	Without ulceration
T2b	>1.0–2.0 mm	With ulceration
T3	>2.0–4.0 mm	Unknown or unspecified
T3a	>2.0–4.0 mm	Without ulceration
T3b	>2.0–4.0 mm	With ulceration
T4	>4.0 mm	Unknown or unspecified
T4a	>4.0 mm	Without ulceration
T4b	>4.0 mm	With ulceration

Used with permission of the American Joint Committee on Cancer (AJCC), Chicago, Illinois. The original and primary source for this information is the AJCC Cancer Staging Manual, eighth edition (2017) published by Springer International Publishing (Gershenwald JE, Scolyer RA, Hess KR, et al, Melanoma of the skin. In: Amin MB, Edge SB, Greene FL, et al, eds. AJCC Cancer Staging Manual. 8th ed. New York: Springer International Publishing; 2017:563-5854).

Table 3
N category (regional metastasis) criteria for cutaneous melanoma

N Category	Number of Tumor-Involved Regional Lymph Node	Presence of In-Transit, Satellite, and/or Microsatellite Metastases
NX	Regional nodes not assessed (eg, SLN biopsy not performed, regional nodes previously removed for another reason) Exception: When there are no clinically detected regional metastases in a pT1 cM0 melanoma, assign cN0 instead of pNx	No
N0	No regional metastases detected	No
N1	One tumor-involved node or in-transit, satellite, and/or microsatellite metastases with no tumor-involved nodes	
N1a	One clinically occult (ie, detected by SLN biopsy)	No
N1b	One clinically detected	No
N1c	No regional lymph node disease	Yes
N2	Two or 3 tumor-involved nodes or in-transit, satellite, and/or microsatellite metastases with 1 tumor-involved node	
N2a	Two or 3 clinically occult (ie, detected by sentinel lymph node [SLN] biopsy)	No
N2b	Two or 3, at least 1 of which was clinically detected	No
N2c	One clinically occult or clinically detected	Yes
N3	Four or more tumor-involved nodes or in-transit, satellite, and/or microsatellite metastases with 2 or more tumor-involved nodes, or any number of matted nodes without or with in-transit, satellite, and/or microsatellite metastases	
N3a	Four or more clinically occult (ie, detected by SLN biopsy)	No
N3b	Four or more, at least 1 of which was clinically detected, or presence of any number of matted nodes	No
N3c	Two or more clinically occult or clinically detected and/or presence of any number of matted nodes	Yes

Used with permission of the American Joint Committee on Cancer (AJCC), Chicago, Illinois. The original and primary source for this information is the AJCC Cancer Staging Manual, eighth edition (2017) published by Springer International Publishing (Gershenwald JE, Scolyer RA, Hess KR, et al. Melanoma of the skin. In: Amin MB, Edge SB, Greene FL, et al, eds. AJCC Cancer Staging Manual. 8th ed. New York: Springer International Publishing; 2017:563-5854).

SURGICAL TREATMENT

Wide local excision is the recommended treatment for head and neck melanomas and involves removal of all tissue to the level of the fascia, which is typically preserved unless involved by tumor. The NCCN guidelines for margins for cutaneous melanoma in the head and neck do not differ from other regions. Margins are based on Breslow depth of the primary lesion.[21]

- A melanoma in situ, a margin between 0.5 cm to 1.0 cm is recommended.
- A melanoma with a Breslow depth less than or equal to 1.0 mm, a 1.0 cm margin is recommended.
- A melanoma with a Breslow depth between 1.0 mm and 2.0 mm, a margin of 1.0 cm to 2.0 cm is recommended.
- A melanoma with a Breslow depth between 2.0 mm and 4.0 mm, a margin of 2.0 cm is recommended.
- A melanoma with a Breslow depth greater than 4.0 mm, a margin of 2.0 cm is recommended.

Wide margins can pose several treatment challenges in the head and neck region and must take into account anatomic complexity, functional considerations, proximity to vital structures, and cosmetic appearance. The NCCN recognizes these limitations and comments that peripheral resection margins may be modified to accommodate individual anatomic or functional considerations. The safety and efficacy of narrower surgical margins have not been prospectively studied in randomized controlled trials and may increase the risk for margin positivity and/or local recurrence.[21]

Table 4
M category (distant metastasis) criteria for cutaneous melanoma

M Category	Anatomic Site	LDH Level
M0	No evidence of distant metastasis	Not applicable
M1	Evidence of distant metastasis	See below
M1a	Distant metastasis to skin, soft tissue including muscle, and/or nonregional lymph node	Not recorded or unspecified
M1a(0)		Not elevated
M1a(1)		Elevated
M1b	Distant metastasis to lung with or without M1a sites of disease	Not recorded or unspecified
M1b(0)		Not elevated
M1b(1)		Elevated
M1c	Distant metastasis to non-CNS visceral sites with or without M1a or M1b sites of disease	Not recorded or unspecified
M1c(0)		Not elevated
M1c(1)		Elevated
M1d	Distant metastasis to CNS with or without M1a, M1b, or M1c sites of disease	Not recorded or unspecified
M1d(0)		Not elevated
M1d(1)		Elevated

Used with permission of the American Joint Committee on Cancer (AJCC), Chicago, Illinois. The original and primary source for this information is the AJCC Cancer Staging Manual, eighth edition (2017) published by Springer International Publishing (Gershenwald JE, Scolyer RA, Hess KR, et al. Melanoma of the skin. In: Amin MB, Edge SB, Greene FL, et al, eds. AJCC Cancer Staging Manual. 8th ed. New York: Springer International Publishing; 2017:563-5854).

The gold standard for histologic assessment of excised melanoma is use of permanent sections. Frozen sections carry a false negative rate of 5% to 10% and they are not recommended.[24] Consider delay of complex reconstruction or wound closure until histologic margin assessment is complete. Risk factors for upstaging include location in cosmetically or functionally sensitive areas, partial preoperative biopsies, older patient age and non-lentigo maligna histologic subtypes.[20]

Mohs micrographic surgery (MMS) is not recommended for primary treatment of invasive cutaneous melanoma. It may be considered selectively for minimally invasive melanomas when standard margins cannot be achieved in anatomically constrained areas.[21] Large lentigo maligna lesions with an in situ diagnosis may be addressed with MMS. Another option is to use the technique of multiple punch biopsies around the margin of the larger lesion with indistinct borders. This will help to obtain a negative margin when dealing with lesions with indistinct borders. It is also acceptable to place a nonadherent dressing on the open wound and reconstruct the defect after the final pathology is available.

INDICATIONS FOR SENTINEL LYMPH NODE INVESTIGATION

The Multicenter Selective Lymphadenectomy Trial I (MSLT-I) compared wide excision and nodal observation with lymphadenectomy for nodal relapse (observation group) to wide excision and SLNB, with immediate lymphadenectomy for nodal metastases detected on biopsy (biopsy group). Mean 10-year disease-free survival rates were significantly improved in the biopsy group in patients with intermediate-thickness melanomas, defined as 1.20 to 3.50 mm and thick melanomas, defined as greater than 3.50 mm. Sentinel node biopsy–based staging of intermediate-thickness or thick primary melanomas provides important prognostic information and has become standard of care. Biopsy-based management prolongs disease-free survival for all patients and prolongs distant disease–free survival and melanoma-specific survival for patients with nodal metastases from intermediate-thickness melanomas.[25]

The NCCN recommends that SLNB should be discussed and offered for patients with higher-risk stage IB (>1 mm thick or 0.76–1.0 mm thick with ulceration or mitotic rate $\geq$1 per mm^2) or stage II melanoma. Conventional risk factors such as ulceration, high mitotic rate, and lymphovascular invasion are very uncommon in melanomas 0.75 mm thick or less. In the rare event that a conventional high-risk feature is present, the decision about SLNB should be left to the patient and the treating physician. For patients with stage IA melanomas that are 0.76 to 1.0 mm thick without ulceration, and with mitotic rate 0 per mm^2, SLNB should be considered in the appropriate clinical context.[21] Another consideration for SLNB in IA lesions are biopsy specimens that are broadly positive at the deep margin. Thus, the true depth of invasion cannot be determined.

UNIQUE PROBLEMS OF HEAD AND NECK SENTINEL NODE TECHNIQUES

Lymphatic drainage of the head and neck is variable and complex. Aberrant drainage patterns are seen in 24% to 70% of head and neck melanomas and multiple drainage basins are seen in 50% of cases.[26] In rare cases, no lymphatic drainage is seen on preoperative lymphoscintigraphy.[27]

Traditional SLNB technique includes lymphoscintigraphy. Radioactive colloid is injected 2 to 4 hours before the procedure, and a nuclear medicine scan is performed to determine the number and location of nodal basins.[3] This is particularly helpful in head and neck melanomas that may be at risk for bilateral lymphatic drainage when the lesion is located midline. In cases in which there is no visualization of the SLN on lymphoscintigraphy at time of wide local excision, intraoperative injections of radioactive colloid can be considered to identify the SLN intraoperatively. In one study in which no lymphatic drainage was seen on preoperative lymphoscintigraphy, an SLN was found intraoperatively in 64% of cases using this technique.[9]

The melanoma and nodal basin may be in close proximity in the head and neck region and background from the primary injection may overlap with the field of radioactivity of the SLN. Some surgeons use a lower dose of radiotracer when the primary site is near the nodal basin.[27] When there is overlap in the field, the primary lesion may be excised first with appropriate margins so the gamma probe can be used effectively to identify an SLN.[20]

Single-photon emission computed tomography scan (SPECT) aids in identification of SLN in the head and neck. Compared with standard lymphoscintigraphy, SPECT/CT was found to be superior, locating higher number of positive sentinel nodes per patient and higher rate of disease-free survival especially for lesions in the head and neck and should be considered when performing SLNB.[28]

In the operating room, vital blue dye can be injected into the dermis surrounding the primary lesion to aid in identification of the SLN but depends on surgeon preference. The absorptive clearance of blue dye from the dermis can vary widely, and persistently blue dermal bleeding from surgical sites can have some aesthetic implications. The blue dye may diffusely stain the tissue around the resection site. When the nodal basin is in close proximity to the primary site, the dye may lose its effectiveness, so it is recommended to use a maximum 1 mL of dye in the head and neck.[9] The combination of intraoperative hand-held gamma probe and isosulfan blue improved the identification of SLNs in the head and neck to 96% from 93% for intraoperative hand-held gamma probe alone or 73% for isosulfan blue alone[29] (**Fig. 1**A, B).

Indocyanine green can also assist in localization of SLN and has similar or improved rates of nodal localization when compared with vital blue dye. It provides similar lymphatic staining and the additional benefit of being identified using near-infrared spectroscopy imaging rather than direct visualization.[27]

Approximately 25% to 30% of head and neck melanomas drain to lymph nodes within the parotid bed.[23] When SLNB is in the parotid region, a preauricular incision and facial nerve monitor is recommended. Potential injury to the facial nerve has led some surgeons to advocate superficial parotidectomy over the mapping procedure.[10] However, in experienced hands, the sentinel node can be readily identified and excised without any deficits in facial nerve function (**Figs. 2A, B, 3**).

TREATMENT OF LYMPH NODES BASED ON SENTINEL LYMPH NODE BIOPSY

Traditionally, SLNB was used as a staging modality and all patients with positive SLN returned to the operating room for completion lymph-node dissection. Multicenter Selective Lymphadenectomy Trial II (MSLT-II), published in June 2017, specifically evaluated the need for immediate completion lymph-node dissection after positive SLNB. They found a similar 3-year melanoma-specific survival between completion lymph-node dissection within 140 days from positive biopsy and observation with ultrasound surveillance of

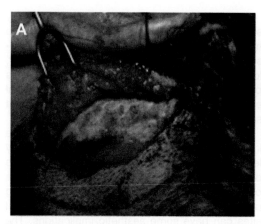
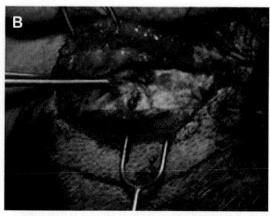

Fig. 1. (*A*) Streak of blue dye in the mastoid area within the lymphatic channel leading to sentinel lymph node. (*B*) Lymph node stained blue.

the affected nodal region. They did find that the immediate completion lymph-node dissection group experienced slightly improved disease-free survival (68% vs 63% *P* = .05) and improved regional control following immediate completion lymph-node dissection versus observation alone (92% vs 77%, *P*<.001). No significant between-group difference in distant metastasis–free survival was detected. Regional control in the head and neck may be more important than other anatomic locations given the critical structures within this region including the trachea, esophagus, cranial nerves, and major vessels. Adverse events were more common among patients after completion lymph-node dissection than among patients in the observation group. A total of 24.1% of the patients in the dissection group and 6.3% of those in the observation group reported

lymphedema (*P*<.001). Other common complications include wound dehiscence and infection.[30]

Melanomas of the anterolateral scalp, temple, lateral forehead, lateral cheek, and ear anterior to the external auditory canal drain via the parotid nodal basin to the jugular lymph node chain.[3] Most nodes are located in the superficial lobe. Approximately two-thirds of glands have nodes in the superficial lobe only and one-third have nodes in the deep and superficial lobes. The superficial nodes drain the pinna, scalp, eyelids, facial skin, and lacrimal glands. The deep nodes, when present, drain the middle ear nasopharynx and soft palate.[31,32] A superficial parotidectomy versus total may be indicated when completion lymph-node dissection is performed. In stage III melanoma, in which metastatic melanoma involves the parotid nodal basin, superficial

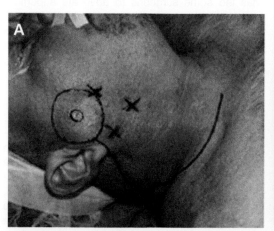
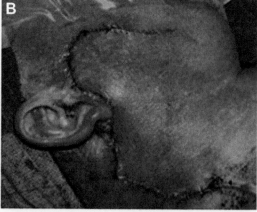

Fig. 2. (*A*) Melanoma primary located directly over the parotid gland. Note location of sentinel nodes in close proximity to the primary tumor. (*B*) The incision for resection of the primary tumor was incorporated with the incision to access the sentinel nodes. The incision was designed as a standard parotidectomy incision so that it can be used if the patient needed a completion parotidectomy and upper neck dissection.

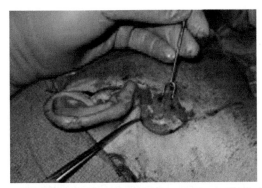

Fig. 3. Note the isosulfan blue injected in the helical rim and an intra parotid node with blue pigmentation. Again, a portion of a parotidectomy incision is used to access the sentinel nodes.

parotidectomy had higher rates of parotid bed melanoma recurrence and recurrence resulting in significant facial nerve functional deficit when compared with total parotidectomy.[33] Melanomas located on the posterior scalp and occiput posterior to the external auditory canal can drain to postauricular, suboccipital, and posterior triangle nodes. These nodal basins are not addressed during modified radical neck dissections, so adjustments may need to be made to address these regions when completion lymph-node dissection is indicated.[34]

SUMMARY

Cutaneous melanoma in the head and neck accounts for 25% of all melanomas. Lentigo maligna melanoma and desmoplastic melanoma have higher incidence in the head and neck region. The NCCN guideline recommendations for surgical margins and SLNB in head and neck melanoma are the same as other cutaneous melanomas but may require case-by-case modifications depending on the location and structures involved in and around the suggested margins. Lymphatic drainage in the head and neck is variable and complex. SPECT/CT has been found to be superior, locating a higher number of positive sentinel nodes per patient and a higher rate of disease-free survival especially for lesions in the head and neck when compared with standard lymphoscintigraphy. The recent MSTL-II trial has shown improvement in regional control and slight improvement in disease-free survival in completion lymph-node dissection versus observation after positive SLNB, but there was no difference in melanoma-specific survival.

CLINICS CARE POINTS

- Incidence of melanoma is continuing to increase and cutaneous melanoma in the head and neck accounts for 25% of all melanomas.

- Lentigo maligna melanoma and desmoplastic melanoma have higher incidence in the head and neck region.

- The NCCN guideline recommendations for cutaneous melanoma surgical margins and SLNB remain unchanged for head and neck melanoma but may require case-by-case modifications depending on the location of the melanoma and structures involved in and around the suggested margins.

- Lymphatic drainage in the head and neck is variable and complex, and SPECT has been shown to help identify SLNs in the head and neck region.

- The recent MSTL-II trial has shown improvement in regional control and slight improvement in disease-free survival in completion lymph-node dissection versus observation after positive SLNB, but there was no difference in melanoma-specific survival.

- Regional control in the head and neck may be more important than other anatomic locations given the critical structures within this region.

DISCLOSURE

The authors have nothing to disclose.

REFERENCES

1. Siegel RL, Miller KD, Jemal A. Cancer statistics, 2018. CA Cancer J Clin 2018;68(1):7–30.

2. Lentsch EJ, Myers JN. Melanoma of the head and neck: current concepts in diagnosis and management. Laryngoscope 2001;111(7):1209–22.

3. Schmalbach C, Durham A, Johnson T, et al. Management of cutaneous head and neck melanoma. In: Flint P, Francis H, Haughey B, et al, editors. Cummings otolaryngology: head and neck surgery. 7th edition. Elsevier; 2021. p. 1124–37.

4. Tseng WH, Martinez SR. Tumor location predicts survival in cutaneous head and neck melanoma. J Surg Res 2011;167(2):192–8.

5. Zenga J, Nussenbaum B, Cornelius LA, et al. Management controversies in head and neck melanoma: a systematic review. JAMA Facial Plast Surg 2017; 19(1):53–62.

6. Košec A, Rašić I, Pegan A, et al. Sex- and site-related significance in cutaneous head and neck

melanoma [published online ahead of print, 2019 Sep 23]. Ear Nose Throat J 2019;100(5):343–9.

7. Kraft S, Granter SR. Molecular pathology of skin neoplasms of the head and neck. Arch Pathol Lab Med 2014;138(6):759–87.

8. International Agency for Research on Cancer Working Group on Artificial Ultraviolet (UV) Light and Skin Cancer. The association of use of sunbeds with cutaneous malignant melanoma and other skin cancers: a systematic review [published correction appears in Int J Cancer. 2007 Jun 1;120(11):2526]. Int J Cancer 2007;120(5):1116–22.

9. Newell GR, Sider JG, Bergfelt L, et al. Incidence of cutaneous melanoma in the United States by histology with special reference to the face. Cancer Res 1988;48(17):5036–41.

10. Haenssle HA, Hoffmann S, Buhl T, et al. Assessment of melanoma histotypes and associated patient related factors: basis for a predictive statistical model. J Dtsch Dermatol Ges 2015;13(1):37–45.

11. Cockerell CJ. The pathology of melanoma. Dermatol Clin 2012;30(3):445–68.

12. Crowson AN, Magro C, Mihm MC Jr. Unusual histologic and clinical variants of melanoma: implications for therapy. Curr Oncol Rep 2007;9(5):403–10.

13. Anderson WF, Pfeiffer RM, Tucker MA, et al. Divergent cancer pathways for early-onset and late-onset cutaneous malignant melanoma. Cancer 2009;115(18):4176–85.

14. Vikey AK, Vikey D. Primary malignant melanoma, of head and neck: a comprehensive review of literature. Oral Oncol 2012;48(5):399–403.

15. Fadaki N, Li R, Parrett B, et al. Is head and neck melanoma different from trunk and extremity melanomas with respect to sentinel lymph node status and clinical outcome? Ann Surg Oncol 2013;20(9):3089–97.

16. Bachar G, Tzelnick S, Amiti N, et al. Patterns of failure in patients with cutaneous head and neck melanoma. Eur J Surg Oncol 2020;46(5):914–7.

17. Keung EZ, Gershenwald JE. The eighth edition American Joint Committee on Cancer (AJCC) melanoma staging system: implications for melanoma treatment and care. Expert Rev Anticancer Ther 2018;18(8):775–84.

18. Lachiewicz AM, Berwick M, Wiggins CL, et al. Survival differences between patients with scalp or neck melanoma and those with melanoma of other sites in the Surveillance, Epidemiology, and End Results (SEER) program. Arch Dermatol 2008;144(4): 515–21.

19. Karimipour DJ, Schwartz JL, Wang TS, et al. Microstaging accuracy after subtotal incisional biopsy of cutaneous melanoma. J Am Acad Dermatol 2005; 52(5):798–802.

20. Etzkorn JR, Sharkey JM, Grunyk JW, et al. Frequency of and risk factors for tumor upstaging after wide local excision of primary cutaneous melanoma. J Am Acad Dermatol 2017;77(2):341–8.

21. Coit DG, Thompson JA, Albertini MR, et al. Cutaneous melanoma, version 2.2019, NCCN clinical practice guidelines in oncology. J Natl Compr Canc Netw 2019;17(4):367–402.

22. Janz TA, Neskey DM, Nguyen SA, et al. Is imaging of the brain necessary at diagnosis for cutaneous head and neck melanomas? Am J Otolaryngol 2018;39(5): 631–5.

23. Gershenwald JE, Scolyer RA, Hess KR, et al. Melanoma staging: evidence-based changes in the American Joint Committee on Cancer eighth edition cancer staging manual. CA Cancer J Clin 2017; 67(6):472–92.

24. Morton DL, Cochran AJ, Thompson JF, et al. Sentinel node biopsy for early-stage melanoma: accuracy and morbidity in MSLT-I, an international multicenter trial. Ann Surg 2005;242(3):302–13.

25. Morton DL, Thompson JF, Cochran AJ, et al. Final trial report of sentinel-node biopsy versus nodal observation in melanoma. N Engl J Med 2014; 370(7):599–609.

26. O'Brien CJ, Uren RF, Thompson JF, et al. Prediction of potential metastatic sites in cutaneous head and neck melanoma using lymphoscintigraphy. Am J Surg 1995;170(5):461–6.

27. Pavri SN, Gary C, Martinez RS, et al. Nonvisualization of sentinel lymph nodes by lymphoscintigraphy in primary cutaneous melanoma: incidence, risk factors, and a review of management options. Plast Reconstr Surg 2018;142(4):527e–34e.

28. Stoffels I, Boy C, Pöppel T, et al. Association between sentinel lymph node excision with or without preoperative SPECT/CT and metastatic node detection and disease-free survival in melanoma. JAMA 2012;308(10):1007–14.

29. Patel SG, Coit DG, Shaha AR, et al. Sentinel lymph node biopsy for cutaneous head and neck melanomas. Arch Otolaryngol Head Neck Surg 2002;128(3):285–91.

30. Faries MB, Thompson JF, Cochran AJ, et al. Completion dissection or observation for sentinel-node metastasis in melanoma. N Engl J Med 2017; 376(23):2211–22.

31. Bialek EJ, Jakubowski W, Zajkowski P, et al. US of the major salivary glands: anatomy and spatial relationships, pathologic conditions, and pitfalls. Radiographics 2006;26(3):745–63.

32. Chason HM, Downs BW. Anatomy, head and neck, parotid gland. In: StatPearls. Treasure Island, FL: StatPearls Publishing; 2020.

33. Wertz AP, Durham AB, Malloy KM, et al. Total versus superficial parotidectomy for stage III melanoma. Head Neck 2017;39(8):1665–70.

34. Goepfert H, Jesse RH, Ballantyne AJ. Posterolateral neck dissection. Arch Otolaryngol 1980;106(10): 618–20.

Lentigo Maligna

Jacob D. Franke, BS[a], Katlyn M. Woolford, BS[a],
Michael W. Neumeister, MD, FRCSC[b],*

KEYWORDS

- Lentigo Maligna • Lentigo Maligna Melanoma • Melanoma in situ

KEY POINTS

- Lentigo maligna (LM) is a melanocytic neoplasm that classically presents in elderly patients as a slowly growing macule on sun-exposed skin.
- LM is the most common melanoma in situ, accounting for 79 to 83% of all cases, and its incidence has been increasing in recent decades.
- LM has a good prognosis but may progress to lentigo maligna melanoma (LMM). Surgical excision is the mainstay of treatment, but traditional margins of 0.5 centimeters may not be adequate and result in recurrence.

INTRODUCTION

Lentigo maligna (LM) is a melanocytic neoplasm found on chronically sun-exposed areas of the body, particularly the head and neck (**Fig. 1**). It commonly occurs in the elderly and has been referred to as a "senile freckle."[1] It has also been termed "Hutchinson melanotic freckle," as it was first described by John Hutchinson in 1892.[2] LM is defined as melanoma in situ and thus confined to the epidermis.[3,4] LM lesions that invade the dermis are termed lentigo maligna melanoma (LMM), 1 of the 4 subtypes of malignant melanoma.[5]

CAUSE

Melanoma has one of the highest somatic mutation rates of all malignancies.[6] Chronic ultraviolet radiation (UR) has been strongly associated with lentigo melanoma.[7,8] One study reported that LMM associations with UR were greatest for individuals born in locations with high levels of UR and continued to reside there throughout adulthood, indicating an accumulative effect.[9] Chronic UR induces melanocyte proliferation and causes oxidative damage that results in mutations of several genes, including BRAF, KIT, and NRAS.[10,11] LM development has also been attributed to UR damage of follicular stem cells.[12] Furthermore, UR has been shown to decrease immune surveillance through immunosuppression of T-cell reactions.[4,13] In addition to UR, LM has been associated with nonpermanent hair dyes, x-ray irradiation, and estrogen/progesterone.[5] Several genetic conditions are associated with LM, including porphyria cutanea tarda, oculocutaneous albinism, xeroderma pigmentosum, and Werner syndrome.[14]

EPIDEMIOLOGY

LM is the most common melanoma in situ, as it comprises 79% to 83% of all cases.[15,16] LMM accounts for 4% to 15% of all melanomas and 10% to 26% of melanomas of the head and neck.[5] LM and LMM predominantly occur in older Caucasian adults with peak incidence occurring between 65 and 80 years of age, but cases have been reported in young adults as well (**Fig. 2**).[5,17,18] The incidence of LM and LMM has been increasing in recent decades. In the Netherlands, the LM incidence rate increased from 0.72 to 3.84 cases/100,000 person-years between 1989 and 2013, whereas the LMM incidence rate increased from 0.24 to 1.19 cases/100,000 person-years in the same time period.[19] Similar trends have been reported in Denmark and Austrialia.[20,21] Age-specific data

[a] Southern Illinois University, School of Medicine, 747 N. Rutledge Street, Springfield, IL 62702, USA;
[b] Department of Surgery, The Elvin G Zook Endowed Chair - Institute for Plastic Surgery, Southern Illinois University, 747 N Rutledge Street #3, Springfield, IL 62702, USA
* Corresponding author.
E-mail address: mneumeister@siumed.edu

Clin Plastic Surg 48 (2021) 669–675
https://doi.org/10.1016/j.cps.2021.06.007
0094-1298/21/© 2021 Elsevier Inc. All rights reserved.

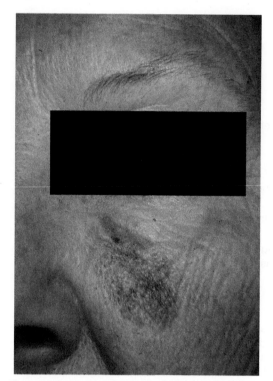

Fig. 1. A classic case of lentigo maligna on the face of an elderly woman.

from California reported large increases in the incidence of LM and LMM from 1990 to 2000. LM diagnoses increased 52% for adults aged 45 to 64 years and 96% for adults 65 years of age or older. LMM incidence increased 88% for individuals 45 to 64 years of age and 105% for individuals 65 years of age or older.[22] The evidence suggests that rates of LM and LMM are increasing faster than any other melanoma subtypes.[19,22] However, there is uncertainty if the data indicate a true increase in incidence or if it is the result of increased awareness and surveillance.[23]

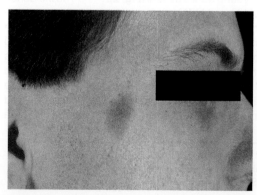

Fig. 2. Despite most commonly occurring in the elderly, this pigmented macule on the face of a young man is consistent with lentigo maligna.

PRESENTATION AND DIAGNOSIS

LM presents clinically as an asymmetric, slowly growing macule on sun-exposed skin (**Fig. 3**). Most of the cases occur in the head and neck, but extrafacial cases can occur on the arms, back, and legs.[5,24] Classically, LM seems as a patch with poorly defined borders and varied pigmentation, with shades from light brown to black.[5] Rarely, LM can present as an amelanotic lesion, appearing as a gradually expanding erythematous patch.[25] Lesions are typically asymptomatic and rarely ulcerated, but advanced tumors may bleed or become painful and itchy.

LM can be challenging to diagnose, because it is often mistaken for other pigmented lesions. Differential diagnoses include solar lentigo, seborrheic keratoses, pigmented actinic keratosis, benign lichenoid keratosis, or pigmented basal cell carcinoma.[26] Excisional biopsy remains the gold standard for diagnosis of LM.[27] Punch biopsies are also used to diagnose LM, because the lesions are often large and found on the face and neck. Punch biopsies of at least 5 mm in diameter are necessary to minimize sampling error.[28,29] Forty-eight percent of lesions are greater than 10 mm in diameter at biopsy.[30] Smaller lesions can be removed through an excisional biopsy. On histology, LM is characterized by the

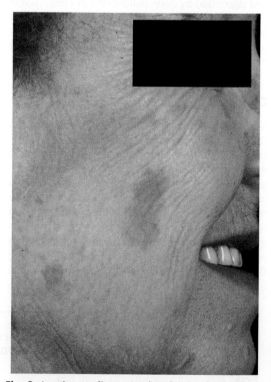

Fig. 3. Lentigo maligna on the cheek of an elderly woman with solar-damaged skin.

proliferation of atypical melanocytes at the dermal-epidermal junction. Extension of melanocytes into periadnexal structures is a common finding.[5] Pagetoid spread, common in the superficial spreading subtype of melanoma, infrequently occurs.[31] Findings of chronic sun damage are typically present, including solar elastosis, increased pigmentation of basal keratinocytes, atrophy of the epidermis, and variable melanocyte hyperplasia, which makes detecting early LM difficult.[32] The melanocytes are often singly arranged in the stratum basale layer, but organized nests of melanocytes and multinucleated melanocytes may be present as well.[32] Immunohistochemistry staining with S100, MART-1, MITF, and Sox10 can aid in reaching a definitive diagnosis.[33]

Although histology remains the diagnostic method of choice, several other diagnostic tools exist including dermoscopy, confocal reflectance microscopy (CRM), and Wood's light examination. Dermoscopy has been reported to have a sensitivity of 89% and a specificity of 98% for the detection of early LM.[34] Dermoscopy can be helpful in distinguishing LM from solar lentigo (SL).[35] SL, commonly called a liver spot, is an irregular pigmented macule on sun-damaged skin that results from keratinocyte and melanocyte hyperplasia without melanocytic atypia or nests.[36] Dermoscopic findings of LM include asymmetric pigmented follicular openings, angulated lines, and gray dot granules.[4,37] CRM is a noninvasive imaging method that uses a 100x microscopy objective to detect tissue architecture at the cellular level.[38] RCM can aid in the diagnosis of hypopigmented lesions without the need for a biopsy, but it is inadequate to evaluate for invasive lesions. RCM is also used to delineate LM margins before surgery and to monitor recurrence following treatment.[39,40] RCM features consistent with LM and LMM include large pagetoid cells greater than 20 μm, nonedged papillae, atypical cells at the dermoepidermal junction, melanophages in the superficial dermis, and follicular localization of atypical cells.[41] The Wood's lamp emits ultraviolet light at wavelengths between 320 and 400 nm. The shorter wavelengths are unable to penetrate the dermis and are absorbed by epidermal melanin. Lesions of the epidermis containing increased melanin fluoresce, which helps delineate the borders between LM and normal skin.[42,43]

PROGNOSIS AND STAGING

LM is benign but has the potential to develop into LMM. The risk of progression from LM to LMM is unknown, but reported rates have varied widely, between 5% and 50%.[44,45] Recently, a study from Australia estimated that the risk of progression was 3.5% per year, which equates to an average time of 28.3 years for LM to progress to LMM.[46] However, cases of progression to LMM in less than 6 months have also been reported.[47] Although no clinical or histologic predictors of progression have been identified, it is proposed that the risk of malignant transformation may be proportional to LM size (**Fig. 4**).[48] Overall, the prognosis for LM is excellent. LMM tends to be thinner than other subtypes of melanoma at presentation, which results in more favorable outcomes, but there is no difference in survival when controlling for thickness of tumor invasion.[5,14] One study reported the 5-year disease-related survival rates for LM and LMM were 100% and 97.1%, respectively.[49] TNM criteria based on the American Joint Committee on Cancer Staging Manual is used to stage LMM, as it is for all melanomas.[50]

TREATMENTS

There are a variety of surgical and nonsurgical methods used to treat LM, although surgical

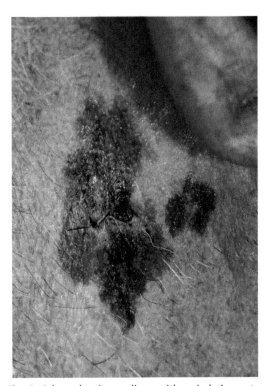

Fig. 4. A large lentigo maligna with varied pigmentation and poorly defined borders that progressed to lentigo maligna melanoma. The diagnosis was made with biopsy.

excision remains the gold standard for care, as it allows for the confirmation of histologically negative margins and results in lower recurrence rates.[51] As the most common location for LM to arise is the neck and face, a tissue sparing technique is best suited for both aesthetics and functionality. Treatment should be initiated as early as possible and several factors should be taken into consideration when determining the best treatment modality: the patient's age, overall health, comorbidities, life expectancy, size and location of the lesion, accessibility of treatment, and patient preferences.[52]

Subclinical extension of LM is common, making it difficult for the lesion to be completely excised. Traditionally margins of 0.5 cm have been used for melanoma in situ, although there is growing evidence that this is inadequate for LM. When traditional excisional methods are performed, LM has an 8% to 20% recurrence rate.[15] One study demonstrated that 0.5 cm margins were adequate in less than 50% of cases, with 53 of the 92 cases requiring safety margins greater than 0.5 cm to achieve complete clearance.[53] Another study of more than 1500 cases of LM treated with Mohs micrographic surgery (MMS) indicated that margins of 0.6 cm had a clearance rate of 79%, whereas 1.2 cm margins yielded a clearance rate of 97% and a recurrence rate of 0.26%.[54] Multiple surgical techniques have been proposed for the treatment of LM including MMS, geometric staged excision, and the spaghetti technique.

In 1941, Frederic Edward Mohs introduced the MSS. It involves excision of the tumor with histologic examination of horizontal and vertical sections to get a 3-dimensional study of the tumor.[55] To examine 100% of the surgical margins, concentric disclike samples are removed, processed, and evaluated intraoperatively. When all margins are histologically confirmed negative, the wound is repaired. Recurrence rates of LM have been demonstrated to be 1.8% to 1.9% when treated with MMS and 5.8% to 5.9% when treated with wide local excision (WLE) by several institutions that perform both MMS and WLE for LM.[56,57] Advantages of this technique include minimal removal of surrounding normal tissue and decreased cost of treatment with removal of the lesion and repair done on the same day.

Staged excision has also been shown to be efficacious in the treatment of LM with a recurrence rate of 1.7%.[58] In this technique a geometric shape is drawn around the demarcated lesion with margins of 0.3 to 0.5 cm. The shape is then excised, processed, and sent for evaluation, and the patient is sent home with a pressure dressing on the wound. Ideally, evaluation of the lesion is completed within 24 hours, allowing the patient to return to the clinic the following day. If the margins are negative, the defect is repaired. If the margins are positive, further stages are excised. One study found that staged excision was associated with a significantly lower recurrence rate and no difference in the final size of the surgical defect when compared with MMS.[59] Similar to the geometric staged excision is the variant "spaghetti technique," which has a reported recurrence rate of 4.76%.[60] This technique involves the removal of a thin strip of skin 0.2 cm wide (the "spaghetti" strand), circumscribing the central demarcated lesion that is left in place. The linear defect is then sutured, and the "spaghetti" strand sent for evaluation. The patient returns at a later date when evaluation of the sample is complete, and further strips of skin are removed until the margins are negative, at which point the central lesion is removed and the defect repaired, avoiding a large open wound.

Although surgical excision is the mainstay of treatment, there are multiple nonsurgical options for those that prefer not to undergo surgery or are otherwise poor surgical candidates, particularly the elderly with comorbidities. Imiquimod 5% cream is a topical immunomodulator that has been reported as a potential second-line treatment for LM, although data on its efficacy have been mixed. Imiquimod's clinical clearance rate is 46% to 78%, and the histologic clearance rate is 37% to 76%.[61,62] Other topical agents including azelaic acid and 5-fluorouracil cream have also been suggested as possible therapeutic modalities. Grenz rays are a type of radiation therapy commonly used in the treatment of LM and have reported cure rates of 86% to 95%.[15] Radiotherapy has good tolerance and generally favorable cosmetic results but does increase risk of squamous cell carcinoma. Cryotherapy has also been used to treat LM, as melanocytes are susceptible to cold-induced damage. Reported recurrence rates for cryotherapy range from 0% to 40%.[51] Cryotherapy is fast and easy to apply, but healing time is longer and scarring may occur. Laser ablation, electrodesiccation and curettage, and chemical peels have also been proposed and studied for the treatment of LM.

SUMMARY

LM is a slow growing melanocytic neoplasm that has been increasing in incidence in recent decades. Its occurrence on chronically sun-damaged skin and its clinical resemblance to benign lesions can make for a challenging diagnosis. Metastasis may occur if LM is left untreated, so early diagnosis and intervention is key with surgical excision being the gold standard.

CLINICS CARE POINTS

- Lentigo maligna is a melanocytic neoplasm associated with chronic ultraviolet radiation.
- Lentigo maligna presents as a slowly growing macule with poorly defined borders and varied pigmentation. It is most commonly found on the head and neck but extrafacial cases can occur on the arms, legs, and back.
- Lentigo maligna can be difficult to differentiate from other pigmented lesions such as solar lentigo, seborrheic keratoses, and pigmented basal cell carcinoma.
- Punch biopsy of at least 5 millimeters and histology is the diagnostic method of choice for lentigo maligna.
- Lentigo maligna is benign but can progress to lentigo maligna melanoma with reported progression rates varying widely between 5-50%.
- Surgical excision is the gold standard of care, though traditional margins of 0.5 centimeters may not be adequate and result in recurrence rates of 8-20%.

DISCLOSURE

The authors have nothing to disclose.

REFERENCES

1. Kallini JR, Jain SK, Khachemoune A. Lentigo maligna: review of salient characteristics and management. Am J Clin Dermatol 2013;14(6):473–80.
2. van Ruth S, Toonstra J. Eponyms of Sir Jonathan Hutchinson. Int J Dermatol 2008;47(7):754–8.
3. Silvers DN. Focus on melanoma: the therapeutic dilemma of lentigo maligna (Hutchinson's freckle). J Dermatol Surg 1976;2(4):301–3.
4. DeWane ME, Kelsey A, Oliviero M, et al. Melanoma on chronically sun-damaged skin: lentigo maligna and desmoplastic melanoma. J Am Acad Dermatol 2019;81(3):823–33.
5. Cohen LM. Lentigo maligna and lentigo maligna melanoma. J Am Acad Dermatol 1995;33(6): 923–36 [quiz 937-40].
6. Alexandrov LB, Nik-Zainal S, Wedge DC, et al. Signatures of mutational processes in human cancer. Nature 2013;500(7463):415–21.
7. Schreiber MM, Moon TE, Bozzo PD. Chronic solar ultraviolet damage associated with malignant melanoma of the skin. J Am Acad Dermatol 1984;10(5 Pt 1):755–9.
8. Elwood JM, Hislop TG. Solar radiation in the etiology of cutaneous malignant melanoma in Caucasians. Natl Cancer Inst Monogr 1982;62:167–71.
9. Linos E, Li WQ, Han J, et al. Lifetime ultraviolet radiation exposure and lentigo maligna melanoma. Br J Dermatol 2017;176(6):1666–8.
10. Noonan FP, Zaidi MR, Wolnicka-Glubisz A, et al. Melanoma induction by ultraviolet A but not ultraviolet B radiation requires melanin pigment. Nat Commun 2012;3:884.
11. Bastian BC. The molecular pathology of melanoma: an integrated taxonomy of melanocytic neoplasia. Annu Rev Pathol 2014;9:239–71.
12. Bongiorno MR, Doukaki S, Malleo F, et al. Identification of progenitor cancer stem cell in lentigo maligna melanoma. Dermatol Ther 2008;21(Suppl 1):S1–5.
13. Bruhs A, Schwarz T. Ultraviolet radiation-induced immunosuppression: induction of regulatory T cells. Methods Mol Biol 2017;1559:63–73.
14. Smalberger GJ, Siegel DM, Khachemoune A. Lentigo maligna. Dermatol Ther 2008;21(6):439–46.
15. Erickson C, Miller SJ. Treatment options in melanoma in situ: topical and radiation therapy, excision and Mohs surgery. Int J Dermatol 2010;49(5):482–91.
16. Hemminki K, Zhang H, Czene K. Incidence trends and familial risks in invasive and in situ cutaneous melanoma by sun-exposed body sites. Int J Cancer 2003;104(6):764–71.
17. Farshad A, Burg G, Panizzon R, et al. A retrospective study of 150 patients with lentigo maligna and lentigo maligna melanoma and the efficacy of radiotherapy using Grenz or soft X-rays. Br J Dermatol 2002;146(6):1042–6.
18. Durnick A, Stolz W, Landthaler M, et al. Lentigo maligna and lentigo maligna melanoma in young adults. Dermatol Surg 2004;30(5):813–6.
19. Greveling K, Wakkee M, Nijsten T, et al. Epidemiology of lentigo maligna and lentigo maligna melanoma in The Netherlands, 1989-2013. J Invest Dermatol 2016;136(10):1955–60.
20. Toender A, Kjær SK, Jensen A. Increased incidence of melanoma in situ in Denmark from 1997 to 2011: results from a nationwide population-based study. Melanoma Res 2014;24(5):488–95.
21. Youl PH, Youlden DR, Baade PD. Changes in the site distribution of common melanoma subtypes in Queensland, Australia over time: implications for public health campaigns. Br J Dermatol 2013; 168(1):136–44.
22. Swetter SM, Boldrick JC, Jung SY, et al. Increasing incidence of lentigo maligna melanoma subtypes: northern California and national trends 1990-2000. J Invest Dermatol 2005;125(4):685–91.
23. Higgins HW, Lee KC, Galan A, et al. Melanoma in situ: Part I. Epidemiology, screening, and clinical features. J Am Acad Dermatol 2015;73(2):181–90 [quiz 191-2].

24. Cox NH, Aitchison TC, MacKie RM. Extrafacial lentigo maligna melanoma: analysis of 71 cases and comparison with lentigo maligna melanoma of the head and neck. Br J Dermatol 1998; 139(3):439–43.

25. Powell AM, Russell-Jones R. Amelanotic lentigo maligna managed with topical imiquimod as immunotherapy. J Am Acad Dermatol 2004;50(5):792–6.

26. McGuire LK, Disa JJ, Lee EH, et al. Melanoma of the lentigo maligna subtype: diagnostic challenges and current treatment paradigms. Plast Reconstr Surg 2012;129(2):288e–99e.

27. Akay BN, Kocyigit P, Heper AO, et al. Dermatoscopy of flat pigmented facial lesions: diagnostic challenge between pigmented actinic keratosis and lentigo maligna. Br J Dermatol 2010;163(6):1212–7.

28. Al-Niaimi F, Jury CS, McLaughlin S, et al. Review of management and outcome in 65 patients with lentigo maligna. Br J Dermatol 2009;160(1):211–3.

29. Stevens G, Cocherell CJ. Avoiding sampling error in the biopsy of pigmented lesions. Arch Dermatol 1996;132(11):1380–2.

30. Tiodorovic-Zivkovic D, Argenziano G, Lallas A, et al. Age, gender, and topography influence the clinical and dermoscopic appearance of lentigo maligna. J Am Acad Dermatol 2015;72(5):801–8.

31. Kraft S, Granter SR. Molecular pathology of skin neoplasms of the head and neck. Arch Pathol Lab Med 2014;138(6):759–87.

32. Reed JA, Shea CR. Lentigo maligna: melanoma in situ on chronically sun-damaged skin. Arch Pathol Lab Med 2011;135(7):838–41.

33. Kasprzak JM, Xu YG. Diagnosis and management of lentigo maligna: a review. Drugs Context 2015;4: 212281.

34. Schiffner R, Schiffner-Rohe J, Vogt T, et al. Improvement of early recognition of lentigo maligna using dermatoscopy. J Am Acad Dermatol 2000;42(1 Pt 1):25–32.

35. Tanaka M, Sawada M, Kobayashi K. Key points in dermoscopic differentiation between lentigo maligna and solar lentigo. J Dermatol 2011;38(1):53–8.

36. Andersen WK, Labadie RR, Bhawan J. Histopathology of solar lentigines of the face: a quantitative study. J Am Acad Dermatol 1997;36(3 Pt 1):444–7.

37. Samaniego E, Redondo P. Lentigo maligna. Actas Dermosifiliogr 2013;104(9):757–75.

38. Rajadhyaksha M, Grossman M, Esterowitz D, et al. In vivo confocal scanning laser microscopy of human skin: melanin provides strong contrast. J Invest Dermatol 1995;104(6):946–52.

39. Ahlgrimm-Siess V, Massone C, Scope A, et al. Reflectance confocal microscopy of facial lentigo maligna and lentigo maligna melanoma: a preliminary study. Br J Dermatol 2009;161(6):1307–16.

40. Connolly KL, Nehal KS, Busam KJ. Lentigo maligna and lentigo maligna melanoma: contemporary issues in diagnosis and management. Melanoma Manag 2015;2(2):171–8.

41. Guitera P, Pellacani G, Crotty KA, et al. The impact of in vivo reflectance confocal microscopy on the diagnostic accuracy of lentigo maligna and equivocal pigmented and nonpigmented macules of the face. J Invest Dermatol 2010;130(8):2080–91.

42. Mustakallio KK, Korhonen P. Monochromatic ultraviolet-photography in dermatology. J Invest Dermatol 1966;47(4):351–6.

43. Robinson JK. Use of digital epiluminescence microscopy to help define the edge of lentigo maligna. Arch Dermatol 2004;140(9):1095–100.

44. McKenna JK, Florell SR, Goldman GD, et al. Lentigo maligna/lentigo maligna melanoma: current state of diagnosis and treatment. Dermatol Surg 2006; 32(4):493–504.

45. Weinstock MA, Sober AJ. The risk of progression of lentigo maligna to lentigo maligna melanoma. Br J Dermatol 1987;116(3):303–10.

46. Menzies SW, Liyanarachchi S, Coates E, et al. Estimated risk of progression of lentigo maligna to lentigo maligna melanoma. Melanoma Res 2020; 30(2):193–7.

47. Kelly JW. Following lentigo maligna may not prevent the development of life-threatening melanoma. Arch Dermatol 1992;128(5):657–60.

48. Iznardo H, Garcia-Melendo C, Yélamos O. Lentigo maligna: clinical presentation and Appropriate management. Clin Cosmet Investig Dermatol 2020;13: 837–55.

49. Gambichler T, Kempka J, Kampilafkos P, et al. Clinicopathological characteristics of 270 patients with lentigo maligna and lentigo maligna melanoma: data from a German skin cancer centre. Br J Dermatol 2014;171(6):1605–7.

50. Gershenwald JE, Scolyer RA. Melanoma staging: American Joint committee on cancer (AJCC) 8th edition and beyond. Ann Surg Oncol 2018;25(8): 2105–10.

51. McLeod M, Choudhary S, Giannakakis G, et al. Surgical treatments for lentigo maligna: a review. Dermatol Surg 2011;37(9):1210–28.

52. Arlette JP, Trotter MJ, Trotter T, et al. Management of lentigo maligna and lentigo maligna melanoma: seminars in surgical oncology. J Surg Oncol 2004; 86(4):179–86.

53. Agarwal-Antal N, Bowen GM, Gerwels JW. Histologic evaluation of lentigo maligna with permanent sections: implications regarding current guidelines. J Am Acad Dermatol 2002;47(5):743–8.

54. Kunishige JH, Doan L, Brodland DG, et al. Comparison of surgical margins for lentigo maligna versus melanoma in situ. J Am Acad Dermatol 2019;81(1): 204–12.

55. Trost LB, Bailin PL. History of Mohs surgery. Dermatol Clin 2011;29(2):135–9, vii.

56. Nosrati A, Berliner JG, Goel S, et al. Outcomes of melanoma in situ treated with Mohs micrographic surgery compared with wide local excision. JAMA Dermatol 2017;153(5):436–41.

57. Hou JL, Reed KB, Knudson RM, et al. Five-year outcomes of wide excision and Mohs micrographic surgery for primary lentigo maligna in an academic practice cohort. Dermatol Surg 2015;41(2):211–8.

58. Abdelmalek M, Loosemore MP, Hurt MA, et al. Geometric staged excision for the treatment of lentigo maligna and lentigo maligna melanoma: a long-term experience with literature review. Arch Dermatol 2012;148(5):599–604.

59. Walling HW, Scupham RK, Bean AK, et al. Staged excision versus Mohs micrographic surgery for lentigo maligna and lentigo maligna melanoma. J Am Acad Dermatol 2007;57(4):659–64.

60. Gaudy-Marqueste C, Perchenet AS, Taséi AM, et al. The "spaghetti technique": an alternative to Mohs surgery or staged surgery for problematic lentiginous melanoma (lentigo maligna and acral lentiginous melanoma). J Am Acad Dermatol 2011;64(1): 113–8.

61. Marsden JR, Fox R, Boota NM, et al. Effect of topical imiquimod as primary treatment for lentigo maligna: the LIMIT-1 study. Br J Dermatol 2017;176(5): 1148–54.

62. Mora AN, Karia PS, Nguyen BM. A quantitative systematic review of the efficacy of imiquimod monotherapy for lentigo maligna and an analysis of factors that affect tumor clearance. J Am Acad Dermatol 2015;73(2):205–12.

Spitz Nevus
Review and Update

Amanda Brown, BS[a], Justin D. Sawyer, MD[a], Michael W. Neumeister, MD, FRCSC[b],*

KEYWORDS

- Spitz nevus • Atypical Spitz nevus • Spindle and epithelioid cell nevus • Skin neoplasm
- Spitz tumor • Spitzoid lesion • Spitzoid melanoma • Juvenile melanoma

KEY POINTS

- Spitzoid melanocytic lesions encompass a spectrum, from benign Spitz nevi to malignant spitzoid melanoma.
- Histopathologic examination of an atypical Spitz lesion by an expert pathologist is mandatory, often followed by expert consultation with a dermatopathologist.
- Younger patients are more likely to have a benign-behaving Spitz nevus.
- Classic, benign Spitz nevi have neat organizational characteristics, such as symmetry, maturation, and distinct margins.
- Most histopathologic criteria remain poorly predictive in cases that overlap between atypical Spitz nevi and melanoma.

INTRODUCTION

A Spitz nevus is a melanocytic neoplasm of epithelioid and/or spindle melanocytes that usually appears in childhood. These lesions are benign; however, their clinical and microscopic characteristics make them difficult to distinguish from melanoma. Because of this, spitzoid neoplasms have been a subject of controversy among clinicians for decades and remain diagnostically challenging. There are 3 classes of spitzoid neoplasms: typical Spitz nevus, atypical Spitz nevus, and spitzoid melanoma. Atypical or borderline Spitz nevi are rare, and show features of both typical Spitz nevi and melanoma. Although Spitz nevi are considered benign, the clinical, dermoscopic, and histopathologic features of the atypical Spitz nevi overlap with those of distinctly malignant spitzoid melanoma.[1] Atypical lesions are the most controversial regarding diagnosis and treatment because their malignant potential remains unknown. However, there have been reports of typical Spitz nevi that have metastasized and resulted in death.[2] More recently, immunophenotypic and molecular analyses have begun to clarify the subtypes of spitzoid lesions.

The diagnosis of a Spitz nevus must be carefully distinguished from melanoma, because the difference may result in unnecessarily aggressive excision and associated morbidities, excision sites, and donor sites for coverage, particularly in the pediatric population.

EPIDEMIOLOGY

Spitz nevi are estimated to represent less than 1% of all childhood melanocytic nevi, and incidence decreases as the patients age.[3] They most commonly appear in the first 2 decades of life with no predilection for sex. Adulthood Spitz nevi tend to affect young women more than men.[3] The age of those diagnosed with Spitz nevus typically ranges from 1 to 61 years, with a mean age of 22 years[4,5]; however, congenital Spitz nevi have been reported.[6] In comparison, spitzoid malignant melanoma has a mean age at diagnosis of 55 years, ranging from 8 to 90 years.[5] The most commonly affected population is white people;

[a] The Institute for Plastic Surgery, Southern Illinois University School of Medicine, 747 N. Rutledge Street, Springfield, IL 62704, USA; [b] The Institute for Plastic Surgery, Department of Surgery, Southern Illinois University, 747 N. Rutledge Street, Springfield, IL 62704 USA
* Corresponding author.
E-mail address: mneumeister@siumed.edu

Clin Plastic Surg 48 (2021) 677–686
https://doi.org/10.1016/j.cps.2021.06.002
0094-1298/21/© 2021 Elsevier Inc. All rights reserved.

however, rare reports have been described in the African American and Asian populations.[7]

Patient age may influence the differential diagnosis of Spitz nevus versus spitzoid malignant melanoma. However, there is overlap in the age distribution of Spitz nevi and melanoma, and studies have shown that the occurrence of Spitz nevi is common in adults.[4] In addition, the diagnosis of melanoma in prepubescent children is exceedingly rare; however, cases of children misdiagnosed with a Spitz nevus followed by wide metastasis and fatality are well documented in the literature.[8] Attempts have been made to quantify the influence of age on differentiating Spitz nevi from melanoma using the Bayes theorem of probability.[9] Nevertheless, careful examination and histologic findings undermine all probabilistic suggestions, and it is essential to consider these lesions even when they seem improbable.

HISTORY

Spitz tumors were first described in 1910 by Darier and Civatte[10] as a rapidly growing red nodule on the cheek of a young boy, and were later characterized by American pathologist Sophie Spitz, in 1948.[11] Although the pediatric lesions were histologically indistinguishable from melanoma, they typically showed benign clinical behavior, lacking the bellicosity associated with melanoma, prompting her to further study the lesions in children.[12] Of 13 children studied, 1 died of extensively metastasized malignant melanoma, whereas the other 12 had excised lesions without recurrence or metastasis. This report challenged the prior notion that these lesions were unable to metastasize in childhood. Spitz coined the name juvenile melanoma, which was later renamed Spitz nevi in her honor.

On histology, Spitz characterized these benign lesions by epidermal changes such as hyperkeratosis, patchy parakeratosis, large acidophilic cells, giant cells, occasional mitotic figures, pigment located in the superficial part of the lesion, and capillary dilatation in the papillary dermis.[11] In particular, the giant cells were described as a distinguishing feature from malignant melanoma of adults, although giant cells have been reported in some melanomas since that time.[13] In 1953, Allen and Spitz[14] refined the description of pathologic criteria for distinguishing Spitz nevi from melanoma.

CLINICAL PRESENTATION

The Spitz nevus most commonly presents in children but they may appear at any age and are typically located on the face, head, neck, or lower extremities (**Fig. 1**). They tend to grow rapidly, reaching a size of approximately 1 cm within 6 months and remaining static thereafter.[15]

The lesions are uniform in color and may range from nonpigmented or pink, to pigmented with a tan, brown, or black-blue appearance. Classically, Spitz nevi are a flat-topped or dome-shaped, reddish-brown or pink papule. It is important to differentiate the red and pink lesions from hemangiomas. In addition, a pigmented spindle cell nevus of Reed is typically a dark, bluish to black papule.

Spitz nevi are most frequently seen in white people, and less commonly in those of African and Asian descent. Data suggest that the hyperpigmented variant may be more common than other color variants in these populations. A 29-year-long retrospective chart review of African American patients diagnosed with a Spitz nevus revealed the most common presentations among the 11 patients identified were hyperpigmentation (73%) and elevation (82%).[7] An additional review in Korea concluded that 49% of 77 patients with a Spitz nevus had the hyperpigmented variety.[16]

Common clinical features of Spitz nevi include small diameter (<5–6 mm), location on the face or lower extremities, and solitary presentation. However, they may erupt as multiple, grouped lesions, coalesced on a base of macular hyperpigmentation.[17,18] Ulceration of a typical Spitz nevus is rare but may be more associated with traumatic excoriation in the pediatric population.

The term atypical Spitz nevus refers to a lesion showing 1 or more atypical features and often an indeterminate potential of malignancy. These lesions tend to be larger than stereotypical Spitz nevi, often greater than 10 mm in diameter. In addition, the atypical class is more often noted to have irregular borders/topography, or ulceration.

Typical and atypical Spitz nevi are both generally asymptomatic. Uncommonly, the lesions may bleed, itch, flake, peel, or be reported as painful, especially during the initial phase of rapid growth.[15]

DIFFERENTIAL DIAGNOSIS

A comprehensive differential diagnosis list is generated by the broad range of phenotypical presentations of Spitz nevi. The list may be tailored according to the particular presentation encountered; for example, erythematous or nonpigmented lesions that bleed easily are commonly misdiagnosed as a pyogenic granuloma or hemangioma. Other nonmelanocytic lesions that may share clinical features with Spitz nevi include juvenile xanthogranuloma, molluscum contagiosum,

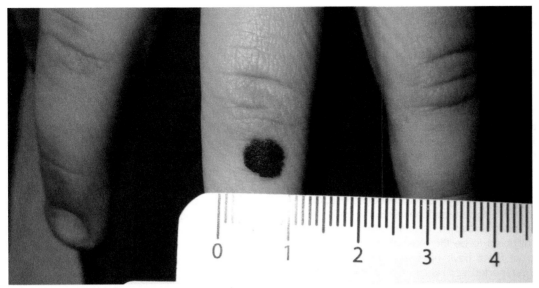

Fig. 1. Spitz nevus on the finger of a 5-year-old child. (*Courtesy of* Joseph Conlon, MD, Springfield, IL.)

and mastocytoma. A melanocytic Spitz nevus may appear similar to a dermatofibroma, acquired or congenital compound nevus, or intradermal nevus. Most of these may be easily distinguished from Spitz nevi on histologic examination; for example, compound nevi lack vertically oriented spindle or epithelioid cells in nests and Kamino bodies.

The histologic differentiation of Spitz tumors from melanoma is a challenging undertaking in dermatopathology. Again, age on presentation is an important, but not absolute, criterion for discernment between these 2 lesions.

DIAGNOSIS

Because of the generally nonspecific gross appearance of Spitz nevi, misdiagnosis is common, as detailed earlier. The diagnosis must be verified via biopsy and pathologic examination. If there is concern for an atypical melanocytic lesion or melanoma, excisional biopsy of the whole lesion is preferred to examine the entire specimen.[1] All biopsies of Spitz nevi should seek confirmatory consultation, because these lesions can lead to metastasis and death, albeit rarely.

A clear consensus does not yet exist for the process of diagnosing Spitz nevi or atypical Spitz lesions. Some clinicians recommend removal for all suspected Spitz nevi in children, whereas others perform partial biopsy or monitor clinically. One survey reports that full-thickness removal by either punch biopsy or excision was chosen by 45% of dermatologists and 96% of plastic surgeons.[19] In children, particularly those less than

12 years old, physicians are more likely to observe the Spitz lesion over time because of the low likelihood of melanoma. A spitzoid lesion appearing in adulthood is generally more alarming, because these are less likely to be a benign Spitz lesion. Each case should be considered in a collaborative effort to ensure the best diagnosis and to avoid overly aggressive treatment, especially in the pediatric population.

DERMOSCOPIC FEATURES

Dermoscopy is often used to evaluate pigmented skin lesions and can be a useful tool in the diagnosis of Spitz nevi. Spitz nevi typically display a starburst pattern caused by peripheral radial lines or pseudopods. The starburst pattern is present in more than 50% of Spitz nevi. The diagnostic sensitivity of the starburst pattern is reported to be 96%.[20]

A globular pattern is observed in approximately 20% of Spitz nevi.[20] These appear as evenly distributed brown globules or large dots. Dotted vessels may be observed within the globules. A symmetric gray-blue color may be noted in the center of the lesion. A classic (pink/red) Spitz nevus may reveal a similar pattern of rounded structures with dotted vessels on a background of little pigmentation.

Dermoscopic recognition of a characteristic starburst or globular pattern may support the diagnosis of a pigmented Spitz nevus. Dermoscopy plays an important role in refining the differential diagnosis of Spitz nevus and melanoma; however, atypical Spitz nevi are often indistinguishable from melanoma. It is still necessary to perform a biopsy or excision for patients with suspicious clinical manifestations or atypical patterns.

PATHOLOGY

The Spitz nevus can be categorized histopathologically as junctional, intradermal, or, in most cases, compound.[7,21] Symmetric, well-circumscribed histology favors the diagnosis of a benign, typical Spitz nevus (**Fig. 2**). The histologic hallmark of a typical Spitz nevus is the presence of epithelioid and/or spindle melanocytes, usually arranged in nests at the base of the elongated rete ridges (**Fig. 3**). The nests are regularly spaced within the uniformly hyperplastic epidermis. Spindle cells are classically considered to be the most abundant cell type in typical Spitz nevi; however, some investigators have reported epithelioid cells as the most abundant cell type.[22,23] Other classic features of Spitz nevi include vertical orientation of melanocytes within the nests, referred to as the bundles-of-bananas or raining-down pattern.[24]

The epithelioid melanocytes of a Spitz nevus are typically large with nuclei that may be appear round, irregularly shaped, or multilobulated. The epithelioid cells are typically more cuboidal compared with the elongated spindle cells. Both epithelioid and spindle melanocytes have abundant cytoplasm that may appear opaque. The mitotic rate in Spitz nevi is low, usually less than $2/mm^2$. Mitoses are rare or absent in the deep dermis.

Features that may appear in both melanoma and typical Spitz nevi include pagetoid growth of melanocytes (upward spreading) and Kamino bodies.[22] Eosinophilic hyaline globules, or Kamino bodies (**Fig. 4**), were historically pathognomonic for Spitz nevi; however, their occurrence was later reported in melanoma (ie, similar globules appear in 2%–26% of melanomas).[25,26] These globules are often situated above the tips of the dermal papillae. Studies have revealed that the globules are composed largely of basement membrane, notably types IV and VII collagen and laminin.[26] Kamino bodies are far more commonly found in Spitz nevi; however, this is no longer pathognomonic for Spitz.

In comparison, distinguishing factors that favor the diagnosis of melanoma, include epidermal atrophy, asymmetry, and abnormal mitosis with a dermal mitotic rate greater than $2/mm^2$.[27] The diagnosis of a benign lesion requires a constellation of findings and is not based on any single finding.

ATYPICAL SPITZ NEVUS PATHOLOGY

A Spitz tumor with 1 or more atypical features, but not enough to qualify as a melanoma, is termed an atypical Spitz nevus. On histology, the intraepidermal features of an atypical Spitz nevus include asymmetry, variation in cell orientation, absent or few Kamino bodies, irregular spacing of nests, presence of coalescing or bridging nests, and significant degrees of melanocyte cytologic atypia.[27,28] Atypical features recognized in the dermis may include increased cellularity, lack of maturation of cells, deep extension to the lowermost dermis or subcutis, presence of mitoses, and disordered infiltration of collagen. Because of the overlapping similarities of benign and malignant pathologies, prediction of biological behavior is most difficult with this spitzoid variant. By definition, these lesions display features that are atypical or borderline, thus a diagnostic consensus is difficult to achieve and there is currently a lack of objective criteria for predicting their malignant potential.[28]

PATHOLOGIC SUBTYPES OF SPITZ NEVUS
Desmoplastic Spitz Nevus

The desmoplastic Spitz nevus is a rare variant of spitzoid lesions that was first described in 1975.[29] This uncommon melanocytic lesion bears histologic similarities to certain benign lesions, such as dermatofibroma, or malignant neoplasms, such as desmoplastic malignant melanoma, thus expanding the differential diagnosis compared with a typical Spitz nevus. If the patient is African American, the differential may also include keloidal nodule.[30] The desmoplastic Spitz nevus is characterized by dermal proliferation of large epithelioid and/or spindle melanocytes within a desmoplastic stroma, comprising thick, eosinophilic collagen bundles. Also known as a sclerotic variant, these lesions are clinically firm or indurated because of marked dermal fibrosis, similar to a scar, that accompanies the nevus.

The eosinophilic stroma often resembles that of dermatofibroma or neurofibroma[31]; however, it may be distinguished by the presence of melanocytes and positive immunohistochemical staining for S100 protein and antibody HMB-45. It is differentiated from a typical Spitz nevus by a lack of Kamino bodies, increased dermal collagen, and presence of ganglionlike epithelioid cells. Junctional activity, nesting, and pigmentation are usually absent. In addition, the symmetry of the lesion, presence of mature melanocytes, and general cell cohesiveness are distinguishing factors from desmoplastic malignant melanoma.

One case study reported the development of 2 desmoplastic Spitz nevi in a 28-year-old woman after receiving a multicolored arm sleeve tattoo.[32] Both lesions appeared in red ink, 1 after 8 to

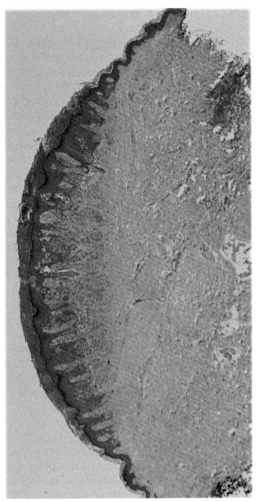

Fig. 2. At low power, the lesion is symmetric and well circumscribed (hematoxylin-eosin [H&E], original magnification ×20). (*Courtesy of* Morgan Wilson, MD, Springfield, IL.)

12 months and the second developed 3 years later. She denied history of similar lesions; thus, the emergence is less easily dismissed as coincidental. Perhaps a chemical property of the red ink or mechanical trauma from the tattoo gun triggered an inflammatory response, initiating the development of desmoplastic nevi. In addition, there are reports of melanoma, among other cutaneous malignancies, developing within the margins of a tattoo; however, this is the first report of a Spitz variant and the strength of association remains uncertain.[33]

Childhood Versus Adult Spitz Nevus

Several large series have documented that more than half of patients diagnosed with Spitz nevi

are less than 20 years old.[34] Children are much more likely to develop Spitz nevi than melanomas, whereas the converse is true for adults. In general, clinicians are more likely to recommend excision of a spitzoid lesion for adults because of the correlation of increasing age and melanoma, whereas children less than 10 to 12 years old may be closely monitored.

Desmoplastic Spitz nevi are more common in young adults, with a mean age at diagnosis reported as 28.2 years, versus the mean age at diagnosis of desmoplastic melanoma at 75 years.[35] Melanoma in children is exceedingly rare; however, atypical lesions occur and some may be misdiagnosed melanomas.[12] The classic ABCDE (Asymmetry, Border irregularity, Color variation, Diameter ≥ 6 mm, and Evolution over time) criteria for melanoma occur in only 40% of children less than 10 years old with melanoma.[36]

Interestingly, 1 study found that adults with history of a Spitz nevus had increased likelihood of developing a separate primary melanoma, possibly suggesting a general predilection to melanocytic neoplasia and the need for periodic total-body skin examinations.[37] Whether this association exists in childhood Spitz nevi is yet to be determined.

ANCILLARY TESTS

The histologic distinction between atypical Spitz nevus and spitzoid melanoma is difficult. Immunohistochemical markers and/or genetic testing that reveals the presence (or absence) of certain chromosomal variations can be helpful in distinguishing the two. Spitz lesions have been evaluated with a throng of melanocytic markers, including S-100, Melan-A/Mart-1, HMB-45, and apoptosis regulators, including Ki-67, cyclin D1, p15, and p16.[38,39] These tools are helpful in combination with clinical and histologic features for challenging cases; however, their power in predicting the biological behavior of atypical Spitz nevi is uncertain and requires continued evaluation with larger studies.

Ki-67 is a nuclear protein expressed most highly during mitosis that has been helpful in the distinction of benign Spitz nevi from malignant melanoma. The expression of Ki-67 correlates with the risk stratification of Spitz tumors, with a low index typical of a benign nevus and a higher index in a melanoma.[40]

HMB-45 is a melanogenesis protein used to assess the maturation and depth of a lesion. Typically, expression of this protein decreases toward the base of Spitz lesions, whereas melanoma shows a more uniform distribution.[41] This marker has high sensitivity for melanoma (92%); however,

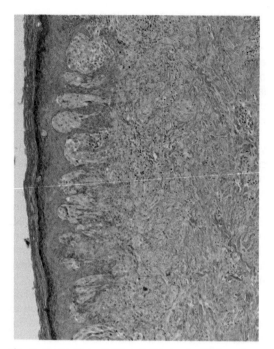

Fig. 3. Nests of vertically oriented, spindled melanocytes are noted between elongated rete ridges (H&E, original magnification ×100). (*Courtesy of* Morgan Wilson, MD, Springfield, IL.)

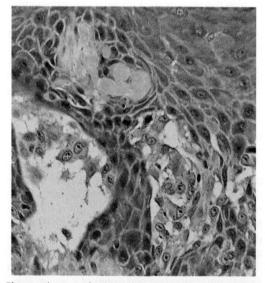

Fig. 4. The neoplastic melanocytes have large, oval nuclei with prominent nucleoli. Within the overlying epidermis, there is a pale, eosinophilic globule (Kamino body) (H&E, original magnification ×400) (*Courtesy of* Morgan Wilson, MD, Springfield, IL.)

it does not react with spindle cell melanomas or desmoplastic melanomas.[42]

An antibody panel consisting of p16, Ki-67, and HMB-45 has been reviewed as a discriminatory tool in atypical spitzoid tumors versus spitzoid melanoma. One retrospective study introduced a grading scale, known as the PKH (p16-Ki-67-HMB45) score, and found significantly higher scores associated with melanoma.[39]

PRAME (preferentially expressed antigen in melanoma) is a melanoma-associated antigen isolated by autologous T cells in patients with melanoma. This marker has shown utility in the distinction of melanoma from some benign melanocytic lesions. A recent study found that, out of 140 cutaneous melanocytic nevi, 86.4% were completely negative for PRAME; however, the 13.6% of nevi that were immunoreactive included some benign and atypical Spitz lesions.[43] Although it is not common for Spitz lesions to be immunoreactive,[44] knowledge of the PRAME expression pattern in indefinite histopathologic or spitzoid lesions is currently limited.

In addition to Ki-67 and HMB-45, other markers with increased expression in melanoma include p53, cyclin D1, and p21.[41] Most of these significant differences are related to cell-cycle dysregulation and high mitotic activity.

MOLECULAR STUDIES

Abnormal DNA contents have been detected in various Spitz lesions. Whole-genome analysis by comparative genomic hybridization (CGH) revealed that a minority (approximately 20%) of Spitz nevi have amplification of chromosome 11p (a genome area housing the *HRAS* gene).[45] This feature is not commonly seen in melanoma; however, *HRAS* has been correlated to some spitzoid melanomas and therefore may have lower specificity for benign Spitz nevi.[46,47] Further, *HRAS*-positive Spitz nevi typically show increased expression of p16 and cyclinD1 via immunohistochemistry. A study of 16 atypical Spitz tumors with array CGH showed that nearly all chromosomal variations present were not seen in melanoma,[48] suggesting that atypical Spitz nevi may be distinguishable from melanoma genetically.

In contrast with CGH, fluorescence in situ hybridization (FISH) probes specific loci on chromosomes to show gains or losses via a fluorescent tag. FISH analysis is a helpful ancillary diagnostic tool for confirming melanomas, and 1 study found that 4 probes targeting chromosomes 6p25, 6-centromere, 6q23, and 11q13 showed 86.7% sensitivity and 95.4% specificity of the validation cohort.[49] Although FISH may be useful in diagnosing melanoma,[50] this technique is increasingly discouraged in the evaluation of atypical Spitz lesions. In 1 study, FISH failed to identify a fatal, metastatic, atypical Spitz tumor because of lack of expressing the most common aberrations in melanoma involving chromosomes 6 and 11p.[48] Thus, a comprehensive full-genome evaluation offers greater sensitivity and specificity than currently available FISH probes in identifying Spitz lesions with uncertain biological behavior.

An autosomal dominant inactivating mutation in the BAP1 (BRCA1-Associated Protein 1) gene has been associated with increased susceptibility to several tumors, including atypical Spitz tumors, cutaneous melanoma, uveal melanoma, and mesothelioma.[51] Sometimes referred to as BAP1-inactivated melanocytic tumors, these tumors usually show BRAF (protein kinase B-raf) mutations, which are typically absent in Spitz tumors.

TREATMENT OF SPITZ NEVUS

Most practitioners continue to biopsy all suspected Spitz nevi out of concern for melanoma. A consensus-based algorithm for management of spitzoid lesions was proposed in 2017.[1] According to this algorithm, the lowest-risk lesion is symmetric, in a patient less than 12 years old, nonnodular, with a starburst pattern; these lesions may be closely monitored and removed if asymmetric evolution or other concerning features develop. Lesions with concern for atypia or melanoma are recommended to be removed with 3-mm to 5-mm margins. Confirmed atypical Spitz lesions with positive margins should undergo reexcision to attain clear margins. Removal of the entire lesion reduces the risk of recurrence.[2] Clinical follow-up with superficial node palpation is recommended at least once per year for 3 years. Higher-risk lesions, including dermatoscopically asymmetric lesions with spitzoid features (both flat/raised and nodular) should be excised to rule out melanoma with wide, 1-cm margins.

The ancillary testing to establish a diagnosis and treatment plan can be time consuming and delay therapy. When the behavior of a biopsied lesion cannot be predicted with certainty or if there is poor interobserver agreement, these patients should be evaluated with their best interests in mind. All patients should have regular follow-ups to check for changes or recurrences regardless of treatment plan.

SENTINEL LYMPH NODE BIOPSY

The controversy in determining the biological potential of an atypical Spitz lesion arises from histopathologic changes beyond what would be expected for a Spitz nevus, but without fulfilling the criteria of melanoma. The sentinel lymph node biopsy was proposed as a possible solution to this problem, based on the notion that melanocytic cells in the sentinel lymph nodes show malignant potential. However, melanocytic cell deposits are frequently found in the sentinel nodes of patients with atypical Spitz tumors and their prognosis remained substantially better than that of patients with melanoma and positive sentinel lymph nodes.[52,53] A systematic review of 541 patients with atypical Spitz tumors found that presence of a positive sentinel lymph node was not associated with an unfavorable outcome.[52] Therefore, the peculiar ability of an atypical Spitz nevus to spread to nearby lymph nodes does not necessarily prove malignancy. In summary, complete excision with clear margins and careful follow-up are sufficient for atypical Spitz tumors, especially in pediatric patients.

EVOLUTION OF SPITZ NEVUS

Evolution is a well-known characteristic of Spitz nevi. Dermoscopy is an important tool used to follow the morphologic changes of these lesions. They typically show an initial phase of rapid growth lasting approximately 6 months, followed by a stagnant period.[15] Following this, the most common evolution seems to be involution, occurring in about 80% of Spitz nevi[21]; however, the proper diagnosis is impossible to confirm without biopsy and histopathologic evaluation by a dermatopathologist. Both pigmented and nonpigmented forms can regress partially or completely.[15]

One study with clinical follow-up data showed evolution of the dermoscopic pattern in 21 of 27 nevi (68%), whereas a stable pattern was noted in the remaining 6 (22%).[20] The evolution could include changes in features, size, and color. Of dermoscopic patterns, a common evolution is transformation from starburst or globular pattern to a brown homogeneous pattern. In addition, these lesions revealed a sequential evolution pattern from globular, to starburst, then to a homogeneous pattern, whereas other lesions showed progression from globular directly to a homogenous pattern. Notably, the absence of evolution supports a diagnosis of Spitz nevus because of the near-universal finding of evolution in pediatric and adult melanomas.[20]

PROGNOSIS

To help determine whether an atypical Spitz tumor is at medium, moderate, or high risk of metastasis, a grading system based on the patient's age and a subset of morphologic characteristics was proposed 2 decades ago.[54] In summary, patients less than 10 years old, lesions less than 10 mm, absent subcutaneous involvement, absent ulceration, and 0 to 5 mm^2 of mitotic activity show the best prognosis. Spitz nevi with typical features on presentation and biopsy have the most favorable prognosis. Age is one of the main criteria to discriminate Spitz lesions with indolent behavior from atypical Spitz nevi with greater risk of malignancy and melanoma. However, age should not be overly relied on to diagnose benign versus malignant lesions, and all diagnoses of Spitz nevi should seek confirmatory consultation because of the uncommon ability for the lesions to lead to metastasis and death.[8]

One longitudinal study investigated the long-term outcome of 144 patients with typical or atypical Spitz nevi and found that none developed metastasis after a median follow-up of 9 years.[37] Other studies investigating long-term outcomes have reached similar conclusions.[53,55] However, 6 of the 144 developed a separate melanoma, suggesting a potential increased risk of melanoma in those with history of Spitz nevus. This association is yet to be fully elucidated. In general, with regard to the prognosis in the case of typical Spitz nevi with low-risk clinical features, it is reasonable to be cautiously optimistic.

SUMMARY

Spitzoid melanocytic lesions encompass a spectrum, from benign Spitz nevi to malignant spitzoid melanoma. Benign biological behavior of a Spitz lesion can usually be determined via light microscopy when typical features are found. The clinical relevance of Spitz nevi lies within the continuous challenge in distinguishing atypical Spitz features from melanoma. Histopathologic examination of an atypical Spitz lesion by an expert pathologist is mandatory, often followed by expert consultation with a dermatopathologist. Recent advances in immunohistochemistry and molecular studies will continue to provide more answers as more patients are examined.

CLINICS CARE POINTS

- Clinicians are more likely to recommend excision of a spitzoid lesion for adults because of the correlation of increasing age and

melanoma, whereas children less than 10 to 12 years old may be closely monitored.

- The diagnosis of a Spitz nevus must be carefully distinguished from melanoma, because the difference may result in unnecessarily aggressive excision and associated morbidities.

- Lesions with concern for atypia or melanoma are recommended to be removed with 3-mm to 5-mm margins. Confirmed atypical Spitz lesions with positive margins should undergo reexcision to attain clear margins.

- The best prognosis is shown by patients who are less than 10 years old with lesion less than 10 mm, absent subcutaneous involvement, absent ulceration, and 0 to 5 mm^2 of mitotic activity.

DISCLOSURE

The authors have nothing to disclose.

REFERENCES

1. Lallas A, Apalla Z, Ioannides D, et al. Update on dermoscopy of Spitz/Reed naevi and management guidelines by the International Dermoscopy Society. Br J Dermatol 2017;177(3):645–55.
2. Luo S, Sepehr A, Tsao H. Spitz nevi and other spitzoid lesions part II. Natural history and management. J Am Acad Dermatol 2011;65(6):1087–92.
3. Dika E, Ravaioli GM, Fanti PA, et al. Spitz nevi and other spitzoid neoplasms in children: overview of incidence data and diagnostic criteria. Pediatr Dermatol 2017;34(1):25–32.
4. Cesinaro AM, Foroni M, Sighinolfi P, et al. Spitz nevus is relatively frequent in adults: a clinicopathologic study of 247 cases related to patient's age. Am J Dermatopathol 2005;27(6):469–75.
5. Lott JP, Wititsuwannakul J, Lee JJ, et al. Clinical characteristics associated with Spitz nevi and spitzoid malignant melanomas: the Yale University spitzoid neoplasm repository experience, 1991 to 2008. J Am Acad Dermatol 2014;71(6):1077–82.
6. Schaffer JV. Update on melanocytic nevi in children. Clin Dermatol 2015;33(3):368–86.
7. Farid YI, Honda KS. Spitz nevi in African Americans: a retrospective chart review of 11 patients. J Cutan Pathol 2021;48(4):511–8.
8. Barnhill RL, Argenyi ZB, From L, et al. Atypical Spitz nevi/tumors: lack of consensus for diagnosis, discrimination from melanoma, and prediction of outcome. Hum Pathol 1999;30(5):513–20.
9. Vollmer RT. Patient age in Spitz nevus and malignant melanoma: implication of Bayes rule for differential diagnosis. Am J Clin Pathol 2004;121(6):872–7.

10. Darier J, Civatte J. Naevus ou naevo-carci nome chez un nourisson. Bull Soc Fanc Derm 1910;21:61-3.

11. Spitz K, Piliang M, Mostow E. Sophie Spitz: a woman ahead of her time. Int J Womens Dermatol 2019; 5(3):190-1.

12. Spitz S. Melanomas of childhood. Am J Pathol 1948; 24(3):591-609.

13. Kim HY, Yoon JH, Cho EB, et al. A case of spitzoid melanoma. Ann Dermatol 2015;27(2):206-9.

14. Allen AC, Spitz S. Malignant melanoma; a clinico-pathological analysis of the criteria for diagnosis and prognosis. Cancer 1953;6(1):1-45.

15. Voloshynovych M, Rosendahl C, Girnyk G, et al. Clinical evolution of Spitz nevi. Galacian Med J 2020;27(2).

16. Kim YC, Do JE, Bang D, et al. Spitz naevus is rare in Korea. Clin Exp Dermatol 2010;35(2):135-9.

17. Boone SL, Busam KJ, Marghoob AA, et al. Two cases of multiple spitz nevi: correlating clinical, histologic, and fluorescence in situ hybridization findings. Arch Dermatol 2011;147(2):227-31.

18. Mazzurco J, Menssen K, Schapiro B, et al. Eruptive disseminated Spitz nevi in a 26-year-old African-American woman. Int J Dermatol 2012;51(10):1270-1.

19. Metzger AT, Kane AA, Bayliss SJ. Differences in treatment of Spitz nevi and atypical Spitz tumors in pediatric patients among dermatologists and plastic surgeons. JAMA Dermatol 2013;149(11):1348-50.

20. Emiroglu N, Yildiz P, Biyik Ozkaya D, et al. Evolution of Spitz nevi. Pediatr Dermatol 2017;34(4):438-45.

21. Argenziano G, Agozzino M, Bonifazi E, et al. Natural evolution of Spitz nevi. Dermatology 2011;222(3): 256-60.

22. Verardino GC, Rochael MC. Spitz nevi in the classic histopathological pattern–lamb in wolf's clothing. An Bras Dermatol 2015;90(1):91-5.

23. Requena C, Requena L, Kutzner H, et al. Spitz nevus: a clinicopathological study of 349 cases. Am J Dermatopathol 2009;31(2):107-16.

24. Hillen LM, Van den Oord J, Geybels MS, et al. Genomic landscape of spitzoid neoplasms impacting patient management. Front Med (Lausanne) 2018;5:344.

25. Kamino H, Flotte TJ, Misheloff E, et al. Eosinophilic globules in Spitz's nevi. New findings and a diagnostic sign. Am J Dermatopathol 1979;1(4):319-24.

26. Venkatesh D, Smitha T. Kamino bodies. J Oral Maxillofac Pathol 2019;23(1):17-8.

27. Crotty KA, Scolyer RA, Li L, et al. Spitz naevus versus Spitzoid melanoma: when and how can they be distinguished? Pathology 2002;34(1):6-12.

28. Harms KL, Lowe L, Fullen DR, et al. Atypical spitz tumors: a diagnostic challenge. Arch Pathol Lab Med 2015;139(10):1263-70.

29. Reed RJ, Ichinose H, Clark WH, et al. Common and uncommon melanocytic nevi and borderline melanomas. Semin Oncol 1975;2:119-47.

30. Yu J, Jen MV, Yan AC, et al. Angiomatoid and desmoplastic Spitz nevus presenting as a keloidal nodule. Pediatr Dermatol 2018;35(4):e228-30.

31. Sherrill AM, Crespo G, Prakash AV, et al. Desmoplastic nevus: an entity distinct from spitz nevus and blue nevus. Am J Dermatopathol 2011;33(1): 35-9.

32. Saunders BD, Nguyen M, Joo JS, et al. Desmoplastic intradermal spitz nevi arising within red tattoo ink. Dermatol Online J 2018;24(11):13030/qt15r7x0pt.

33. Paprottka FJ, Krezdorn N, Narwan M, et al. Trendy tattoos-maybe a serious health risk? Aesthetic Plast Surg 2018;42(1):310-21.

34. Tlougan BE, Orlow SJ, Schaffer JV. Spitz nevi: beliefs, behaviors, and experiences of pediatric dermatologists. JAMA Dermatol 2013;149(3):283-91.

35. Nojavan H, Cribier B, Mehregan DR. Desmoplastic Spitz nevus: a histopathological review and comparison with desmoplastic melanoma. Ann Dermatol Venereol 2009;136(10):689-95.

36. Saiyed FK, Hamilton EC, Austin MT. Pediatric melanoma: incidence, treatment, and prognosis. Pediatr Health Med Ther 2017;8:39-45.

37. Sepehr A, Chao E, Trefrey B, et al. Long-term outcome of Spitz-type melanocytic tumors. Arch Dermatol 2011;147(10):1173-9.

38. Ma SA, O'Day CP, Dentchev T, et al. Expression of p15 in a spectrum of spitzoid melanocytic neoplasms. J Cutan Pathol 2019;46(5):310-6.

39. Garola R, Singh V. Utility of p16-Ki-67-HMB45 score in sorting benign from malignant Spitz tumors. Pathol Res Pract 2019;215(10):152550.

40. Kapur P, Selim MA, Roy LC, et al. Spitz nevi and atypical Spitz nevi/tumors: a histologic and immunohistochemical analysis. Mod Pathol 2005;18(2): 197-204.

41. Garrido-Ruiz MC, Requena L, Ortiz P, et al. The immunohistochemical profile of Spitz nevi and conventional (non-Spitzoid) melanomas: a baseline study. Mod Pathol 2010;23(9):1215-24.

42. Weedon D. Weedon's skin pathology. 3rd Ed. London (UK): Churchill Livingstone, ISBN 9780702034855; 2010. p. 706-56.

43. Lezcano C, Jungbluth AA, Nehal KS, et al. PRAME expression in melanocytic tumors. Am J Surg Pathol 2018;42(11):1456-65.

44. Raghavan SS, Wang JY, Kwok S, et al. PRAME expression in melanocytic proliferations with intermediate histopathologic or spitzoid features. J Cutan Pathol 2020;47(12):1123-31.

45. Ali L, Helm T, Cheney R, et al. Correlating array comparative genomic hybridization findings with histology and outcome in spitzoid melanocytic neoplasms. Int J Clin Exp Pathol 2010;3(6): 593-9.

46. van Engen-van Grunsven AC, van Dijk MC, Ruiter DJ, et al. HRAS-mutated Spitz tumors: a

subtype of Spitz tumors with distinct features. Am J Surg Pathol 2010;34(10):1436–41.

47. Wan X, Liu R, Li Z. The prognostic value of HRAS mRNA expression in cutaneous melanoma. Biomed Res Int 2017;2017:5356737.

48. Raskin L, Ludgate M, Iyer RK, et al. Copy number variations and clinical outcome in atypical spitz tumors. Am J Surg Pathol 2011;35(2):243–52.

49. Gerami P, Jewell SS, Morrison LE, et al. Fluorescence in situ hybridization (FISH) as an ancillary diagnostic tool in the diagnosis of melanoma. Am J Surg Pathol 2009;33(8):1146–56.

50. Wiesner T, Kutzner H, Cerroni L, et al. Genomic aberrations in spitzoid melanocytic tumours and their implications for diagnosis, prognosis and therapy. Pathology 2016;48(2):113–31.

51. Murali R, Wiesner T, Scolyer RA. Tumours associated with BAP1 mutations. Pathology 2013;45(2):116–26.

52. Lallas A, Kyrgidis A, Ferrara G, et al. Atypical Spitz tumours and sentinel lymph node biopsy: a systematic review. Lancet Oncol 2014;15(4):e178–83.

53. Caraco C, Mozzillo N, Di Monta G, et al. Sentinel lymph node biopsy in atypical Spitz nevi: is it useful? Eur J Surg Oncol 2012;38(10):932–5.

54. Spatz A, Calonje E, Handfield-Jones S, et al. Spitz tumors in children: a grading system for risk stratification. Arch Dermatol 1999;135(3):282–5.

55. Cerrato F, Wallins JS, Webb ML, et al. Outcomes in pediatric atypical spitz tumors treated without sentinel lymph node biopsy. Pediatr Dermatol 2012;29(4):448–53.

Melanoma of the Hands and Feet (With Reconstruction)

Alexis M. Ruffolo, MD[a],*, Ashwath J. Sampath, MD[b],
Jeffrey H. Kozlow, MD, MS[c], Michael W. Neumeister, MD[a]

KEYWORDS

• Melanoma • Subungual melanoma • Reconstruction

KEY POINTS

- Melanoma of the hand and foot has a worse prognosis than cutaneous melanomas at other sites, possibly due to delayed diagnosis and anatomic challenges to treatment.
- Acral lentiginous melanoma is the most common type of melanoma on acral skin, characterized by a radial growth phase evolving to a vertical growth phase.
- Melanoma of the hand and foot is primarily treated with surgical excision and reconstruction.
- Reconstruction of the hand and foot after excision of melanoma should restore anatomy while maximizing preservation of function.

IMPORTANCE OF HAND AND FOOT MELANOMA

While melanoma only comprises 4% of all dermatologic cancers, it accounts for 80% of the deaths.[1] Incidence of melanoma has been rising throughout the world in recent decades. In the United States, incidence rates have increased 1.8% annually from 2012 to 2016.[2] Meanwhile, stage and thickness at the time of diagnosis have improved leading to a slower increase in mortality than incidence.[1] Melanomas of the hand and foot have a worse prognosis compared with melanomas in other anatomic regions. It is hypothesized that the poor prognosis of hand and foot melanomas may be due to the aggressive nature of acral lentiginous melanoma (ALM), which is the most common subtype found in the hand and foot, or delayed treatment resulting from a diagnosis late in the clinical course.[3] In addition,

compared with other types of cutaneous hand malignancies, melanoma is the least frequent, but with higher rates of lymph node metastasis and death.[4] The scarcity and heterogeneity of studies regarding hand and foot melanoma limit the development of definitive diagnostic and therapeutic guidelines.

The care of a patient with melanoma of the hand or foot is provided through many physicians including primary care physicians, dermatologists, surgical oncologists, and plastic surgeons whose services must be coordinated to diagnose, biopsy, and treat in a timely manner.

Melanomas of the hand and foot are primarily treated surgically. The hand and foot both provide an anatomic treatment challenge. There is a limited subcutaneous layer in the hand with underlying structures that are relatively superficial and at risk of involvement by melanoma or at risk of damage with surgical excision of the melanoma.

No conflict of interest.
No funding sources have supported this work.
[a] Division of Plastic Surgery, Southern Illinois University School of Medicine, 747 N Rutledge Street #3, Springfield, IL 62702, USA; [b] Department of Internal Medicine, St. Louis University School of Medicine, 1201 S Grand Boulevard, St Louis, MO 63104, USA; [c] Section of Plastic and Reconstructive Surgery, University of Michigan School of Medicine, 1500 East Medical Center Drive, Ann Arbor, MI 48109, USA
* Corresponding author. 747 N Rutledge Street #3, Springfield, IL 62702.
E-mail address: aruffolo57@siumed.edu

Clin Plastic Surg 48 (2021) 687–698
https://doi.org/10.1016/j.cps.2021.05.009

Moreover, the hand is specialized and structurally unique, and reconstruction of hand soft-tissue defects must take into account the need to restore and protect function.[4] The challenges of melanoma on the foot include the importance of weight-bearing on the plantar surface combined with overall demands placed on the soft tissues with ambulation.

This review will highlight the major histologic subtypes of melanoma found on the hand or foot, the typical topical distribution, prognosis, and surgical management.

MAJOR HISTOLOGIC SUBTYPES OF MELANOMA

There are six major histologic subtypes of melanoma.[5]

Superficial spreading melanoma is the most common variant. This subtype presents most commonly on the back in males and on the leg in females. It is histologically characterized by atypical epithelioid melanocytes, found alone or in clusters, scattered throughout the epidermis (referred to as "buckshot scatter"). Superficial spreading melanoma tumor cells have abundant cytoplasm, nuclear pleomorphism, and prominent nucleoli.

Nodular melanoma presents as a rapidly enlarging nodule. It is histologically characterized by a dermal mass of dysplastic tumor cells with upward epidermal invasion but with minimal adjacent epidermal spread or horizontal growth. Nodular melanoma tumor cells are round and epithelioid with hyperchromatic nuclei.

Lentigo maligna melanoma (LMM) occurs in chronically sun-exposed skin—scalp, face, neck—and presents as a slowly enlarging, irregularly shaped, and pigmented macule. LMM is a precursor lesion and form of melanoma in situ. On histology, both dermal and epidermal changes are present. Most notably, there is variable epidural atrophy and proliferation of dysplastic melanocytes at the dermoepidermal junction with extension into the adnexal structures, with solar elastosis and presence of melanophages and small foci of lymphocytes in the dermis.

Lentiginous melanoma is a newly classified, slowly progressive melanoma that presents in sun-damaged skin of the trunk and limbs. Histologically there is lentiginous hyperplasia as well as focal junctional nests of melanocytes with varying cytologic atypia and pagetoid spread of single melanocytes.

Desmoplastic melanoma is a slow growing, often nonpigmented lesion that typically occurs (>50%) in the head and neck. Histologically desmoplastic melanoma is characterized by tumor cells which produce a fibromucinous matrix.

ALM presents as a slow-growing flat patch of discolored skin arising on the palms, soles, or beneath the nail. Histologically ALM is characterized by a proliferation of atypical melanocytes along the dermoepidermal junction in a lentiginous pattern.

Of the major histologic subtypes, ALM followed by superficial spreading and nodular melanoma are the most frequent to occur in any acral location.[6,7]

TOPICAL DISTRIBUTION

Several studies have assessed the frequency of melanoma of the hand and foot. Of the melanomas that occur on the hand, the most common location is subungual, followed by the dorsal surface of the hand, and then the palmar surface.[3,8] In the foot, the most common location is the plantar surface, followed by the dorsal surface, and then the subungual area.[9] Subungual melanoma (SM) most commonly affects the thumb and great toe.[10]

Frequency of melanoma cited in the literature for the hands and feet is as follows: 3% on the subungual region of the hand, 3% on the foot, and 1% to 9% on the plantar surface of the foot in Caucasian populations, with higher percentages in Asian and African populations.[11]

ACRAL LENTIGINOUS MELANOMA

While all subtypes of melanoma can be found on the hand or feet, ALM is most critical to review. ALM is a distinct subtype of melanoma found on acral skin. ALM is often confused with acral melanoma, but ALM and acral melanoma should be distinguished from each other. Acral melanoma constitutes any histologic subtype of melanoma that occurs on acral sites: palmar, plantar, subungual, or dorsal aspects of the hand and foot.

ALM accounts for 2% to 3% of all melanomas and is the most common type of melanoma on acral skin.[12] First described by Reed, ALM appears as an asymmetric brown macule or path with irregular borders and varied pigmentation.[13] The standard ABCDE (asymmetric shape, border, color, diameter, evolution) criterion has not been studied for ALM, and the acronym CUBED (colored, uncertain, bleeding, enlarged, delayed) has been proposed to assist in assessing suspicious lesions on the foot or nail.[14] ALM is characterized by lentiginous (radial) growth phase evolving over a period of months to years to a dermal (vertical) growth phase. Classic risk factors for the other subtypes of melanoma including sun exposure, fair skin type, family or personal history of melanoma, and pre-existing melanocytic nevi are not applicable to ALM. Studies, specifically in Asia, have suggested mechanical stress and trauma as risk factors for ALM.[3,15,16] ALM is commonly believed to have an ethnic predilection for African American individuals.[12] However, one study found little difference in the incidence of ALM between blacks and whites. Rather, the proportional difference was believed to be due to a decreased incidence of melanoma on skin surfaces other than the soles of the feet in African Americans.[3]

Standard ABCDE acronym for cutaneous melanoma of the foot and nail	
A	Asymmetry (half of lesion not symmetrical from other half)
B	Border (irregular, ragged, or indistinct border)
C	Color (Lesion has more than one color present.)
D	Diameter (Lesion has diameter >6 mm.)
E	Evolution (any change in lesion in terms of size, shape, or color)

CUBED acronym for foot melanoma. Presence of two or more of the listed features warrants referral to a specialist	
C	Colored lesions where any part is not skin color
U	Uncertain diagnosis
B	Bleeding lesion on the foot or under the nail (includes chronic granulation tissue)
E	Enlargement or deterioration of a lesion or ulcer despite therapy
D	Delay in healing of any lesion beyond 2 mo

SUBUNGUAL MELANOMA

Special consideration is given to SM due to the unique anatomy of the nail unit (**Fig. 1**). The subungual area features poor differentiation between papillary and reticular dermis, minimal subcutaneous fat, and only dermal collagen separating the nail matrix from the underlying distal phalanx.[7,17] As a result, the Breslow depth and Clark level,

both frequently used to determine appropriate management of cutaneous melanoma, are difficult to measure.[17]

Most SMs present as longitudinal melanonychia, or a longitudinal band of brown pigment in the nail plate (**Fig. 2**).[18] This pigmented band has a wide differential diagnosis, including blood, infection, exogenous pigment, and benign and malignant melanotic processes. The most common cause of longitudinal melanonychia in adults is melanocytic activation. In children, the most common cause is benign melanocytic nevi.[18] The wide differential of longitudinal melanonychia contributes to an often late diagnosis or misdiagnosis, and therefore late treatment, of SM.

When diagnosing SM, consider the "ABC rule for SM"[19,20]:

Age: peak incidence in 5th-7th decades of life
African Americans, Asians, and Native Americans with higher frequency of SM
Brown/black coloration
Breadth of 3+ mm and variegated borders
Change in nail band or lack of change in nail morphology despite treatment
Digit affected: thumb, index finger, great toe
Extension of pigment onto proximal or lateral nail fold (Hutchinson's sign)
Family or personal history of melanoma

Patients who possess features that are concerning for possible malignant melanoma of the nail should undergo biopsy. In addition, if a nail bed lesion has not changed significantly after 4 to 6 weeks, a biopsy should be performed. Biopsy techniques include matrix punch biopsy, tangential (shave) biopsy, lateral or midline longitudinal excision, or en bloc excision of all nail tissues.[7,18] If there is a high level of clinical suspicion of invasive melanoma, the biopsy should be excisional.[7,18] Accurate biopsies are critical for staging as initial biopsies may underestimate the depth if performed by providers who are not comfortable with anatomy of the hand or foot. While melanoma of any histologic subtype may present in the subungual area, the most common is ALM.[7]

AMELANOTIC MELANOMA

A relatively large proportion of melanomas that appear in the nail apparatus of the hands and feet are amelanotic (15%–65%).[21]

Amelanotic melanoma is a subtype of cutaneous melanoma which is devoid of melanin, and there is little to no pigment on visual inspection.[22,23] A review of the literature indicates that the frequency of amelanotic melanoma represents

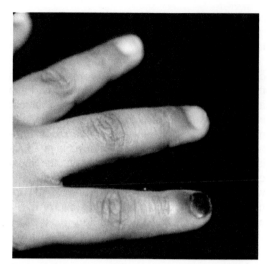

Fig. 1. Subungual melanoma of the index finger.

roughly 2% to 10% of melanomas.[22,23] Discrepancies exist regarding the epidemiologic data because some studies define amelanotic melanoma as melanomas with no clinically visible pigment while others define amelanotic melanoma as melanomas that lack melanin in the cytoplasm of tumor cells on histologic examination.[23] Amelanotic melanoma has been described in all major histologic subtypes. Risk factors for amelanotic melanoma include Caucasian, sun-sensitive phenotype (ie, Fitzpatrick skin type I with red hair), presence of actinic keratoses, oculocutaneous albinism, freckling, and older age. The relationship between sex and amelanotic melanoma is uncertain.[23]

Prompt diagnosis of amelanotic melanoma is a great challenge in further reducing deaths. Lesions do not follow the conventional ABCDE algorithm

because they visually lack pigment.[22] Moreover, the appearance of amelanotic melanomas varies and can mimic benign and malignant conditions including hemangioma, basal cell carcinoma, squamous cell carcinoma, pyogenic granuloma, Merkel cell carcinoma, and others.[24,25] The importance of improving detection of amelanotic melanoma is highlighted by the fact that these lesions present with thicker Breslow thickness, higher mitotic rate, more frequent ulceration, higher tumor stage, and lower survival than pigmented melanomas.[23,25]

Classically, amelanotic melanoma distribution is associated with sun-exposed areas including the dorsal aspect of the hand.[23] Wee and colleagues found that the anatomic distribution of amelanotic melanoma was more common in sun-exposed areas, along with an association with other sites including the plantar aspect of the foot and ungual region of the hand.[22] Moreover, lesions found in the plantar aspect of the foot and ungual region of the hand were associated with tumors that were thicker than other regions.[22]

PROGNOSIS OF MELANOMA OF THE HANDS AND FEET

Numerous studies have found that hand and foot melanomas have a worse prognosis compared with cutaneous malignant melanomas at other sites.[12,26,27] Many studies have attributed this to increased tumor thickness and advanced stage at the time of diagnosis.[26,27] However, inconsistencies exist in the literature regarding the prognostic value of Breslow thickness and ulceration, the two major prognostic factors related to the primary tumor in cutaneous melanomas, in hand and foot melanomas. One systematic review attributes the inconsistencies to the variations in the

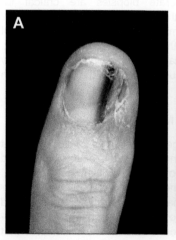
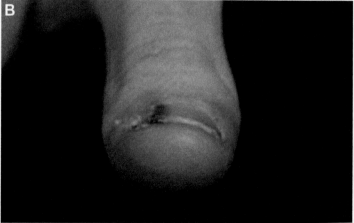

Fig. 2. Subungual melanoma presenting as longitudinal melanonychia.

lower frequencies of BRAF mutations, constitutive activation of phosphatidyl inositol 3 kinase signaling, and tumorigenesis gene amplifications.[12] However, it is unknown whether these intrinsic characteristics result in a more aggressive melanoma.[12]

SM carries a worse prognosis. Diagnosis is typically delayed, so lesions have increased Breslow thickness at the time of diagnosis.[10] Clark level is difficult to determine in a subungual site because of the paucity of soft tissue between the nail matrix and the underlying distal phalanx. Factors found to be associated with worse overall survival include Breslow thickness, Clark level, and positive sentinel lymph node. Specifically, tumor depths greater than 3.0 mm are associated with worse outcomes.[28] Another study found ulceration and lack of pigmentation to be significant prognostic indicators.[29] SM have poorer responses to immunotherapies, so targeted therapies are uncommonly a treatment option, which also contributes to a poorer prognosis.

TREATMENT (SURGICAL MANAGEMENT)
Melanoma of the Hands and Feet

Melanoma of the hands and feet requires a multifaceted approach to management and reconstruction due to the functionality and anatomy of the hands and feet. Importantly, the criteria for sentinel lymph node biopsy are the same for the hand and foot as they are for the remainder of the cutaneous skin. Surgeons should feel comfortable operating in the popliteal fossa and epitrochlear region given the potential for mapping to these regions from the distal extremity. Preoperative nuclear medicine injections can be performed proximal to the lesion, especially for subungal locations. Due to the sensitivity of the injection site, it has been our experience that digital blocks may improve the patient experience with this procedure.

The location of the lesion, in addition to the type (ie, subungual vs cutaneous) largely determines the method of primary resection and which reconstruction options are viable. Dorsal cutaneous lesions are typically treated with wide local excision and often are able to be closed primarily because of the amount of redundant skin present. Full-thickness skin graft (FTSG) or split-thickness skin graft can be used for larger defects where primary closure is not possible.[30] Cutaneous lesions of the volar surface are also frequently excised by wide local excision; however, the volar skin is less mobile and redundant, so primary closure is less frequently an option.[30] In this situation, skin grafts, local tissue rearrangement, regional flaps, or free tissue transfer may be performed.

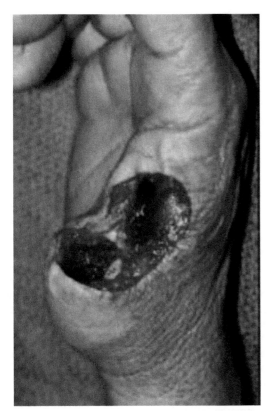

Fig. 3. Cutaneous melanoma of the thumb treated with amputation.

thickness of the epidermis and dermis in acral sites and surgical procedures that lead to fragmented specimens, making it difficult to accurately determine Breslow's thickness.[3] While another study noted that the average depth of melanomas of the nail apparatus at the time of diagnosis is substantially thicker than other anatomic regions and is partially responsible for the poorer prognosis.[21] Furthermore, ulceration may have less prognostic value in hand and foot melanomas than in other cutaneous melanomas because its mechanism may be related to trauma and less related to proliferative cell activity and/or overexpression of *c-myc*.[3] Additional adverse prognostic factors include amelanotic melanomas, subungual tumors, and positive sentinel lymph node biopsy.[4]

With regard to ALM, there is conflicting evidence on whether this subtype contributes to a worse prognosis. The literature assessing prognosis while controlling for tumor thickness is contradictory. Studies have found lower survival rates in ALM than in other cutaneous malignant melanomas, which supports the hypothesis that there are different biological characteristics (ie, genetic pathways) in the development of each melanoma subtype. It is known that ALMs have significantly

Special consideration is given to melanoma that occurs on the digits, including SM. Similar to cutaneous melanomas of other regions of the body, cutaneous melanomas of the digits are typically treated with wide local excision or amputation, depending on the depth of the lesion (**Fig. 3**).[31] Because there is limited excess skin of the digits, skin grafting or local tissue transfer is often required for closure. The unique anatomy of the nail apparatus, and close proximity to the underlying distal phalanx, makes wide resection of the lesion difficult. In a study published by Sinno and colleagues which included 35 patients with primary melanoma of the hand, most patients with cutaneous melanoma underwent wide local excision with primary closure or FTSG.[30] Patients with SM underwent amputation at the most distal interphalangeal (DIP) joint or wide local excision, with reconstruction using local advancement flaps, FTSG, or primary closure.[30]

Subungual Melanoma

Historically, the primary method of treatment of SM is amputation, because it is thought to be an especially aggressive malignancy. Many studies have investigated the optimal level of amputation, with evidence predominately favoring amputation at the DIP joint in the hand and at the metatarsophalangeal (MTP) joint in the foot.[29,32–34] Although it has been our experience that the level of amputation is dictated partly by institutional practices. Preservation of digit length and functional activity are important factors and pose a particular challenge in the excision and reconstruction of SM.[31]

In a single-center, retrospective chart review of 124 patients with SM of the hand or foot, Nguyen and colleagues advocated for function-preserving amputations of the thumb by removing the nail bed and partially amputating a portion of the distal phalanx to leave the flexor pollicis longus and extensor pollicis longus intact. This preserves interphalangeal (IP) joint function, as well as leaves the neurovascular bundle intact to allow sensation of the thumb pad.[33] The authors found that distal amputations with histologically free margins were not significantly associated with overall survival, disease-specific survival, or progression-free survival when compared with proximal resections after adjusting for Breslow depth.[33] The study defined distal amputation in the hand as resection through the DIP joint in fingers and through the IP joint in thumbs. In the foot, distal amputations were defined as those distal to and including the MTP joint.

In addition, O'Leary and colleagues concluded amputation of SM should be performed at the DIP level for the fingers and at the IP level in the

thumb.[32] They reported no incidence of recurrent disease in a retrospective study of 51 patients with primary SM of the hand when amputated at these levels.[32] The authors also found no benefit to overall 5-year survival from elective node dissection in patients with lesions of intermediate thickness (0.76 mm to 4 mm) and no detectable lymph node involvement.[32] Similarly, Quinn and colleagues found no significant difference in local recurrence rates in patients with amputation proximal or distal to the IP joint in the thumb or proximal or distal to the middle phalanx in other digits in a retrospective chart review of 38 patients.[29]

More recently, amputation of the digit involved in SM has been challenged, and the proper surgical treatment is debatable especially as preservation of digit length and functionality is emphasized. A recent review conducted by Cochran and colleagues that involved all cases within literature, including case reports, involving amputation and/or wide local excision for the treatment of SM concluded that aggressive amputation at higher levels is likely not warranted in SM, and melanoma in situ can likely be treated appropriately with wide local excision.[31] The review highlighted the lack of randomized, prospective, or comparative studies in literature and was unable to draw concrete recommendations.

Role of Mohs Micrographic Surgery

The surgical treatment of melanoma has evolved over the last 50 years. Often found in advanced stages, hand and foot melanoma was traditionally managed with amputation and wide local excision. While amputations achieve clear margins, the loss of a digit carries functional consequences that may affect quality of life. Moreover, wide local excisions can unintentionally leave residual tumor at the excisional margins and carry high local recurrence rates when compared with amputation. Recent studies have highlighted the use of Mohs micrographic surgery (MMS) as a treatment modality. The technique involves excision of the primary lesion, followed by complete microscopic evaluation of lateral and deep margins, while maintaining precise anatomic orientation of the tissue.[21]

Compared with other surgical options, MMS allows for tissue conservation and optimal margin control in a functionally sensitive area and provides a high cure rate. MMS allows surgeons to evaluate 100% of the peripheral margin compared with 1% of the peripheral margin in WLE.[35] Maintaining function and cosmesis of the hands, feet, and digits after MMS can be difficult and may require skin grafts and/or flaps to close the defect.

Multiple studies have demonstrated the advantages of MMS for melanoma including cure rates similar to wide local excision and the low rates of marginal recurrence.[36–38] Zitelli and colleagues treated 533 melanomas with MMS and found a local recurrence rate of only .5% with a mean follow-up greater than 5 years.[36] Similarly, Stigall and colleagues treated 882 patients with trunk and proximal extremity melanomas with MMS and found a local recurrence rate of only .1% with a mean follow-up of 5 years.[37]

However, owing to the infrequency of hand and foot melanomas, there are few studies describing treatment of hand and foot melanomas with MMS and those that are published focus on digital melanomas. The largest study, a retrospective chart review conducted by Terushkin and colleagues, concluded that MMS conserves function by avoiding amputation and offers a low local recurrence rate for digital melanomas.[35] Fifty-five of the 57 patients avoided amputation during a mean follow-up of 6.5 years, and the 5- and 10-year melanoma-specific survival rates were 95% and 82.6%, respectively.[35]

Similarly, Brodland reported that 13 of 14 patients who underwent MMS for treatment of SM were spared amputation.[21] Three patients had local recurrence which was successfully re-excised. During a mean follow-up of 7.7 years, the melanoma-specific survival rate was 79% which compared favorably with the 38% to 61% survival reported in literature for similar tumors.[21,39]

Several other studies and case reports containing fewer than 10 patients have been published regarding treatment of digital melanoma with MMS all of which showed low rates of local recurrence.[40–43]

While the data suggest that the use of MMS may be beneficial for treatment of digital melanomas, the topic is controversial. In particular, Nguyen and colleagues argued against the use of MMS for patients with SM because of its unique histologic characteristics.[33] As nodular and superficial spreading melanoma subtypes demonstrate isolated cell nests with decreasing numbers in the periphery, the authors believe there will be incomplete histologic evaluation if treated with MMS. Of note, these claims were based on theory rather than evidence, as none of the 124 cases of SM reviewed in their study were treated with MMS.

Reconstruction

Reconstruction of the hand and foot possess unique challenges. The timing of reconstruction must take in to account the status of margins, as flaps which may impact the identification of margins should not be performed until margin status is confirmed.

The challenge of reconstructing defects of the hand lies within the need to restore anatomy while maximizing preservation of function. The anatomy of the hand is complex, providing the ability to receive tactile stimulus and react with precise fine motor movements. Each region of the hand has its own unique soft-tissue needs that allow the area to function at its highest level.

Soft-tissue reconstruction of the hand can be split into three parts—fingertips, digits, and hand. Fingertip and digital reconstruction typically relies on adjacent tissue from the digit itself, adjacent digits, or the dorsal or palmar hand. Tissues from distant sources (abdomen or toe pulp) are another option when local flaps are insufficient. The distinct anatomy of the soft tissue of the dorsal and palmar surfaces of the hand should be considered when choosing a reconstructive option. The palmar hand has glamorous skin that must be durable enough to withstand significant shear forces when grasping or holding objects. The dorsal hand possesses thin skin that provides coverage of gliding extensor tendons. Planned reconstruction takes into account the characteristics of the defect (size, shape, and location), availability of donor sites, and goals of reconstruction (**Table 1**).

The challenges of reconstructing defects of the foot are similar to those of the hand because both function and anatomy must be restored. The dorsal foot is composed of thin, pliable skin with a delicate layer of subcutaneous adipose tissue. The skin of the dorsal foot is limited, and defects can less frequently be treated by local tissue rearrangement. As such, tissue from other parts of the body must be transferred. The transferred tissue is often bulky, and the patient must undergo further operations to have the tissue thinned.

The plantar surface of the foot possesses the unique capability of bearing weight, which allows the sole of the foot to withstand large compressive forces. This is due to the deformability and thickness of the tissue—the epidermal layer alone is 1.4 mm thick compared with 0.1 mm in other anatomic regions. In addition, the plantar surface provides the protective sensation necessary to reposition while standing and to redistribute weight during ambulation. Reconstruction of defects of the sole of the foot should provide durable soft-tissue coverage and allow the patient to bear weight and ambulate. Similar to the hand, planned reconstruction takes into account the characteristics of the defect (size, shape, and location),

Table 1
Reconstructive options for defects of the hand

Distal Fingertip Reconstruction

Volar V-Y advancement flap	• Defects <1.5 cm oriented in the dorsal oblique or transverse fashion • Flap length is 1.5–2 times the width (Width is limited to that of the nail bed.) • Durable, glabrous, sensate skin • Complications include cold intolerance, scarring, sensory changes
Lateral V-Y advancement flap	• Dorsal oblique and transverse oriented defects • Durable, glabrous, sensate skin • Limited by flap advancement of only .5–.75 cm
Thenar crease flap	• Flap involves skin from volar aspect of thumb at the level of metacarpal phalangeal joint. Digit with fingertip defect is flexed down toward elevated flap which is sutured in place • Requires delayed division (2–3 wk) • Insensate and may result in flexion contractures of recipient finger

Fingertip and distal finger reconstruction

Homodigital and heterodigital flaps	• Axial flaps that are elevated in anterograde or retrograde fashion • Requires careful attention to digital nerves so sensation of the digital aspect of donor finger is not compromised
Thoracoepigastric flap	• Very uncommon to close fingertip injuries with thoracoepigastric flap. Small flaps are raised on trunk to which fingertips are sutured. • Requires delayed division (2–3 wk). Patient must hold their arm across abdomen during this time. • Bulky, insensate flap
Free toe pulp flap	• Free tissue transfer of lateral aspect of great toe • Requires technical skills of fine microsurgery • Complications include thrombosis in anastomosed vessels, poor sensibility recovery, or neuroma formation • Requires patients to be hospitalized for 5–7 d until the fate of flap is known • Durable, glabrous, sensate skin

Distal thumb reconstruction

Volar advancement (Moberg) flap	• Most often used for defects of the distal thumb • Offers up to 2 cm of advancement • Durable, well-vascularized, glabrous, sensate skin • Multiple modifications have been made to provide a little more advancement

Volar and dorsal finger reconstruction

Dorsal metacarpal artery flap	• Most often used for defects of the volar aspect of the thumb

	• Versatile flap that is able to cover the volar aspect of the thumb, dorsal aspect of the thumb, and hand • Reverse dorsal metacarpal artery flap can cover the dorsal or volar aspect of the digits and even fingertip • Sensate skin
Volar and dorsal digit reconstruction	
Cross finger flap	• Used for defects of the volar and dorsal aspects of the digits including the fingertip • Uses skin and subcutaneous tissue on dorm of adjacent finger at level of middle phalanx • Requires delayed division (2–3 wk) • Sensory nerves can be incorporated into the flap to provide sensation • Donor site is covered with a split-thickness skin graft
First web space soft-tissue defect	
Fascial or fasciocutaneous flap	• Contractures of the first web space led to significant impairment of function • Muscle flaps should be avoided due to bulkiness • Lateral arm flap provides appropriate width, depth, and length • Lateral arm flap should not be used if the donor site cannot be closed primarily due to the significant morality associated with grafting this area
Dorsal and palmar hand reconstruction	
Local and regional flaps	• Wide array of local and regional flaps for coverage of hand defects • Rely on flow from radial and ulnar artery, thus patients must have intact palmar arch • Muscle flap offers stable coverage but is bulky if not stretched out before insetting • Fasciocutaneous flaps may be bulky in obese patient • Most patients will require secondary procedures • Fasciocutaneous flaps are easier to elevate and inset than fibrotic muscle or fascial flaps

Table 2
Reconstructive options for defects of the foot

Dorsal foot without bone exposure	
Skin grafting	
Dorsal foot with bone exposure	
Local tissue rearrangement	• V-Y flaps • Transposition and rotational flaps
Distally based sural artery flap	• Well studied, versatile, reconstructive option in patients with soft-tissue defect of dorsal foot • Requires no microsurgical technique
Plantar foot	
Integra	• Allows for granulation tissue to form • Allows for a split-thickness skin graft to be used after formation of granulation tissue
Reverse sural flap	• Well-studied method for coverage of foot defects • More distal reconstructions achieved by harvesting form contralateral calf • May be fascia or muscle graft • Prone to edema and congestion
Instep flap	• Provides non-weight-bearing glabrous tissue from medial plantar region for adjacent defects • Sensation is preserved in flap
Local tissue rearrangement	• Appropriate for small defects • V-Y flaps • Transposition, rotational, unilobed, bilobed cutaneous flaps
Intrinsic muscle flaps	• Infrequently used for plantar reconstruction because of the availability of other suprafascial and fasciocutaneous reconstructions and the resultant loss of function with the sacrifice of a muscle • Can cause postoperative gait abnormality
Toe island flap	• Small cutaneous flap based on proper digital artery • Limited to small defects • Sensation preserved in flap
Fillet toe flap	• Functionless toe undergoes removal of skeletal elements for plantar defect proximal to donor site • Size of flap depends on the digit that is sacrificed

availability of donor sites, and goals of reconstruction (**Table 2**).

CLINICS CARE POINTS

- When assessing lesions on the foot or nail, the acronym CUBED (colored, uncertain diagnosis, bleeding, enlargement or ulceration, delay in healing beyond 2 months) may be used in addition to the standard ABCDE (asymmetric shape, border, color, diameter, evolution).

- Most subungual melanomas (SMs) present as longitudinal melanonychia. When diagnosing SM, use the "ABC rule for SM." Any features concerning for malignant melanoma of the nail require a biopsy.

- When treating melanoma of the hand and foot, consider both the anatomy and function of the region.

- When planning reconstruction, take into account the characteristics of the defect (size, shape, location), availability of donor sites, and goals of reconstruction.

REFERENCES

1. Miller AJ, Mihm MC. Melanoma. N Engl J Med 2006; 355(1):51–65.
2. Melanoma incidence and mortality, United States—2012–2016. U.S. Cancer Statistics Data Briefs, No. 9. July 2019
3. Durbec F, Martin L, Derancourt C, et al. Melanoma of the hand and foot: epidemiological, prognostic and genetic features. A systematic review. Br J Dermatol 2012;166(4):727–39.
4. Maciburko SJ, Townley WA, Hollowood K, et al. Skin cancers of the hand: a series of 541 malignancies. Plast Reconstr Surg 2012;129(6):1329–36.
5. Smoller BR. Histologic criteria for diagnosing primary cutaneous malignant melanoma. Mod Pathol 2006;19(2):S34–40.
6. Dwyer PK, Mackie RM, Watt DC, et al. Plantar malignant melanoma in a white Caucasian population. Br J Dermatol 1993;128(2):115–20.
7. Tan K-B, Moncrieff M, Thompson JF, et al. Subungual melanoma: a study of 124 cases highlighting features of early lesions, potential pitfalls in diagnosis, and guidelines for histologic reporting. Am J Surg Pathol 2007;31(12):1902–12.
8. Dubrow R, Flannery JT, Liu WL. Time trends in malignant melanoma of the upper limb in Connecticut. Cancer 1991;68(8):1854–8.
9. Ishihara K, Saida T, Otsuka F, et al. The Prognosis and Statistical Investigation Committee of the Japanese Skin Cancer Society. Statistical profiles of malignant melanoma and other skin cancers in Japan: 2007 update. Int J Clin Oncol 2008;13(1):33–41.
10. Blessing K, Kernohan NM, Park KG. Subungual malignant melanoma: clinicopathological features of 100 cases. Histopathology 1991;19(5):425–9.
11. Bennett DR, Wasson D, MacArthur JD, et al. The effect of misdiagnosis and delay in diagnosis on clinical outcome in melanomas of the foot. J Am Coll Surg 1994;179(3):279–84.
12. Bradford PT, Goldstein AM, McMaster ML, et al. Acral lentiginous melanoma: incidence and survival patterns in the United States, 1986-2005. Arch Dermatol 2009;145(4). https://doi.org/10.1001/archdermatol.2008.609.
13. Reed RJ. New concepts in surgical pathology of the skin. Hoboken: Wiley; 1976.
14. Bristow IR, de Berker DA. Development of a practical guide for the early recognition for malignant melanoma of the foot and nail unit. J Foot Ankle Res 2010;3:22.
15. Jung HJ, Kweon S-S, Lee J-B, et al. A clinicopathologic analysis of 177 acral melanomas in Koreans: relevance of spreading pattern and physical stress. JAMA Dermatol 2013;149(11):1281–8.
16. Melanomas and mechanical stress points on the plantar surface of the foot | NEJM. Available at: https://www-nejm-org.ezp.slu.edu/doi/full/10.1056/NEJMc1512354. Accessed October 24, 2020.
17. Ovid. Surgical management of subungual melanoma: Mayo clinic experience of 124 cases. Available at: http://ovidsp.dc2.ovid.com.ezp.slu.edu/ovid-a/ovidweb.cgi?. Accessed October 22, 2020.
18. Mannava KA, Mannava S, Koman LA, et al. Longitudinal melanonychia: detection and management of nail melanoma. Hand Surg 2013;18(01):133–9.
19. Levit E, Kagen M, Scher R, et al. The ABC rule for clinical detection of subungual melanoma☆, ☆☆. J Am Acad Dermatol 2000;42(2):269–74.
20. Kamyab K, Abdollahi M, Nezam-Eslami E, et al. Longitudinal melanonychia in an Iranian population: a study of 96 patients. Int J Womens Dermatol 2016; 2(2):49–52.
21. Brodland DG. The treatment of nail apparatus melanoma with Mohs micrographic surgery. Dermatol Surg 2001;27(3):269–73.
22. Wee E, Wolfe R, Mclean C, et al. Clinically amelanotic or hypomelanotic melanoma: anatomic distribution, risk factors, and survival. J Am Acad Dermatol 2018;79(4):645–51.e4.
23. Gong H-Z, Zheng H-Y, Li J. Amelanotic melanoma. Melanoma Res 2019;29(3):221–30.
24. Pizzichetta MA, Talamini R, Stanganelli I, et al. Amelanotic/hypomelanotic melanoma: clinical and

dermoscopic features. Br J Dermatol 2004;150(6): 1117–24.

25. Koch SE, Lange JR. Amelanotic melanoma: the great masquerader. J Am Acad Dermatol 2000; 42(5 Part 1):731–4.

26. Rex J, Paradelo C, Mangas C, et al. Management of primary cutaneous melanoma of the hands and feet: a clinicoprognostic study. Dermatol Surg 2009; 35(10):1505–13.

27. Bello DM, Chou JF, Panageas KS, et al. Prognosis of acral melanoma: a series of 281 patients. Ann Surg Oncol 2013;20(11):3618–25.

28. Nunes LF, Mendes GLQ, Koifman RJ. Subungual melanoma: a retrospective cohort of 157 cases from Brazilian National Cancer Institute. J Surg Oncol 2018;118(7):1142–9.

29. Quinn MJ, Thompson JE, Crotty K, et al. Subungual melanoma of the hand. J Hand Surg 1996;21(3): 506–11.

30. Sinno S, Wilson S, Billig J, et al. Primary melanoma of the hand: an algorithmic approach to surgical management. J Plast Surg Hand Surg 2015;49(6): 339–45.

31. Cochran AM, Buchanan PJ, Bueno RA, et al. Subungual melanoma: a review of current treatment. Plast Reconstr Surg 2014;134(2):259–73.

32. O'Leary JA, Berend KR, Johnson JL, et al. Subungual melanoma. A review of 93 cases with identification of prognostic variables. Clin Orthop 2000;(378): 206–12.

33. Nguyen JT, Bakri K, Nguyen EC, et al. Surgical management of subungual melanoma: Mayo clinic experience of 124 cases. Ann Plast Surg 2013;71(4): 346–54.

34. Martin DE, English JC, Goitz RJ. Subungual malignant melanoma. J Hand Surg 2011;36(4):704–7.

35. Terushkin V, Brodland DG, Sharon DJ, et al. Digit-Sparing Mohs surgery for melanoma. Dermatol Surg 2016;42(1):83–93.

36. Zitelli JA, Brown C, Hanusa BH. Mohs micrographic surgery for the treatment of primary cutaneous melanoma. J Am Acad Dermatol 1997;37(2 Pt 1): 236–45.

37. Stigall LE, Brodland DG, Zitelli JA. The use of Mohs micrographic surgery (MMS) for melanoma in situ (MIS) of the trunk and proximal extremities. J Am Acad Dermatol 2016;75(5):1015–21.

38. Valentín-Nogueras SM, Brodland DG, Zitelli JA, et al. Mohs micrographic surgery using Mart-1 immunostains in the treatment of invasive melanoma and melanoma in situ. Dermatol Surg 2016;42(6):733–44.

39. Muchmore JH, Krementz ET, Carter RD, et al. Regional perfusion for the treatment of subungual melanoma. Am Surg 1990;56(2):114–8.

40. Husain Z, Allawh RM, Hendi A. Mohs micrographic Surgery for digital melanoma and nonmelanoma skin cancers. Cutis 2018;101(5):346-352.

41. Loosemore MP, Morales-Burgos A, Goldberg LH. Acral lentiginous melanoma of the toe treated using Mohs surgery with sparing of the digit and subsequent reconstruction using split-thickness skin graft. Dermatol Surg 2013;39(1 Pt 1):136–8.

42. Banfield CC, Dawber RP, Walker NP, et al. Mohs micrographic surgery for the treatment of in situ nail apparatus melanoma: a case report. J Am Acad Dermatol 1999;40(1):98–9.

43. High WA, Quirey RA, Guillén DR, et al. Presentation, histopathologic findings, and clinical outcomes in 7 cases of melanoma in situ of the nail unit. Arch Dermatol 2004;140(9):1102–6.

Melanoma in Pregnancy and Pediatrics

Michael R. Romanelli, MD, MA[a], Alaa Mansour, MS3[b], Allyne Topaz, MD[a],
Danielle Olla, MD[a],*, Michael W. Neumeister, MD, FRCSC[c]

KEYWORDS

- Melanoma • Pediatrics • Pregnancy • Pediatric melanoma • Pregnancy-associated melanoma

KEY POINTS

- Diagnosis and management of melanoma during pregnancy must take into account several considerations including safe imaging modalities, choice of tracer dye, trimester, positioning of the patient, choice of anesthesia, antiseptic, and postoperative care.
- The survival rate of pregnant and nonpregnant women diagnosed with melanoma is the same, and transplacental and fetal metastases of melanoma are rare but often fatal to the infant.
- Pediatric melanoma may present similar to an adult subtype, a transformation from a congenital melanocytic nevus, or as a spitzoid melanoma, and it is treated with wide local excision with adjuvant therapy in advanced forms of disease.

PREGNANCY-ASSOCIATED MELANOMA

Incidence

It is estimated that one-third of malignancies in women occur in their childbearing years. Melanoma is more common than breast, endocrine, or gynecologic cancers in pregnant women. The incidence of melanoma during pregnancy is low, however, at around 0.05% to 0.1% of pregnancies, similar to nonpregnant women.[1] The incidence varies geographically, with a predominance in equatorial nations. Overall, the data do not suggest that pregnancy worsens the prognosis of melanoma, nor is pregnancy contraindicated in patients with a previous history of melanoma. Clinicians should note, however, that melanoma recurrence is more likely in the first 2 to 3 years following the original diagnosis and treatment; therefore families should understand the ramifications of pregnancy on melanoma. There are some articles reporting a poorer prognosis in pregnancy-associated melanoma, but many scientists believe the cases are too heterogeneous and the numbers are too low to draw substantial conclusions. Theories for a poorer prognosis include delayed diagnosis because of unawareness of natural pigment changes during pregnancy, greater lymphogenesis, higher than normal levels of pregnancy-associated plasma protein-A, increased natural growth factors that feed tumor growth, hormone effects, or enhanced maternal-fetal immune tolerance.[2]

Diagnosis and Staging

Diagnosing melanoma during pregnancy is similar to that of any patient population.[3] Lesions with changes in symmetry, borders, color, diameter, or new nevi identified during pregnancy should be carefully evaluated by a health care provider. Concerning lesions warrant dermatologic evaluation.[4] Morphologic changes in color, size, irregularity of borders, or pigment regression should have an excisional biopsy with 1 to 2 mm margins at any stage of the pregnancy. Small excisional procedures under local anesthesia using

[a] Institute for Plastic Surgery, Southern Illinois University, 747 North Rutledge Street #3, Springfield, IL 62702, USA; [b] Southern Illinois University School of Medicine, 747 North Rutledge Street #3, Springfield, IL 62702, USA; [c] Department of Surgery, Institute for Plastic Surgery, Southern Illinois University, 747 North Rutledge Street #3, Springfield, IL 62702, USA
* Corresponding author.
E-mail address: dolla41@siumed.edu

Clin Plastic Surg 48 (2021) 699–705
https://doi.org/10.1016/j.cps.2021.06.004

lidocaine, bupivacaine, and prilocaine with or without epinephrine are considered safe during pregnancy. Although animal studies have demonstrated epinephrine induced uterine artery spasm, this has not been observed in people. Histopathology confirms the diagnosis of melanoma with Breslow thickness, mitotic rate, regression, and ulceration status of the tumor as vital parameters in evaluating melanoma invasiveness.[5]

The staging of melanoma consists of 3 basic components: primary tumor size (T), regional lymph nodes (N), and metastasis (M). Imaging can be key in staging melanoma. Radiation during pregnancy imposes fetal risk, and as such ultrasonography and magnetic resonance imaging (MRI) are encouraged. Magnetic field and high temperatures of MRI have been associated with neonatal sensorineural hearing loss and miscarriages. Therefore, MRI is avoided during the first trimester. Low-dose computed tomography (CT) scan or CT scan with lead shielding may also be utilized if required.

Sentinel lymph node mapping and biopsies using technetium are considered safe to be performed during pregnancy when performed under local anesthesia. Sentinel lymph node biopsy (SLNB) should be considered when Breslow thickness is greater than 0.76 mm, there is regression of 50% to 75% of the original hyperpigmentation, and Clarke's level 4 lesions and ulceration are present.[1] A radiation dose of less than 5 mGy is encountered during the sentinel node mapping. The International Commission on Radiological Protection recommends radiation doses less than 100 mGy to the fetus to mitigate malformations, microcephaly, intellectual disability, fetal growth disturbances, and pregnancy loss from the radiation exposure.[2,6] Theoretically, the fetal cancer risk, such as leukemia, could be higher with radiation exposure. Technetium 99 is preferred during pregnancy as tracer dye for SLNB. There is less systemic spread and lower risk of anaphylactic reaction than isosulfan blue and less teratogenicity than methylene blue.[1] Clinicians should weigh the potential risks but given the low in utero dose, the standard of care as per nonpregnant women is often followed.

Following a comprehensive literature review, Gill and colleagues suggested the recommendations in **Box 1** for pregnant patients needing positron emission tomography (PET) or PET/CT scans:

safely performed under local anesthesia at any point during pregnancy with margins based on Breslow depth of the primary lesion as recommended by the National Comprehensive Cancer Network (NCCN) guidelines.[1] Full obstetric history is essential, and the patient's obstetrician should be made aware.

Procedures requiring anesthesia such as wide local excision, SLNB, and lymph node dissections should be performed during the second trimester (13 to 24 weeks), and may be delayed postpartum in avoidance of anesthesia. Surgery should be avoided during the first trimester to avoid early pregnancy loss and during the third trimester to avoid preterm delivery. Operative delay may potentially impact the prognosis of melanoma, and the risks and benefits should be discussed extensively with the patient for an informed decision to be made.

During surgery, certain pregnancy-related considerations require attention. Patient positioning should be 30° left lateral tilt to prevent aortocaval compression. Normal physiologic changes of pregnancy, such as increased urinary frequency, acid reflux, and joint laxity, can be resolved by encouraging urination preoperatively, changing positions periodically, and head lifting.

Antiseptic choices, including baby shampoo, alcohol, and chlorhexidine-based solutions are safe during pregnancy. Povidone-iodine is deferred given the risk of fetal hypothyroidism, and hexachlorophene is contraindicated because of its toxicity to the fetal central nervous system.

Immunotherapy and targeted therapy have shown promise in the treatment of melanoma at large, although obstetric and fetal complications remain unknown.[7] The fetus has well known immune tolerance toward the maternal immune system. Targeted drugs such as BRAF inhibitors carry risks of teratogenicity. Checkpoint inhibitors against CTLA4 and PD1, such as ipilimumab, have been used to treat melanoma during pregnancy.[8] Risks include miscarriage, stillbirth, and preterm birth. Many conventional melanoma oncologic agents such as interferon alpha and cyclophosphamide are contraindicated in pregnancy, and all agents require consideration of future pregnancy planning and breastfeeding. The decision to utilize these medications is individualized, requiring an informed decision.

Management

Treatment of melanoma during pregnancy does not differ from the treatment of melanoma outside of pregnancy.[3] Excision of melanoma can be

Prognosis

Historically, pregnancy was believed to negatively impact the prognosis of melanoma. Studies, however, show no difference in the prognosis between recurrence rates and potential ramifications of having melanoma during pregnancy. Although stand protocols have not been developed, a past history of a thin melanoma is believed to offer low risk. Patients with high-risk melanoma are advised to reconsider plans for future pregnancy for 2 to 5 years.[1]

Metastasis of high-risk melanoma during pregnancy has been reported in only 30 placental metastasis described in the literature.[2,11-14] Most studies demonstrate that transplacental metastasis often does not affect the child, as most patients deliver healthy, unaffected children.[15,16] Only 8 cases of fetal involvement have been reported in the literature.[11,12] Six of those 8 patients, however, died within their first year of life. Underreporting may contribute to the low reported rates of placental involvement, as most placentas are not sent for pathology. Recent studies correlating tumor proliferation activity and staging of pregnancy-associated melanoma reveal no impact of pregnancy on tumor progression for early-stage melanoma.[17]

Early stage melanoma has no negative impact on obstetric or neonatal outcomes in pregnant women.[15,18] Pregnant patients with advanced melanoma show tendencies toward preterm delivery, low birth weight, higher cesarean section rate and miscarriages.[3]

During pregnancy with advanced melanoma, reports of up to 25% metastasis to the placenta have been reported. Experimental studies in pregnant mice with advanced melanoma revealed concerning enhancement of tumor growth, angiogenesis, lymph angiogenesis, lymphatic metastasis, and reduction in overall survival.[19] Thus, for patients with a history of advanced or current metastatic melanoma, the placenta must be carefully examined, and long-term neonatal follow-up is required to investigate any evidence of metastatic melanoma.

Summary

Knowledge of melanoma in pregnancy continues to evolve. The exact incidence of melanoma during pregnancy is unknown. As women more commonly delay pregnancy to later age, melanoma during pregnancy will likely increase. After adjusting for age, melanoma incidence is the same between pregnant and nonpregnant women. Diagnosis and management follow nonpregnant algorithms with certain additional considerations during pregnancy. Small localized melanoma can be excised at any stage of pregnancy with local anesthesia. Procedures requiring general anesthesia such as lymph node dissections should be

pregnant and nonpregnant women in the early stages of melanoma.[9,10]

Melanoma recurrence depends on the staging of melanoma. Early stage melanoma with less than 0.5 mm Breslow thickness has a 1% to 3% recurrence rate within the first 5 years. However, more advanced melanoma with greater than 4 mm thickness has a greater than 50% recurrence rate within the first 2 years. Patients with any grade melanoma should be advised about performed in the second trimester or delayed until postpartum if possible to decrease risks of general anesthesia to the fetus. Immunotherapy and targeted therapy have shown promise, although obstetric and fetal complications remain unknown. Localized melanoma prognosis during pregnancy does not differ from the prognosis of nonpregnant women, and future pregnancy planning does not demand delay. Advanced melanoma tends toward preterm delivery, low birth weights, higher cesarean section rates, and early pregnancy loss. Transplacental and fetal metastases are rare, especially in early stage melanoma, but may be as high as 25% in advanced stages.

PEDIATRICS MELANOMA
Incidence

Malignant melanoma in children and adolescents is a rare disease annually, affecting approximately 1 in 1,000,000 under the age of 20 years. Pediatric melanoma accounts for 1.3% of all melanomas.[20] Incidence increases with age in the pediatric demographic.[21] The highest incidence in the pediatric population presents among ages 15 to 19 years, accounting for 73% to 79% of pediatric melanomas.[22] Although teenage years show a female predominance, younger age groups are predominantly male.[23] From 1970 to 2009, pediatric melanoma incidence increased,[24] although recent literature suggests decreasing trends between 2000 and 2010. This may be partly attributable to public health measures encouraging the use of sunscreen and sun exposure awareness in the pediatric population.[21]

Risk Factors

Most melanoma cases in the pediatric population arise de novo. Risk factors include excessive exposure to ultraviolet light, propensity to sunburn, and an inability to tan. Patients of Caucasian descent with fair hair, blue eyes, and fair Fitzpatrick skin type remain prone to melanoma. Positive family history is associated with a fourfold increase in the risk of childhood melanoma.[25,26]

Pre-existing conditions account for roughly 25% of pediatric patients with melanoma.[27] Patients with large or giant congenital melanocytic nevi (CMN), although rare, present with a lifetime risk of melanoma transformation, with higher risks earlier in life. Large CMNs present with a risk of malignant transformation between 1% and 5%, whereas giant CMNs confer greater risks of 5% to 20%. If CMNs are accompanied by smaller satellite nevi, transformation risk increases to 10% to 15%.[28]

Another rare condition commonly associated with pediatric melanoma is xeroderma pigmentosum (XP). XP is an autosomal-recessive disorder resulting in an inability to repair ultraviolet light-induced damage. Patients with this condition are 2000 times more likely to develop melanoma than age-matched children without XP.[29] Children with immunodeficiency syndromes also present with an increased risk of acquiring melanoma, with rates up to sixfold that of patients without immunodeficiency.[30]

Clinical Presentation

The division of melanoma in children is usually divided into in utero, birth, childhood, and adolescence. In utero is primarily of transplacental origin, whereas after that inciting factors include melanoma from giant congenital nevus, neurocutaneous melanosis, and de novo melanoma. As the child ages, atypical melanocytic neoplasms play an increasing role in melanoma formation. Melanomas in children often present as thicker lesions with a higher positivity of sentinel lymph nodes but better prognosis than melanomas in adults. The overall 10-year survival of melanomas in children is around 70% to 80%. Melanoma in children may resemble an amelanotic lesion similar in appearance to a wart, pyogenic granuloma, or dermatofibroma rather than an evolving mole. Accordingly, the traditional ABCDE mnemonic designed to characterize a lesion's asymmetry, border irregularity, color variability, diameter greater than 6 mm, and evolving criteria has been modified to ABCD to more aptly describe melanoma in the pediatric population as Amelanotic, Bleeding, "Bump" with uniform Color, arising De novo ,and any Diameter. This atypical presentation often results in a delay in diagnosis and treatment.[31]

Diagnosis

Diagnosis via tissue dermatohistopathology obtained by biopsy or wide local excision should be performed by an experienced dermatopathologist given broad histopathologic variability. Diagnoses are complicated by histologic similarities with Spitz nevi, dysplastic nevi, halo nevi, and CMN.[32] Features suggestive of malignancy include Breslow depth, mitotic rate, ulceration, margin status, and the presence of microsatellites. The utility of SLNB has been widely debated, with proponents arguing the benefits observed in adult studies may outweigh the risks. Accordingly, SLNB may assist in diagnosis when histologic findings are ambiguous such as controversial spitzoid melanocytic lesions.[33] When compared with adults, pediatric patients have a higher incidence of sentinel lymph node metastases but have a lower incidence of recurrence.[34] SLNBs are frequently positive in pediatric patients (55%–66%) and given the associated morbidity of the procedure, many question the need for the procedure.[34] Complete lymph node dissection increases morbidity, and is not recommended in the pediatric population.[35]

Treatment

Wide local excision is the mainstay of treatment for pediatric melanoma as in adult patients. Margins are based on Breslow depth of the primary lesion as recommended by the NCCN guidelines.[36]

- A melanoma in situ, a margin between 0.5 cm to 1.0 cm is recommended.
- A melanoma with a Breslow depth less than or equal to 1.0 mm, a 1.0 cm margin is recommended.
- A melanoma with a Breslow depth between 1.0 mm and 2.0 mm, a margin of 1.0 cm to 2.0 cm is recommended.
- A melanoma with a Breslow depth between 2.0 mm and 4.0 mm, a margin of 2.0 cm is recommended.
- A melanoma with a Breslow depth greater than 4.0 mm, a margin of 2.0 cm is recommended.

Adjuvant therapy in the pediatric population is controversial given limited data, and is traditionally reserved for advanced disease with ulceration, increased Breslow depth, and positive SLNB. Generally speaking, adjuvant therapies are tolerated by children as they are in adults. The importance of prevention cannot be understated; avoidance of extended sun exposure, use protective clothing, and use of sunscreen remain imperative.

Prognosis and Survival

The American Joint Committee on Cancer (AJCC) staging used for prognosis of adult cutaneous melanomas is applicable to pediatric adult subtype melanomas based on tumor thickness, mitotic rate, ulceration, and nodal metastases. Unfortunately, the AJCC criteria do not correlate with outcomes in amelanotic lesions, or spitzoid melanoma specifically with regard to Breslow thickness and nodal metastases.[37] Historically, survival of patients with pediatric melanoma was thought to be stage-dependent and similar to adults.[38] Recent literature, however, supports significantly increased melanoma survival in young adults when compared with an adult cohort.[39] Within the pediatric population subset, overall

survival differences in prepubertal patients compared with adolescents was not significant; however, younger ages frequently showed thicker tumors and increased risk of lymph node metastases.[40] Although survival rates are generally higher in pediatric cohorts, maternal melanoma transplacental metastases in the fetus are frequently lethal.[12]

Discussion

Current knowledge of pediatric melanoma is limited given the rare incidence. Accordingly, pediatric melanoma studies are not as extensive as the adult population. Although the incidence of melanoma has been increasing overall, studies have shown it has been decreasing in the pediatric population, likely given extensive public health measures. Pediatric melanoma may present similarly as in an adult; however, it can transform from a congenital melanocytic nevus, or present as a spitzoid-type melanoma. Diagnosis is often challenged by the difference in clinical presentation relative to adults, and variation in histopathology. Treatment is primarily based on wide local excision, and adjuvant therapeutic regimens for adults have undergone recent trials to identify their potential use in the pediatric population. Early clinical detection, correct diagnosis, and treatment are critical for survival.

CLINICS CARE POINTS

- During pregnancy, changes in any nevus should be examined carefully, especially for those in the abdomen, back, and breast.
- Diagnosis and management of melanoma during pregnancy are the same as in nonpregnant patients with several considerations.
- Technetium 99 is preferred during pregnancy as a tracer dye.
- Excisional biopsy with 1 to 2 mm margin can be done safely at any time during the pregnancy with local anesthesia.
- Wide local excision, SLNB and lymph node dissection may be indicated based on the staging. Trimester considerations, positioning of the patient, choice of anesthesia, antiseptic, and postoperative care should be considered for the pregnant patient.
- Immunotherapy has shown excellent responses in pregnant patients with melanoma,

with a patient-tailored approach. Oncologic agents are not without risk to the fetus and have future considerations postpartum.

- The survival rate of pregnancy-associated melanoma is the same in nonpregnant women diagnosed with melanoma.

- Pediatric melanoma affects approximately 1 in 1,000,000 children and incidence increases with age.

- Most pediatric melanoma cases arise de novo, while pre-existing conditions account for 25% of cases.

- Clinically, pediatric melanoma presents as either similar to an adult subtype, transformation from a congenital melanocytic nevus, or spitzoid melanoma.

- Giant congenital melanocytic nevi present with a 5% to 20% risk of transformation.

- Wide local excision is the primary form of treatment, and adjuvant therapy may be indicated in advanced forms of disease.

DISCLOSURE

The authors have nothing to disclose.

REFERENCES

1. Salvini C, Scarfì F, Fabroni C, et al. Melanoma and pregnancy. G Ital Dermatol Venereol 2017;152(3): 274–85.

2. Still R, Brennecke S. Melanoma in pregnancy. Obstet Med 2017;10(3):107–12.

3. de Haan J, Lok CA, de Groot CJ, et al. Melanoma during pregnancy: a report of 60 pregnancies complicated by melanoma. Melanoma Res 2017; 27(3):218–23.

4. Richtig G, Byrom L, Kupsa R, et al. Pregnancy as a driver for melanoma. Br J Dermatol 2017;177(3): 854–7.

5. Li JN, Nijhawan RI, Srivastava D. Cutaneous surgery in patients who are pregnant or breastfeeding. Dermatol Clin 2019;37(3):307–17.

6. Gill MM, Sia W, Hoskinson M, et al. The use of PET/CT in pregnancy: a case report of malignant parathyroid carcinoma and a review of the literature. Obstet Med 2018;11(1):45–9.

7. Burotto M, Gormaz JG, Samtani S, et al. Viable pregnancy in a patient with metastatic melanoma treated with double checkpoint immunotherapy. Semin Oncol 2018;45(3):164–9.

8. Johnson DB, Sullivan RJ, Menzies AM. Immune checkpoint inhibitors in challenging populations. Cancer 2017;123(11):1904–11.

9. Silipo V, De Simone P, Mariani G, et al. Malignant melanoma and pregnancy. Melanoma Res 2006; 16(6):497–500.

10. Byrom L, Olsen CM, Knight L, et al. Does pregnancy after a diagnosis of melanoma affect prognosis? Systematic review and meta-analysis. Dermatol Surg 2015;41(8):875–82.

11. Driscoll MS, Martires K, Bieber AK, et al. Pregnancy and melanoma. J Am Acad Dermatol 2016;75(4): 669–78.

12. Alexander A, Samlowski WE, Grossman D, et al. Metastatic melanoma in pregnancy: risk of transplacental metastases in the infant [published correction appears in J Clin Oncol 2010;28(22):3670]. J Clin Oncol 2003;21(11):2179–86.

13. Berk-Krauss J, Liebman TN, Stein JA. Pregnancy and melanoma: recommendations for clinical Scenarios. Int J Womens Dermatol 2018;4(2):113–5.

14. Todd SP, Driscoll MS. Prognosis for women diagnosed with melanoma during, before, or after pregnancy: weighing the evidence. Int J Womens Dermatol 2017;3(1):26–9.

15. Mendizábal E, De León-Luis J, Gómez-Hidalgo NR, et al. Maternal and perinatal outcomes in pregnancy-associated melanoma. Report of two cases and a systematic literature review. Eur J Obstet Gynecol Reprod Biol 2017;214:131–9.

16. Jeremić J, Jeremić K, Stefanović A, et al. Pregnancy associated with melanoma and fetal anomalies: a case report and review of literature. Clin Exp Obstet Gynecol 2015;42(3):386–7.

17. Merkel EA, Martini MC, Amin SM, et al. A comparative study of proliferative activity and tumor stage of pregnancy-associated melanoma (PAM) and non-PAM in gestational age women. J Am Acad Dermatol 2016;74(1):88–93.

18. Bannister-Tyrrell M, Roberts CL, Hasovits C, et al. Incidence and outcomes of pregnancy-associated melanoma in new South wales 1994-2008. Aust N Z J Obstet Gynaecol 2015;55(2):116–22.

19. Khosrotehrani K, Nguyen Huu S, Prignon A, et al. Pregnancy promotes melanoma metastasis through enhanced lymphangiogenesis. Am J Pathol 2011; 178(4):1870–80.

20. Wong JR, Harris JK, Rodriguez-Galindo C, et al. Incidence of childhood and adolescent melanoma in the United States: 1973-2009. Pediatrics 2013; 131(5):846–54.

21. Campbell LB, Kreicher KL, Gittleman HR, et al. Melanoma incidence in children and adolescents: decreasing trends in the United States. J Pediatr 2015;166(6):1505–13.

22. de Vries E, Steliarova-Foucher E, Spatz A, et al. Skin cancer incidence and survival in European children and adolescents (1978-1997). Eur J Cancer 2006; 42(13):2170–82.

23. Lange JR, Palis BE, Chang DC, et al. Melanoma in children and teenagers: an analysis of patients from the national cancer data Base. J Clin Oncol 2007;25(11):1363–8.

24. Austin MT, Xing Y, Hayes-Jordan AA, et al. Melanoma incidence rises for children and adolescents: an epidemiologic review of pediatric melanoma in the United States. J Pediatr Surg 2013;48(11):2207–13.

25. Whiteman DC, Valery P, McWhirter W, et al. Risk factors for childhood melanoma in Queensland, Australia. Int J Cancer 1997;70(1):26–31.

26. Berg P, Wennberg AM, Tuominen R, et al. Germline CDKN2A mutations are rare in child and adolescent cutaneous melanoma. Melanoma Res 2004;14(4):251–5.

27. Pappo AS. Melanoma in children and adolescents. Eur J Cancer 2003;39(18):2651–61.

28. Krengel S, Hauschild A, Schäfer T. Melanoma risk in congenital melanocytic naevi: a systematic review. Br J Dermatol 2006;155(1):1–8.

29. Downard CD, Rapkin LB, Gow KW. Melanoma in children and adolescents. Surg Oncol 2007;16(3):215–20.

30. Tracy ET, Aldrink JH. Pediatric melanoma. Semin Pediatr Surg 2016;25(5):290–8.

31. Cordoro KM, Gupta D, Frieden IJ, et al. Pediatric melanoma: results of a large cohort study and proposal for modified ABCD detection criteria for children. J Am Acad Dermatol 2013;68(6):913–25.

32. Wechsler J, Bastuji-Garin S, Spatz A, et al. Reliability of the histopathologic diagnosis of malignant melanoma in childhood. Arch Dermatol 2002;138(5):625–8.

33. Gamblin TC, Edington H, Kirkwood JM, et al. Sentinel lymph node biopsy for atypical melanocytic lesions with spitzoid features. Ann Surg Oncol 2006;13(12):1664–70.

34. Roaten JB, Partrick DA, Bensard D, et al. Survival in sentinel lymph node-positive pediatric melanoma. J Pediatr Surg 2005;40(6):988–92.

35. Palmer PE 3rd, Warneke CL, Hayes-Jordan AA, et al. Complications in the surgical treatment of pediatric melanoma. J Pediatr Surg 2013;48(6):1249–53.

36. Coit DG, Thompson JA, Albertini MR, et al. Cutaneous melanoma, version 2.2019, NCCN clinical practice guidelines in oncology. J Natl Compr Canc Netw 2019;17(4):367–402.

37. Paradela S, Fonseca E, Pita-Fernández S, et al. Prognostic factors for melanoma in children and adolescents: a clinicopathologic, single-center study of 137 Patients. Cancer 2010;116(18):4334–44.

38. Saenz NC, Saenz-Badillos J, Busam K, et al. Childhood melanoma survival. Cancer 1999;85(3):750–4.

39. Lasithiotakis K, Leiter U, Meier F, et al. Age and gender are significant independent predictors of survival in primary cutaneous melanoma. Cancer 2008;112(8):1795–804.

40. Moore-Olufemi S, Herzog C, Warneke C, et al. Outcomes in pediatric melanoma: comparing prepubertal to adolescent pediatric patients. Ann Surg 2011;253(6):1211–5.

Mucosal Melanoma

Danielle Olla, MD[a],*, Michael W. Neumeister, MD, FRCSC[b]

KEYWORDS

- Melanoma • Mucosal melanoma • Head and neck mucosal melanoma

KEY POINTS

- Mucosal melanoma (MM) is a rare cancer representing less than 1% of all malignant melanomas with a 5-year survival of only 25%.
- Surgical resection with clear margins is the mainstay of treatment but is influenced by the tumor size, functional considerations, and proximity to vital structures.
- Although not well defined given the rarity of MM, there is a role for radiation and systemic therapy in the treatment of this disease.

INTRODUCTION

First described in 1856, mucosal melanoma (MM) is a rare but aggressive cancer arising in melanocytes within ectodermal mucosa.[1] Melanocytes derive from neural crest cells and migrate through embryonic mesenchyme to their final destination. Most melanocytes are located in the epidermis and dermis but are encountered in various extracutaneous sites such as eyes, mucosal tissue, and leptomeninges.[2] The function of melanocytes in the mucosal membranes is not well understood, but antimicrobial and immunologic cellular functions are proposed.[3] The pathogenesis of MM is unknown. MM rarely carries the oncogenic mutations in BRAF that are frequently found in cutaneous melanoma. Studies have found mutations or increased copy number of KIT mutations in MM.[3]

Incidence

MM represents less than 1% of all malignant melanomas. Compared to an increasing incidence of cutaneous melanoma, the incidence of MM remains stable. The highest incidence of MM is in the head and neck region (55.4%), followed by anus and rectum (23.8%), female reproductive tract (18%), and the urinary tract mucosa (2.8%).[4]

The median age at diagnosis is 70 years for MM, decades later than for cutaneous melanomas.[1] Sixty-five percent of patients are older than 60 years, and less than 3% are younger than 30 years. MM is twice as frequent in women.[1] Female predominance is most apparent given higher rates in genital tract melanomas, while no difference exists in rates between genders for extragenital MM.

Risk Factors

Risk factors for MM have not been identified given their rare incidence. Studies have not found any association to human papilloma viruses, human herpes viruses, and polyomavirus.[1] Unlike cutaneous melanoma, ultraviolet light exposure is not considered a risk factor given their anatomic site of origin.[5] Formaldehyde has been suggested as a risk factor for sinonasal mucosal melanoma (SMM) after reported cases in workers exposed to this chemical. Smoking has been suggested as a risk factor in oral MM given the increase in oral pigmented lesions in smokers.[3]

Prognosis

The clinical presentation of MM is often nonspecific and differs in relation to the site of origin. The lack of early and specific signs contributes to late diagnosis and poor prognosis. Compared with a 5-year survival rate of 80.8% in cutaneous melanomas, MM has a 5-year survival of only 25%.[6]

a Institute for Plastic Surgery, Southern Illinois University, 747 N Rutledge Street #3, Springfield, IL 62702, USA;
b Department of Surgery, The Elvin G Zook Endowed Chair - Institute for Plastic Surgery, Southern Illinois University, 747 N Rutledge Street #3, Springfield, IL 62702, USA
* Corresponding author.
E-mail address: dolla41@siumed.edu

Clin Plastic Surg 48 (2021) 707–711
https://doi.org/10.1016/j.cps.2021.05.010

Mucosal Melanoma of the Head and Neck

Mucosal melanoma of the head and neck (HNMM) represents 6% of all melanomas of the head and neck. Most HNMMs occur in the nasal cavity, paranasal sinus region, and oral cavity. Local, regional, and distant failures are observed in 81% of patients. The 5-year overall survival rates are low, ranging from 15% to 35%.[7]

Signs and symptoms of MM vary depending on their location. In the sinonasal tract, patients may experience epistaxis, facial pain, and nasal obstruction which is often confused with inflammatory conditions. On endoscopy, there is often a polypoid unilateral lesion with different degrees of pigmentation within the mass. There may be satellite lesions spreading along mucosal and submucosal planes. Most common sites include inferior turbinate/lateral side wall and nasal septum.[3]

The oral cavity is easier to examine so MM may be diagnosed earlier. Oral MMs are often hyperpigmented lesions, but 10% to 30% may present as amelanotic making the diagnosis more challenging. There may also be satellite lesions in oral MMs, and common sites include the hard palate as well as the maxillary and mandibular gums.[3]

Biopsy confirms the diagnosis of MM. Patients require a complete history and physical with complete head and neck examination. CT with contrast and/or MRI with contrast are needed to determine the extent of disease. This is particularly important for sinus disease. Consider chest CT, PET CT, and brain MRI to evaluate for metastasis.

Staging

AJCC cancer staging recognizes two key features in MM.

1. There is a poor prognosis even with a limited primary burden of disease.
2. There is some gradation of survival based on the burden of disease as reflected in the local, regional, and distant extent of disease.

The following staging system was published in the 2021 version of the National Comprehensive Cancer Network (NCCN) guidelines. The staging system begins with T3N0 and reflects the burden of disease:

Primary tumor (T)

- T3 tumors are limited to the mucosa and immediate underlying soft tissue, regardless of thickness or greatest dimension.
- T4 is broken down into T4a and T4b.
  - T4a is a moderately advanced disease involving deep soft tissue, cartilage, bone, or overlying skin

  - T4b is a very advanced disease. Tumor involves brain, dura, skull base, lower cranial nerves, masticator space, carotid artery, prevertebral space, or mediastinal structures.

Regional lymph node (N)

- Nx, Regional lymph nodes cannot be assessed
- N0, No regional lymph node metastasis
- N1, Regional lymph node metastasis present

Distant metastasis (M)

- M0, No distant metastasis
- M1, Distant metastasis

Histologic grade (G)

- There is no recommended histologic grading system at this time

Vulvovaginal Mucosal Melanoma

Melanomas arising from the female urogenital tract account for up to 7% of melanomas in women. They most commonly arise from the vulva, and less than 5% from the vagina.[8] Median age of diagnosis is 66 years, with vaginal MM developing earlier in the sixth and seventh decades, while vulvar MM develops later in the seventh decade.[6] Most patients present with vaginal bleeding, palpable mass, itching, or discharge, but MMs may also be found as a pigmented lesion on routine examination.[9] The 5-year survival rate for vulvovaginal MM is 36% with better outcomes for vulvar MM than for vaginal MM.[6]

Anorectal Mucosal Melanoma

Anorectal MM accounts for less than 1% of all melanoma subtypes.[8] Between 39% and 42% of anorectal melanomas are located within the rectum, one-third in the anal canal, and the remainder have an indeterminate site of origin.[6] The incidence increases with age, and the average age at diagnosis is 68 to 72 years. Unlike other types of MM, anorectal MM has been increasing in frequency. Women are 1.6 to 2.3 times more likely to develop anorectal MM. These primary lesions are often large on presentation with regional nodal metastasis found in 80% of patients at the time of diagnosis.[9] Patients may present with signs of obstruction or bleeding. The 5-year overall survival rate is approximately 20%.[6]

Treatment

Surgical treatment

Surgery is considered the mainstay of treatment for MM. Surgical resection with clear margins may be the aim of treatment, but the ability to achieve this is influenced by the size of the tumor, anatomic complexity, functional considerations, proximity to vital structures, and patient wishes.[3,10] No convincing evidence exists that an aggressive surgical approach improves local control or survival. The role of sentinel lymph node biopsy (SLNB) in MM is under investigation, and the prognostic factor of sentinel lymph nodes have not been established. Given the poor prognosis in respect of distant metastasis in MM, a complete regional lymph node dissection after a positive sentinel lymph node is controversial.[11]

Wide local excision is the favored treated for vulvovaginal MM, but surgical treatment can include vulvectomy, vaginectomy, or total exenteration depending on ability to achieve clear margins.[9] The role of SLNB in not well defined in vulvovaginal MM, but single-photon emission CT integrated with CT may accurately localize sentinel nodes compared with planar lymphoscintigraphy, given the complex anatomy and unpredictable lymph node drainage patterns in the pelvis.[5]

Surgical treatment for anorectal MM with localized disease should undergo sphincter-preserving wide local excision with 1- to 2-cm margins when possible. A more aggressive abdominoperineal resection should be reserved for palliation of localized bulky disease or select patients with local recurrence. SLNB should be considered to determine the need for bilateral inguinal dissections.[9]

Radiation therapy

The role of radiation therapy (RT) in MM has not been evaluated in prospective trials, but cutaneous melanoma randomized trials are considered relevant in MM. Sinonasal mucosal melanomas (SMM) are found in an area that is difficult to reach and achieve negative margins even after surgery, and intensive radiotherapy is important in the treatment of SMM but is only applicable to a small subset of patients because of radiosensitive critical tissues such as cranial nerves and brain stem in close proximity to the primary lesion. High-dose proton beam therapy has been found to be an effective local treatment in SSM and less invasive than surgery with comparable outcomes.[12] High-dose conformal proton beam therapy can deliver high doses of radiotherapy to the residual or primary tumor while minimizing exposure to surrounding tissues.

Postoperative radiation to the primary site is typically indicated to improve local disease control.[13] Adjuvant RT has been associated with improved regional lymph node basin control compared with lymph node dissection alone in patients with high-risk, clinically advanced, lymph node-metastatic melanoma.[14] In inoperable or unresectable cases, RT has provided reasonable local control with systemic therapy.[15]

The NCCN recommends postoperative RT for HNMM for the following high-risk features:[16,17]

- Extranodal extension
- Involvement of two or more neck or intraparotid nodes
- Any node 3 cm or greater
- Neck dissection alone with no further basin dissection
- Recurrence in the neck or soft tissue after surgical resection

Systemic Therapy

MMs are molecularly distinct from cutaneous melanomas with a lower rate of BRAF V6000 alternations, tumor mutational burden, and higher rate of chromosomal aberrations. In metastatic disease with specific mutations, immune checkpoint inhibitors are being used in treatment.[18] Adjuvant systemic therapy for MM is limited, but systemic therapy used for cutaneous melanoma is recommended for MM.[19] Patients with specific mutations may benefit from c-KIT inhibitors.[20] When there is a rare V600 mutation of the BRAF gene, a combination BRAF/MEK inhibitor is recommended.[21] Recent data support incorporating vascular endothelial growth factor receptor (VEGF)-based therapy in the treatment of MM. Studies conducted in China have demonstrated a 43% response rate when VEGF receptor–directed multikinase inhibitor, axitinib, was used in combination with PD-1 inhibitor, toripalimab, in locally advanced or unresectable MMs.[18] These results suggest that VEGF-directed blockade may be uniquely effective in MM. In a recent large prospective randomized open-label phase II trial in patients with advanced untreated MM, patients were given carboplatin plus paclitaxel every 4 weeks with or without bevacizumab, which acts by selectively binding circulating VEGF. The median progression-free survival was improved from 3 to 4.8 months, and the median overall survival was significantly improved from 9 to 13.6 months in the bevacizumab arm.[22] The efficacy of the bevacizumab regimen demonstrates the importance of incorporating VEGF-based therapy in the treatment for patients with MM.

SUMMARY

MM is a rare but aggressive cancer arising in mucosal surfaces most commonly in the head and neck. The clinical presentation is often nonspecific and differs in relation to the site of origin, so often diagnosis is delayed resulting in poor prognosis. MM has a 5-year survival of only 25%. Surgery with negative margins is the mainstay of treatment but dependent on several variables including anatomic location, involved structures, and size of tumor. Although not well defined given the rarity of MM, there is a role for radiation and systemic therapy in the treatment of this disease.

CLINICS CARE POINTS

- Mucosal melanoma is a rare cancer representing less than 1% of all malignant melanomas with a 5-year survival of only 25%.

- Mucosal melanoma is most commonly found in the head and neck, followed by anus and rectum, female reproductive tract, and the urinary tract mucosa.

- The staging for head and neck mucosal melanoma starts with T3N0 given poor prognosis even with a limited primary burden of disease.

- Surgical resection with clear margins is the mainstay treatment, but the ability to achieve this is influenced by the size of the tumor, anatomic complexity, functional considerations, and proximity to vital structures.

- Radiation therapy is recommended postoperatively and can provide reasonable local control in inoperable or unresectable cases.

- Systemic therapy used for cutaneous melanoma is recommended for mucosal melanoma, and in metastatic disease with specific mutations, immune checkpoint inhibitors are being used in treatment.

DISCLOSURE

The authors have nothing to disclose.

REFERENCES

1. Yde SS, Sjoegren P, Heje M, et al. Mucosal melanoma: a literature review. Curr Oncol Rep 2018; 20(3):28.
2. Mihajlovic M, Vlajkovic S, Jovanovic P, et al. Primary mucosal melanomas: a comprehensive review. Int J Clin Exp Pathol 2012;5(8):739–53.
3. Ascierto PA, Accorona R, Botti G, et al. Mucosal melanoma of the head and neck. Crit Rev Oncol Hematol 2017;112:136–52.
4. Li W, Yu Y, Wang H, et al. Evaluation of the prognostic impact of postoperative adjuvant radiotherapy on head and neck mucosal melanoma: a meta-analysis. BMC Cancer 2015;15:758.
5. Tacastacas JD, Bray J, Cohen YK, et al. Update on primary mucosal melanoma. J Am Acad Dermatol 2014;71(2):366–75.
6. Lerner BA, Stewart LA, Horowitz DP, et al. Mucosal melanoma: new Insights and therapeutic options for a unique and aggressive disease. Oncology (Williston Park) 2017;31(11):e23–32.
7. Wushou A, Hou J, Zhao YJ, et al. Postoperative adjuvant radiotherapy improves loco-regional recurrence of head and neck mucosal melanoma. J Craniomaxillofac Surg 2015;43(4):553–8.
8. Carvajal RD, Spencer SA, Lydiatt W. Mucosal melanoma: a clinically and biologically unique disease entity. J Natl Compr Canc Netw 2012; 10(3):345–56.
9. Kottschade LA, Grotz TE, Dronca RS, et al. Rare presentations of primary melanoma and special populations: a systematic review. Am J Clin Oncol 2014;37(6):635–41.
10. Jarrom D, Paleri V, Kerawala C, et al. Mucosal melanoma of the upper airways tract mucosal melanoma: a systematic review with meta-analyses of treatment. Head Neck 2017;39(4): 819–25.
11. Schaefer T, Satzger I, Gutzmer R. Clinics, prognosis and new therapeutic options in patients with mucosal melanoma: a retrospective analysis of 75 patients. Medicine (Baltimore) 2017;96(1): e5753.
12. Fuji H, Yoshikawa S, Kasami M, et al. High-dose proton beam therapy for sinonasal mucosal malignant melanoma. Radiat Oncol 2014;9:162.
13. Trotti A, Peters LJ. Role of radiotherapy in the primary management of mucosal melanoma of the head and neck. Semin Surg Oncol 1993;9(3): 246–50.
14. Agrawal S, Kane JM 3rd, Guadagnolo BA, et al. The benefits of adjuvant radiation therapy after therapeutic lymphadenectomy for clinically advanced, high-risk, lymph node-metastatic melanoma. Cancer 2009;115(24):5836–44.
15. Gilligan D, Slevin NJ. Radical radiotherapy for 28 cases of mucosal melanoma in the nasal cavity and sinuses. Br J Radiol 1991;64(768):1147–50.
16. Bonnen MD, Ballo MT, Myers JN, et al. Elective radiotherapy provides regional control for patients with cutaneous melanoma of the head and neck. Cancer 2004;100(2):383–9.
17. Ballo MT, Bonnen MD, Garden AS, et al. Adjuvant irradiation for cervical lymph node metastases from melanoma. Cancer 2003;97(7):1789–96.
18. Shoushtari AN. Incorporating VEGF blockade into a shifting treatment paradigm for mucosal melanoma [published online ahead of print, 2021 Jan 25]. J Clin Oncol 2021;JCO2000520.

19. Seetharamu N, Ott PA, Pavlick AC. Mucosal melanomas: a case-based review of the literature. Oncologist 2010;15(7):772–81.

20. Hodi FS, Corless CL, Giobbie-Hurder A, et al. Imatinib for melanomas harboring mutationally activated or amplified KIT arising on mucosal, acral, and chronically sun-damaged skin. J Clin Oncol 2013; 31(26):3182–90.

21. Curtin JA, Busam K, Pinkel D, et al. Somatic activation of KIT in distinct subtypes of melanoma. J Clin Oncol 2006;24(26):4340–6.

22. Yan X, Sheng X, Chi Z, et al. Randomized phase II study of bevacizumab in combination with carboplatin plus paclitaxel in patients with previously untreated advanced mucosal melanoma [published online ahead of print, 2021 Jan 14]. J Clin Oncol 2021;JCO2000902.

Emerging Therapies in the Treatment of Advanced Melanoma

Sameer Massand, MD[a], Rogerio I. Neves, MD, PhD, FSSO[b],*

KEYWORDS

• Emerging therapies • Oncolytic therapy • Vaccine therapy • Clinical trials

KEY POINTS

• Although immunotherapy and targeted therapy have established themselves as essential components of melanoma treatment, novel approaches in intratumoral oncolytics, adoptive cell therapy, cytokines, and vaccines have been developed as useful alternatives.
• Immunotherapy and targeted therapy appear to be most effective in combination; their ideal pairing and sequencing are to be determined by the results of ongoing clinical trials.
• The therapies that have revolutionized the adjuvant treatment of melanoma are being applied in the neoadjuvant setting, early results of which demonstrate efficacy.

INTRODUCTION

Melanoma, left untreated, metastasizes readily to lymph nodes and distant organs, rendering itself surgically unresectable and ultimately lethal. Developments in systemic and targeted therapy in the last decade have provided clinicians with an effective arsenal in the management of those melanomas that present in the advanced stages. Beginning with the paradigm-shifting medications ipilimumab, a checkpoint inhibitor, and vemurafenib, a kinase inhibitor that binds specifically to BRAF mutants, these classes of medications have brought about significant advances in management. Patients with advanced disease have effective therapeutic options and with expanding indications.

A rapidly growing body of knowledge of the pathways involved in tumorigenesis has allowed for further development in an array of antineoplastic approaches. Specifically, there are progressively more adept immunomodulators, new targets within tumor pathways for mutation-specific therapy, and combination approaches that allow for optimal synergy. Meanwhile, the nascent fields of vaccine therapy, cytokine therapy, intratumoral oncolytic therapy, and adoptive cell therapy (ACT) provide novel approaches that have as yet been unidentified or unexplored.

IMMUNOTHERAPY

Breakthroughs in immunotherapy for advanced melanoma have been primarily in the form of checkpoint inhibition. Monoclonal antibodies targeting CTLA-4 and PD-1 have been established as effective anticancer agents, specifically in treating melanoma and non–small cell lung cancer (**Table 1**). They are also in development for other cancer types. CTLA-4 and PD-1 receptors are known downregulators of T cell immune function, their inhibition therefore potentiating an immune response.

CTLA-4 Inhibition

Cytotoxic T-lymphocyte antigen 4 (CTLA-4) downregulates T cells and may produce inhibitory signals, allowing for a pathologic immune tolerance. Inhibition of CTLA-4 re-establishes the necessary immune response, making it an effective antitumor

[a] Division of Plastic Surgery, Penn State University, 500 University Drive, H071, Hershey, PA 17033, USA;
[b] Department of Cutaneous Oncology, H. Lee Moffitt Cancer Center and Research Institute, 10920 N McKinley Dr, MKC-4, Tampa, FL 33612, USA
* Corresponding author.
E-mail address: Rogerio.neves@moffitt.org

Clin Plastic Surg 48 (2021) 713–733
https://doi.org/10.1016/j.cps.2021.06.008

Table 1
Summary of immunotherapy agents approved and understudy for the treatment of advanced melanoma

| | | Immunotherapy | | | |
Agent	Mechanism	Relevant Trial Findings	Setting	Administration	FDA Approval
Imiplimab	CTLA-4 inhibitor	NCT00094653: Ipilimumab improved overall survival in patients with metastatic melanoma[1]	Refractory, unresectable melanoma	Intravenous	March 2011
Pembrolizumab	PD-1 inhibitor	KEYNOTE-006: Pembrolizumab demonstrates improved OS vs ipilimumab alone[4] KEYNOTE-054: Pembrolizumab demonstrates improved RFS vs placebo[6]	Unresectable melanoma Adjuvant therapy for Stage III	Intravenous	Dec 2015 Feb 2019
Nivolumab	PD-1 inhibitor	CHECKMATE-067 trial: Nivolumab alone or combined with ipilimumab demonstrated longer PFS than ipilimumab alone[5] CHECKMATE-238 trial: Nivolumab monotherapy is effective in the adjuvant setting[7]	Unresectable stage III-IV melanoma Adjuvant therapy for IIIB-IV melanoma	Intravenous	Dec 2014 Dec 2017
Atezolizumab	PDL-1 inhibitor	IMSPIRE150 trial: Improved PFS in combination with cobimetinib and vemurafenib[14]	Unresectable stage III-IV melanoma	Intravenous	July 2020

agent (**Fig. 1**). Ipilimumab, a monoclonal antibody to CTLA-4, was approved in 2011 by the FDA for its reduction in mortality of advanced melanomas. It carries, however, a high rate of adverse effects, with grade 3 or 4 events affecting 23% of patients.[1] In addition, a significant portion of melanomas goes on to develop resistance to therapy with ipilimumab.

PD-1 Inhibition

T-cell surface molecule programmed death protein-1 (PD-1) binds with PDL-1, a ligand often expressed by tumor cells, leading to reduced T cell proliferation, cytokine production, and T cell survival. This serves as another checkpoint, and therefore another target in immunotherapy. Monoclonal IgG antibodies pembrolizumab and nivolumab have been developed and FDA approved, both in 2014. They have been shown to be effective in ipilimumab-refractory and treatment-naïve unresectable or metastatic melanoma with durable results as established in the KEYNOTE-001(NCT01295827), and since then established efficacy in several settings.[2]

PD-1 inhibition is now first-line therapy for unresectable melanoma, regardless of BRAF-mutation status, after the release of data from the KEYNOTE 002, KEYNOTE-006, and CHECKMATE-067 trials.[3–5] In addition, it is approved for adjuvant treatment of resected stage III or IV melanoma with lymph node involvement after establishing efficacy in the KEYNOTE-054 and CHECKMATE-238 trials using pembrolizumab and nivolumab, respectively.[6,7] Recent data released in 2020 demonstrated sustained results for pembrolizumab at 3 years of median follow-up, with 63.7% of experimental-arm patients and 44.1% of control-arm patients (placebo) maintaining recurrence-free status, and for nivolumab at 4 years of median follow-up, with 77.9% of experimental-arm patients and 76.6% of control-arm patients (ipilimumab) maintaining overall survival (OS).[8,9] Furthermore, the widely awaited results of the CHECKMATE-915 trial (NCT03068455) released in October 2020 demonstrate that dual therapy with nivolumab and ipilimumab did not have any added benefit over monotherapy with nivolumab in adjuvant therapy for stages III and IV melanoma, regardless of subgroup.[10] (**Table 2**) This is in contrast to the previously held notion that combination therapy is more effective in metastatic melanoma.[11]

Given the efficacy of PD-1 inhibition in the adjuvant setting, there is an ongoing study to assess an expanded role in the adjuvant management of high-risk stage II melanoma. The KEYNOTE-716 trial, evaluating pembrolizumab against placebo in this earlier-stage population, is expected to reach primary completion in 2022. These

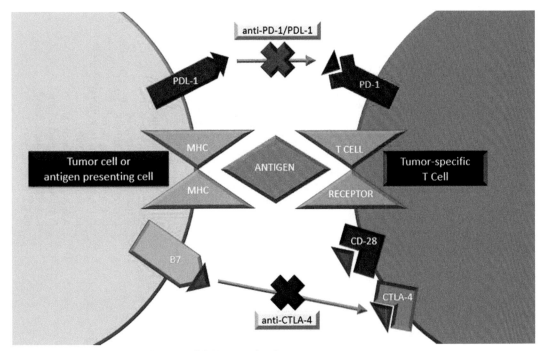

Fig. 1. Basic schematic of checkpoint inhibition mechanism.

Table 2
Relevant ongoing studies in immunotherapy, targeted therapy, combination and sequential therapy, and other emerging therapies, as of March 2021

Identifier	Name	Drugs Tested	Neoadjuvant	Phase	Estimated Completion	Preliminary Results
Immunotherapy						
NCT03068455	An Investigational Immunotherapy Study of Nivolumab Combined With Ipilimumab Compared to Nivolumab by Itself After Complete Surgical Removal of Stage IIIb/c/d or Stage IV Melanoma (CheckMate 915)[58]	Nivolumab + Ipilimumab		III	May-21	Y
NCT02332668	A Study of Pembrolizumab (MK-3475) in Pediatric Participants With an Advanced Solid Tumor or Lymphoma (MK-3475–051/ KEYNOTE-051)[59]	Pembrolizumab		II	Sep-22	Y
NCT03743766	Nivolumab, BMS-936558 in Combination With Relatlimab, BMS-986016 in Patients With Metastatic Melanoma Naïve to Prior Immunotherapy in the Metastatic Setting[60]	Relatlimab		II	Dec-21	N
NCT03776136	A Multicenter, Open-label, Phase 2 Trial to Assess the Efficacy and Safety of Lenvatinib (E7080/MK-7902) in Combination With Pembrolizumab (MK-3475) in Participants With Advanced Melanoma Previously Exposed to an Anti-PD-1/L1 Agent (LEAP-004)[61]	Lenvatinib		II	Jun-21	Y

Targeted therapy

NCT Number	Title	Intervention	Setting	Phase	Date	
NCT01972347	Neoadjuvant Dabrafenib + Trametinib for AJCC Stage IIIB-C BRAF V600 Mutation Positive Melanoma[62]	Dabrafenib + Trametinib	Neoadjuvant	II	May-22	N
NCT02036086	Study of Neo-adjuvant Use of Vemurafenib Plus Cobimetinib for BRAF Mutant Melanoma With Palpable Lymph Node Metastases[63]	Vemurafenib + Cometinib	Neoadjuvant	II	Oct-22	N
NCT02857270	A Study of LY3214996 Administered Alone or in Combination With Other Agents in Participants With Advanced/Metastatic Cancer[64]	LY3214996		I	Sep-21	N

Combination therapy

NCT Number	Title	Intervention	Setting	Phase	Date	
NCT02130466	A Study of the Safety and Efficacy of Pembrolizumab (MK-3475) in Combination With Trametinib and Dabrafenib in Participants With Advanced Melanoma (MK-3475–022/KEYNOTE-022)[65]	Pembrolizumab and Dabrafenib + Cometinib		I/II	Jul-21	Y
NCT02908672	A Study of Atezolizumab Plus Cobimetinib and Vemurafenib vs Placebo Plus Cobimetinib and Vemurafenib in Previously Untreated BRAFv600 Mutation-Positive Patients With Metastatic or Unresectable Locally Advanced Melanoma (IMspire150)[66]	Atezolizumab and Cobimetinib + Vemurafenib		III	Jul-23	Y

(continued on next page)

Table 2
(continued)

Identifier	Name	Drugs Tested	Neoadjuvant	Phase	Estimated Completion	Preliminary Results
NCT03554083	Neoadjuvant Combination Targeted and Immunotherapy for Patients With High-Risk Stage III Melanoma (NeoACTIVATE)[67]	Atezolizumab and Cobimetinib + Vemurafenib	Neoadjuvant	II	Jun-23	N
NCT02858921	Neoadjuvant Dabrafenib, Trametinib and/or Pembrolizumab in BRAF Mutant Resectable Stage III Melanoma (NeoTrio)[68]	Pembrolizumab and Dabrafenib + Cometinib	Neoadjuvant	II	Nov-24	N
NCT02224781	Dabrafenib and Trametinib Followed by Ipilimumab and Nivolumab or Ipilimumab and Nivolumab Followed by Dabrafenib and Trametinib in Treating Patients With Stage III-IV BRAFV600 Melanoma (DREAM-Seq)[69]	Dabrafenib + Trametinib and Ipilimumab + Nivolumab		III	Oct-22	N
NCT02631447	Sequential Combo Immuno and Target Therapy (SECOMBIT) Study (SECOMBIT)[70]	Encorafenib + Binimetinib and Ipilimumab + Nivolumab		II	Dec-21	N
NCT03235245	Immunotherapy with Ipilimumab and Nivolumab Preceded or Not by a Targeted Therapy With Encorafenib and Binimetinib (EBIN)[71]	Encorafenib + Binimetinib and Ipilimumab + Nivolumab		II	Feb-24	N

NCT	Title	Intervention	Setting	Phase	Date	
NCT02902029	Evaluating the Efficacy and Safety of a Sequencing Schedule of Cobimetinib Plus Vemurafenib Followed by Immunotherapy With an Anti- PD-L1 Antibody in Patients With Unresectable or Metastatic BRAF V600 Mutant Melanoma (ImmunoCobiVem)[72]	Vemurafenib + Cometinib and Atezolizumab		II	Jun-22	N
Other therapies						
NCT02211131	Efficacy and Safety of Talimogene Laherparepvec Neoadjuvant Treatment Plus Surgery vs Surgery Alone for Melanoma[73]	T-Vec	Neoadjuvant	II	Apr-22	N
NCT04427306	Neoadjuvant T-VEC in High Risk Early Melanoma[74]	T-Vec	Neoadjuvant	II	May-24	N
NCT02263508	Pembrolizumab With or Without Talimogene Laherparepvec or Talimogene Laherparepvec Placebo in Unresected Melanoma (KEYNOTE-034)[75]	T-Vec		III	Apr-23	N
NCT03567889	Efficacy of Daromun Neoadjuvant Intratumoral Treatment in Clinical Stage IIIB/C Melanoma Patients (Neo-DREAM)[76]	Daromun	Neoadjuvant	III	Dec-24	N
NCT03445533	A Study of IMO-2125 in Combination With Ipilimumab vs Ipilimumab Alone in Subjects With Anti-PD-1 Refractory Melanoma (ILLUMINATE-301)[77]	Tilsotolimod		III	Sep-21	N

(continued on next page)

Table 2
(continued)

Identifier	Name	Drugs Tested	Neoadjuvant	Phase	Estimated Completion	Preliminary Results
NCT02557321	PV-10 in Combination With Pembrolizumab for Treatment of Metastatic Melanoma[78]	PV-10		I/II	Nov-23	N
NCT02983045	A Dose Escalation and Cohort Expansion Study of NKTR-214 in Combination With Nivolumab and Other Anti-Cancer Therapies in Patients With Select Advanced Solid Tumors (PIVOT-02)[79]	Bempegaldesleukin		I/II	Dec-21	Y
NCT03635983	A Study of NKTR-214 Combined With Nivolumab vs Nivolumab Alone in Participants With Previously Untreated Inoperable or Metastatic Melanoma[80]	Bempegaldesleukin		III	Jun-25	N
NCT02360579	Study of Lifileucel (LN-144), Autologous Tumor Infiltrating Lymphocytes, in the Treatment of Patients With Metastatic Melanoma (LN-144)[81]	Lifileucel		II	Dec-24	Y
NCT02410733	Evaluation of the Safety and Tolerability of i.v. Administration of a Cancer Vaccine in Patients With Advanced Melanoma (Lipo-MERIT)[82]	FixVac vaccine		I	May-22	Y

results, too, are widely awaited as they may add an entirely new population to the gradually expanding group of patients who can benefit from PD-1 inhibition.

Finally, PD-1 inhibition is under investigation as a therapy for pediatric solid tumors including pediatric melanoma in the KEYNOTE-051 trial (NCT02332668) results of which are expected in 2022.[12]

PDL-1 Inhibition

Programmed death protein ligand–1, the ligand to PD-1, has been identified as an alternative to PD-1 inhibition with more specificity to cancer processes and therefore, less immunotoxicity. This is supported by a 2019 metanalysis in which Wang and colleagues[13] report a lower rate of severe adverse events in patients receiving PDL-1 inhibitors than those receiving PD-1 inhibitors.

Atezolizumab, a monoclonal antibody to PDL-1, is approved as monotherapy for lung, urothelial, and breast cancer, and since July 2020, is approved in combination with vemurafenib (BRAF inhibitor) and cometinib (MEK inhibitor) for BRAF-V600 mutation-positive unresectable melanoma. This is based on the results of the IMspire150 Trial (NCT02908672), which showed a 15.1-month median progression free survival (PFS) for the experimental group compared with a 10.6-month median PFS for the placebo group. Most adverse events were classified as grade 1 or 2.[14]

Combination Immunotherapy

Combination therapy offers the potential for synergy and therefore a more potent antitumor effect. In many cases, combination therapy has supplanted monotherapy as standard of care, provided that it does not present an unacceptable adverse effect burden.

This is evidenced by the OpACIN trial (NCT02437279) in which neoadjuvant versus adjuvant ipilimumab plus nivolumab was assessed. Although the neoadjuvant combination demonstrated stronger induction of tumor-specific T cells, and maintained a good pathologic response and durable PFS, it had a high toxicity requiring a follow-up study using an alternate dosing schedule.[15] This was done as the OpACIN-neo trial (NCT02977052), which demonstrated high overall response rate (ORR) and pathologic complete response with neoadjuvant low-dose ipilimumab and nivolumab.[16]

Combination therapy with BRAF/MEK inhibition in BRAF mutation-positive melanoma, with MEK inhibition, or with other emerging approaches is addressed in later sections.

Novel Immunotherapies

Despite successes, there remain a significant portion of patients who are unresponsive to checkpoint inhibition, or who grow resistant to it. Several novel immunomodulators have therefore been identified as alternatives.

The lymphocyte-activation gene −3 (LAG-3) is another immune checkpoint molecule that can be manipulated to regulate T cell function. Relatlimab, an anti–LAG-3 monoclonal antibody, is currently undergoing a phase II trial in combination with nivolumab (NCT03743766) for the treatment of immunotherapy-naïve metastatic melanoma and has an estimated completion date of December 2021. Meanwhile, in November 2020, Atkinson and colleagues[17] released phase I results demonstrating encouraging antitumor activity of pembrolizumab plus eftilagimod-alpha, a soluble LAG-3 protein, in patients with metastatic melanoma.

Epacadostat, an IDO1 inhibitor, has been evaluated extensively as another means of enhancing PD-1 inhibitor therapy. By inhibiting the IDO1 enzyme, it prevents downstream progression to an immunosuppressive state in the tumor microenvironment (TME). Attention has shifted away from IDO1 inhibition, however, as phase III results of epacadostat plus pembrolizumab showed no clinical value, and recruitment for a phase III trial evaluating another IDO1 inhibitor, BMS-986205, (NCT03329846) was stopped short far below its anticipated enrollment.[18]

Lenvatinib, a tyrosine kinase inhibitor with suppressive effects on both VEGF and FGF, may hold more promise as an adjunct to PD-1 inhibition. Results of the phase II LEAP-004 trial (NCT03776136) were published at the 2020 ESMO Virtual Congress, demonstrating moderate efficacy in treating late-stage, treatment-refractory melanoma.[19]

Other targets under early investigation are CXCL-10—a small cytokine-line protein that positively affects immunomodulation and tumor suppression, TIM-3—a cell surface receptor that acts as another "checkpoint," and TIGIT—an immunoreceptor that recognizes ligands on tumor cells and mediates T-cell response.[20–22]

TARGETED THERAPY

Whereas immunotherapy incites a broad, systemic response, targeted therapy aims to disrupt pathway aberrations specific to treated cancer. Advances in DNA sequencing and mutation identification in the last decades have offered insight into a spectrum of potential targets. Primarily, the MAP kinase pathway has been discovered as having an outsized role in melanoma. This discovery has burgeoned into a paradigm shift, with MAP kinase targeted therapy serving as a critical component of advanced and unresectable melanoma management.

MAP kinase signaling pathways are complex pathways beginning with many extracellular agents and cascading ultimately to cell proliferation, differentiation, senescence, survival, transformation, and migration.[23] Mutation and subsequent hyperactivation is well established as carcinogenic, and more specifically, melanogenic. Regulation of this pathway serves as the primary objective of targeted therapy in melanoma (**Table 3**).

Specific mutations have been identified as the most common drivers of overactivity in this pathway. BRAF mutations are observed in 50% of melanomas, 90% of which are at codon 600 with substitution of glutamic acid for valine (V600E). RAS mutations are observed in 15% to 28%, MEK mutations in 6% to 7% and typically alongside BRAF mutations, and ERK mutations in less than 1%.

BRAF Inhibitors

Original BRAF inhibitor study was performed using vemurafenib in combination with ipilimumab, and required discontinuation because of hepatic toxicity. With PD-1 inhibitors supplanting anti–CTLA-4 therapy, recent studies have combined BRAF inhibition with PD-1 inhibition instead and offered great results. Vemurafenib and dabrafenib are first-generation BRAF inhibitors, approved following results of the pivotal BRIM-3 trial (NCT01006980) and BREAK-3 trial (NCT01227889).[24,25]

Encorafenib is a second-generation selective kinase inhibitor, approved in 2018 in combination with MEK inhibitor binimetinib for unresectable, BRAF mutation-positive melanoma.

MEK Inhibitors

BRAF inhibitors inherently rely on the presence of a BRAF mutation, limiting their applicability to

Table 3
Summary of targeted therapy agents approved and understudy for the treatment of advanced melanoma

Targeted Therapy					
Agent	Mechanism	Relevant Trial Findings	Setting	Administration	FDA Approval
Vemurafenib	BRAF Inhibitor (first generation)	BRIM-3 trial: Improved PFS and OS with vemurafenib compared to dacarbazine[24]	Unresectable melanoma with BRAF V600 mutation	Oral capsule	Aug 2011
Dabrafenib	BRAF Inhibitor (first generation)	BREAK-3 trial: Improved PFS and OS with vemurafenib compared to dacarbazine.[25]	Unresectable melanoma with BRAF V600 mutation	Oral tablet	May 2013
Encorafenib	BRAF inhibitor (second generation)	COLUMBUS trial: Encorafenib plus binimetinib and encorafenib monotherapy showed favorable efficacy compared with vemurafenib[83]	Unresectable melanoma with BRAF V600 mutation	Oral capsule	June 2018
Trematinib Cobimetinib Binimetinib	MEK Inhibitor	COMBI-d and COMBI-v trials: Combination BRAF/MEK therapy is more effective than monotherapy[26,27]	Unresectable melanoma Neoadjuvant therapy	Oral tablets	May 2013 Dec 2015 June 2018 None

approximately half of all melanomas. This is circumvented by downstream inhibition in the form of MEK inhibition. Trametinib, cobimetinib, and binimetinib have been developed and approved as MEK inhibitors. MEK inhibition monotherapy is fairly limited by inhibition of the MAP-kinase pathway systemically, and resultant toxicity.

BRAF/MEK Inhibition

BRAF and MEK inhibitors demonstrate effective synergy and are primarily used in combination. Results of the COMBI-d (NCT01584648) and COMBI-v (NCT01597908) trials established the clinical superiority of combination therapy, and a pooled long-term follow-up published in 2019 demonstrated that long-term benefit was achieved in approximately one-third of patients with unresectable or metastatic melanoma at the time of enrollment.[4,26,27]

Most recently, BRAF/MEK inhibition therapy has been examined as a potential neoadjuvant therapy. Clinical trials in this follow a wave of case reports and case series exhibiting successful neoadjuvant management of late-stage melanoma with vemurafenib or combination BRAF/MEK inhibition. Perhaps most significant is the result of clinical trial NCT02231775, which examined neoadjuvant dabrafenib + trametinib versus then- standard of care resection and adjuvant therapy. The experimental arm demonstrated significantly improved event-free survival and the study was terminated before completion.[28] A Dutch study termed the REDUCTOR trial trialed the same combination in 17 unresectable melanomas and achieved 35% pathologic complete response, and 14 restagings to resectable disease. Ongoing trials, NCT01972347 and NCT02036086, are evaluating dabrafenib plus trametinib, and vemurafenib plus cometinib, respectively, to provide more evidence of the role of BRAF/MEK inhibition in neoadjuvant therapy. Both trials are expected to release results in 2022.

Novel Targets

BRAF inhibition, as discussed, does not address non-v600 BRAF subtypes, and may actually stimulate the MAP kinase pathway.[29] Recent study has focused on suitable targets for those non-v600 BRAF subtypes, whether RAS or NF-1 mutants or others. In addition, pathway reactivation after initial suppressive response to BRAF/MEK inhibition has been seen via genetic events including new mutations and overexpression of signaling receptors integral to the MAP kinase pathway.[23]

A dual MEK/RAF inhibitor, RO5126766, has been developed, and has the benefit of addressing

RAS-mutated melanomas as well. The clinical study is early, and phase I results across solid tumors demonstrate encouraging antitumor activity and a tolerable adverse effect profile.[30]

An extracellular-signal-regulated kinase (ERK) is a downstream component of the MAP kinase pathway that has emerged as an option for BRAF/MEK inhibition-refractory melanoma and RAS- or NF-1 mutant melanoma and is the subject of multiple clinical trials currently. ERK inhibitors have been found preclinically to have broader efficacy than MEK inhibitors, and early clinical data support their efficacy and tolerance.[31] Several ERK-inhibiting drugs have been developed, including ravoxertinib, LTT462, LY3214996, and ulixertinib. Phase I data demonstrate acceptable safety profiles for ravoxertinib and ulixertinib, and limited clinical efficacy for LTT462.[32] Results of the phase I study NCT02857270 examining LY3214996 are expected to be available in 2021.

The phosphatidylinositol 3-kinase (PI3K) pathway is a separate pathway frequently dysregulated in cancer, including melanoma. It is upregulated following an oncogenic RAS mutation, or as compensation following inhibition of the MAP-kinase pathway because of their interconnectivity. This makes dual blockade for both pathways an appealing treatment approach in advanced melanoma. Dual PI3K and MAP kinase blockade has shown promise in a preclinical setting.[33] However, no PI3K inhibiting agents have yet demonstrated the same efficacy in a clinical setting without significant adverse events.[34]

Other targets within the PI3K pathway include AKT and mTOR. Although several agents have been studied in clinical trials, typically in combination with BRAF/MEK inhibitors, none have yet been identified as providing the same clinical benefit suggested by in vivo studies.[35]

COMBINED IMMUNOTHERAPY AND TARGETED THERAPY

BRAF/MEK inhibition in combination with PDL-1 or PD-1 directed checkpoint inhibition provides similar response rates while prolonging the duration of response. Specifically, BRAF/MEK inhibition has superior OS and PFS in the first 6 months, then after 6 months immunotherapy (combo PD-1+CTLA-4) is superior.[14] A flurry of clinical trials are in the process of establishing the role of combined immunotherapy and targeted therapy.

Preliminary results of the KEYNOTE-022 study (NCT02130466), delivered in December 2020, have demonstrated the superior efficacy of triplet therapy—pembrolizumab plus dabrafenib and trametinib, over placebo plus dabrafenib and trametinib. They do, however, note grade 3 or higher treatment-related AEs in over half of experimental-arm patients.[36] Interestingly, PDL-1 inhibition with atezolizumab plus targeted therapy with vemurafenib and cometinib also demonstrated increased PFS, while maintaining an acceptable adverse event profile. These results are from the IMspire150 trial (NCT02908672), published in June 2020.[14]

Two ongoing trials seek to determine efficacy in the neoadjuvant setting. The NeoACTIVATE trial (NCT03554083) is currently recruiting patients for neoadjuvant treatment with atezolizumab plus cobimetinib or atezolizumab plus vemurafenib and cobimetinib if BRAF-mutation-positive. The NeoTrio trial (NCT02858921) is evaluating pembrolizumab plus dabrafenib and trametinib as neoadjuvant therapy for stage III melanoma. Neither trial is expected to complete before 2023.

As these trials indicate that combination immuno- and targeted therapy may play an outsize role in future therapy, other trials are ongoing to better establish the most effective sequencing and administration of the medications. Two are assessing BRAF/MEK inhibition and CTLA−4/PD-4 inhibition; the DREAMseq trial (NCT02224781) treats patients with either dabrafenib plus trametinib followed by ipilimumab plus nivolumab or ipilimumab plus nivolumab followed by dabrafenib plus trametinib, and the SECOMBIT trial (NCT02631447) follows a similar protocol using encorafenib plus binimetinib instead for its BRAF/MEK inhibition component. The SECOMBIT trial also added a third arm with a "sandwich approach," in which patients receive encorafenib plus binimetinib for 8 weeks, followed by ipilimumab plus nivolumab until disease progression, followed by encorafenib plus binimetinib until disease progression. Preliminary, 2-year results were presented at the 2020 ESMO Virtual Congress and indicated that this third arm achieved the highest PFS.[37]

The EBIN trial (NCT03235245) is recruiting patients to undergo either therapy with encorafenib and binimetinib followed by combination immunotherapy (Ipilimumab and Nivolumab), or immediate combination immunotherapy. ImmunoCobiVen (NCT02902029) seeks to assess the potential sequential benefit of vemurafenib plus cometinib followed by atezolizumab. Both trials are expected to achieve primary completion in 2022.

INTRATUMORAL THERAPY

Intratumoral or intralesional therapy gained attention for its potential ability to treat advanced local disease while minimizing systemic exposure. It was originally introduced in 1988 when its first trial was performed, with an objective response rate of 55% in 20 patients. Since then, checkpoint blockade was reported and widely adopted as the first line of therapy in advanced melanoma, overshadowing intratumoral therapy, which had not yet been widely accepted. In the interim, however, many advances were introduced to improve the response rate.

Intratumoral therapy has many potential benefits. Injection of the tumor itself delivers therapy directly into the TME. Furthermore, abscopal effects have been observed, in which the local injection results in response of distant, untreated lesions, suggestive of a systemic response to the local treatment.[38]

Viral oncolytics have been the primary carrier; however, other mechanisms have been studied as well (**Table 4**). Future studies may focus on patients with melanoma unresponsive to other mainstay therapies, specifically checkpoint blockade.

Talimogene Laherparepvec

Talimogene laherparepvec (T-VEC) is a modified herpes simplex virus designed to preferentially replicate in tumoral cells and stimulate granulocyte macrophage—colony-stimulating factor, leading to tumor cell lysis. It is FDA approved for the treatment of metastatic melanoma based on the results of OPTiM, a phase III clinical trial (NCT00769704), which demonstrated clinical superiority to treatment with granulocyte-macrophage colony-stimulating factor and sargramostim (GM-CSF).[39]

T-VEC has also been found to safely and effectively improve 3-year RFS and OS when used as neoadjuvant therapy followed by surgery versus surgery alone. This interim data from phase II trial NCT02211131 was presented at the 2020 Society for the Immunotherapy for Cancer meeting.[40] Another ongoing phase II trial, NCT04427306, is evaluating T-VEC as neoadjuvant therapy for high-risk early melanoma.

Other future applications of T-VEC will be further established by the results of MASTERKEY-265/KEYNOTE-034 (NCT02263508), a phase III trial evaluating T-VEC in combination with pembrolizumab for unresectable melanoma.

Daromun

Daromun is a combination of two monoclonal antibody-cytokine fusion proteins, darleukin and fibromun. Intratumoral injection of daromun is thought to result in selective delivery of the immunocytokine to tumor sites. Phase II data demonstrated the complete response of 32 injected lesions in 20 patients, and abscopal effect lending

Table 4
Summary of intratumoral agents approved and understudy for the treatment of advanced melanoma

Agent	Mechanism	Relevant Trial Findings	Setting	Administration	FDA Approval
		Intra-tumoral Therapy			
Talimogene Laherparepvec (T-VEC)	Modified herpes simplex virus	OPTiM trial: T-VEC is more effective than GM-CSF treatment alone[39] NCT02211131: Neoadjuvant T-VEC improves 3-year RFS and OS over surgery alone[40]	Recurrent Stage IIIB-IV melanoma Neoadjuvant therapy for early melanoma	Intralesional injection	Oct 2015 None
Daromun	Combination of two monoclonal antibody-cytokine fusion proteins	NCT02076633: Achieves local control with the potential to eradicate advanced melanoma[41] NEODREAM trial: Ongoing trial to assess neoadjuvant use of Daromun[76]	Stage IIIC or IV melanoma Neoadjuvant therapy for Stage IIIB/C melanoma	Intralesional injection	None None
Tilsotolimod	TLR-9 agonist	ILLUMINATE-204 trial: Tilsotolimod effective and well tolerated[42] ILLUMINATE-301 trial: No improvement over ipilimumab alone[77]	Check-point-inhibitor refractory Stage IIIB-IV melanoma	Intralesional injection	June 2017 (Orphan drug status)
CAVATAK (CVA-21)	Injectable form of naturally occurring coxsackie virus	CALM trial: CAVATAK alone demonstrates efficacy[43]	Stage IIIc or IV melanoma	Intralesional injection	None
Canerpaturev (C-REV)	HSV-1 derivative	NCT03153085: C-REV with ipilimumab demonstrates efficacy and tolerance[45]	Stage IIIB-IV melanoma	Intralesional injection	None
PV-10	Injectable rose Bengal sodium	NCT00521053: High rate of complete response as monotherapy[46]	Refractory Stage III-IV melanoma	Intralesional injection	Jan 2007 (Orphan drug status)

complete response to 7/13 noninjected lesions.[41] Neo-DREAM (NCT03567889) is a phase III trial currently recruiting subjects for neoadjuvant therapy with Daromun.

TLR-9

Toll-like receptor-9 (TLR-9) agonism activates the immune response by upregulating type I IFN and dendritic cells (DCs). It is delivered to its target in a virus-like capsule. Data from the phase II ILLUMINATE-204 trial (NCT02644967) were presented at the ESMO Virtual Congress in September 2020. Tilsotolimod, a TLR-9 agonist injected into anti–PD-1-refractory melanoma lesions, demonstrated efficacy and was well tolerated.[42] A phase III study, ILLUMINATE-301 (NCT03445533) is ongoing to establish tilsotolimod as an accessible antimelanoma agent.

CVA-21

CAVATAK (CVA-21) is an injectable form of a naturally occurring coxsackie virus that preferentially infects cells with a high number of I-CAMs such as proliferating tumor cells. It has been studied in the treatment of advanced melanoma as monotherapy (NCT01227551), as combination therapy with ipilimumab (NCT02307149), and as combination therapy with pembrolizumab. All 3 trials showed promising clinical efficacy and tolerable adverse effect profiles.[43]

C-REV

Canerpaturev (C-REV), formerly referred to as HF-10 is another oncolytic virus derived from HSV-1. It

has been shown, in combination with ipilimumab, to have encouraging antitumor activity with a favorable benefit/risk profile in patients with advanced, stage IIIb or later, melanoma.[44,45]

PV-10

PV-10 is an injectable form of rose bengal sodium, which accumulates in tumoral cell lysosomes, avoiding normal cell lysosomes, and causes cell lysis and ensuing immunologic response. It has received orphan drug designation from FDA for treatment in certain melanomas and hepatocellular carcinomas. Early data show a high rate of complete response as monotherapy, and an ongoing trial seeks to establish its use in combination with pembrolizumab (NCT02557321).[46]

CYTOKINE THERAPY

Cytokines have undergone a resurgence as therapeutic techniques in advanced melanoma (**Table 5**). Two decades before this writing, cytokine therapy with interferon alpha (IFN-a) and interleukin-2 (IL-2, or recombinant human aldesleukin) was a widespread approach because of the immunomodulatory effects providing antiproliferation and inhibition of angiogenesis. High levels of toxicity and the more robust efficacy of checkpoint inhibition displaced the use of these agents.

IL-2

Interleukin-2 provides potent CD8 T cell stimulation and downstream antitumor effects. Its

Table 5
Summary of cytokine therapy agents approved and understudy for the management of advanced melanoma

Cytokine Therapy					
Agent	Mechanism	Relevant Trial Findings	Setting	Administration	FDA Approval
Bempegaldesleukin	Prodrug of conjugated IL-2, stimulates T cell response	PIVOT-02 Trial: Bempegaldesleukin plus nivolumab demonstrates prolonged PFS and ORR compared to nivolumab alone[47]	Previously untreated stage IV melanoma	Intravenous	Aug 2019
L19-IL-2	Recombinant human L19 antibody fused to IL-2, adds selective delivery to tumor cells	NCT01055522: L-19-1L-2 plus dacarbazine demonstrates better ORR and PFS than dacarbazine alone[48]	Previously untreated stage IV melanoma	Intravenous	None

administration, however, was notable for relatively low activity in the face of high toxicity. As checkpoint inhibition surfaced, IL-2 lost its appeal as a therapy. Recent advances have re-established its potential use. Bempegaldesleukin is a modified prodrug of aldesleukin, and has been found to have improved tumor exposure while causing less systemic effects. Encouraging phase II data from the PIVOT-02 trial (NCT02983045) were presented at the SITC Meeting in November 2020, with bempegaldesleukin plus nivolumab demonstrating prolonged PFS and ORR in late-stage melanoma as compared with nivolumab alone.[47] A phase III trial assessing the same combination, NCT03635983, is in the recruiting period at the time of this writing.

L19-IL-2

This recombinant human L19 antibody fused with IL-2 is a mechanism to selectively deliver IL-2 into tumor burden. It has been assessed alongside L19-TNF in *Doromun* as described earlier, and also had success alongside dacarbazine in metastatic melanoma patients.[48] It remains a promising adjunct in the resurgence of cytokine therapy.

Others

Several cytokines with varied immunomodulatory effects are under investigation as monotherapies, and more frequently as combination therapies, for the treatment of advanced melanoma. Two notable ones are *IL-15* and *IL-2,* both of which have been examined as therapy for other solid tumors, and are now under investigation in preclinical and early clinical trials as therapeutic agents against advanced melanoma.[49]

ADOPTIVE CELL THERAPY

ACT, like cytokine therapy, has been described for several decades, with the first early trials performed in the 1970s and 1980s. This method, too, has been eclipsed by the successes of checkpoint inhibition. Responses to ACT were often short, and blood analysis within days of administration did not identify circulating administered tumor-infiltrating lymphocytes (TILs). In 2002, it was discovered that preparation of the host with lymphodepleting, nonmyeloablative chemotherapy significantly bolstered the response to ACT.

The process of ACT with TIL involves resection of the melanoma, in vitro identification of tumor-specific lymphocytes and expansion of its colonies, and finally systemic reinfusion to the patient following lymphodepletion (**Table 6**).

One TIL therapy under investigation is lifileucel, in the phase II clinical trial C-144-01 (NCT02360579). Preliminary data were presented at the ASCO 2020 conference, demonstrating efficacy in late-stage melanoma using the TIL therapy, followed by an IL-2 course.[50] The completion of the trial is expected in 2024.

A slightly different ACT approach is that of chimeric antigen receptor (CAR) T-cell therapy. The principle is similar, except that these are systemic T cells obtained through apheresis rather than biopsy or resection. The T cells isolated ex-vivo undergo genetic transduction with a CAR construct, allowing them to target tumor burden on reinfusion. Like TIL, this is enhanced by pretherapeutic

Table 6
Summary of adoptive cell therapy agents approved and understudy for the treatment of advanced melanoma

Adoptive Cell Therapy					
Agent	Mechanism	Relevant Trial Findings	Setting	Administration	FDA Approval
Lifleucel	Autologous tumor-infiltrating leukocytes, obtained via biopsy, expanded ex-vivo and readministered	C-144-01 Trial: Lifleucel followed by an IL-2 course demonstrated efficacy[50]	Refractory stage IIIC or IV melanoma	Single intravenous administration	April 2021 (orphan drug status)
Tisagenlecleucel, Axicabtagene ciloleucel	Same as above, but obtained via apheresis, and transduced with CARs before administration	FDA-approved for other cancer indications[51]	Not yet studied in melanoma	Single IV administration	None

lymphodepletion. Two approved constructs are tisa-genlecleucel and axicabtagene ciloleucel. Optimization and future success of this therapy will rely on the addition of mechanisms to overcome physical barriers in migration to the TME, as well as identification of an ideal target antigen to potentiate antitumor activity once at the tumor site.[51]

VACCINE THERAPY

Vaccine therapy holds one specific advantage over the current standard of care approaches in that checkpoint inhibition and other immunomodulatory and targeted therapies rely on a preexisting immune response to cancer, whereas vaccine therapy can induce an antitumor response that was not spontaneously generated. Vaccine therapy is a promising subfield of antitumor immunotherapy, with recent advancements in design and development (**Table 7**). In general, vaccines have shown lasting immune response rates, up to 100% in some cases, but fail to induce clinically relevant tumor control.

Vaccines contain antigens and adjuvants to elicit activation of dendritic and antigen-specific T cells. The vaccine can be composed of peptides, RNA/DNA, or whole cells, and it is often enhanced with the use of adjuncts. Antigens that are widely used can be melanocytic differentiation antigens (ie, gp100, Melan-A/MART-1), which are expressed on normal melanocytes and therefore potentially autoimmunity inducing, mutated antigens (ie, BRAF, KIT, NRAS), or germline antigens (ie: NY-ESO-1, MAGE-A3), which are present in the placenta or testis as immune-privileged sites, while also being presented by malignant tumors.

Table 7
Summary of immunotherapy agents previously and currently understudy for the treatment of advanced melanoma

Vaccine Therapy					
Agent	Mechanism	Relevant Trial Findings	Setting	Administration	FDA Approval
gp100 Vaccine	Short peptide vaccine	NCT00019682: gp100 plus IL-2 has improved efficacy over IL-2 alone[52]	Stage IIIC or IV melanoma	Single subcutaneous injection	None
6-MHP Vaccine	Short peptide vaccine	MEL-41, MEL-44 trials: Administration of 6-MHP vaccine induces T cell response and improves overall survival[53]	Stage IV melanoma	Single subcutaneous injection	None
MAGE-A3 Vaccine	Long peptide vaccine	DERMA trial: MAGE-A3 did not demonstrate the minimum benefit needed to continue drug development.[54]	Adjuvant therapy for Stage III melanoma	Single subcutaneous injection	None
FixVac (BNT-111) Vaccine	mRNA Vaccine	Lipo-MERIT trial: FixVac alone or in combination with PD-1 inhibitors induces T-cell response and clinical response[55]	Check-point-inhibitor refractory Stage IIIB-IV melanoma	Multiple intravenous injections	None
Autologous DCV	DCV loaded with autologous tumor-associated antigens	MACVAC trial: DCV is associated with minimal toxicity and long-term survival[56]	Stage IIIC or IV melanoma	Multiple subcutaneous injections	None

Abbreviation: DCV, dendritic cell vaccine.

Peptide Vaccines

Peptide vaccines are weak when naked but can have longer effects when combined with adjuvants, as discussed below. The gp100 vaccine is a short peptide vaccine, which has been found to increase peptide-specific T cells in nearly all administered patients (97%), and it has been shown to have improved clinical activity in combination with IL-2 as compared with IL-2 alone in advanced melanoma.[52] 6-melanoma helper peptides (6-MHP) is another short peptide vaccine, which elicits helper T-cell activation in-vivo. It is effective only in HLA-DR allelic patients, and it has been found in both the MEL-41 (NCT00089219) and MEL-44 (NCT00118274) trials to induce T cell response. These two trials combined provided data to determine that OS was improved with administration of the 6-MHP vaccine.[53]

NY-ESO-1 and MAGE-A3 are long peptide vaccines that have similarly been shown to induce an immune response, but not yet a clinical response. DERMA (NCT00796445) was a phase III study evaluating MAGE-A3 as an adjuvant therapy in late-stage melanoma, and did not demonstrate the minimum benefit needed to continue drug development.[54]

RNA/DNA Vaccines

RNA/DNA vaccines can be introduced into APCs through bacterial or viral vectors to mediate effects. These have demonstrated immunogenicity, and until recently, no clinical response had yet been observed. The early results of the Lipo-MERIT trial (NCT02410733) demonstrate a high T-cell activity in addition to clinical response in patients with checkpoint-experienced melanoma who are given either the FixVac vaccine alone, or in combination with PD-1 inhibitors.[55]

DC Vaccines

These follow the same vaccine principles but include DCs for the antigen presentation component. Autologous DCs are isolated from peripheral blood and then pulsed with antigen ex-vivo and administered to the same patient. Results have been mixed, with one trial demonstrating longer survival DC + GM-CSF than tumor cell vaccine.[56] Others showed a lower T cell response.[57]

Adjuncts

Vaccine adjuncts have been introduced as means of potentiating vaccine response. Incomplete Freund's Adjuvant is an oil-based agent allowing for continued exposure. Montanide ISA 51 is one example that has been widely used. TLR-9 agonists have been included to enhance the antigen-specific activation of CD-4 cells. Finally, the combination with GM-CSF attracts and activates DCs and the ensuing immune response.

SUMMARY

Immunotherapy and targeted therapy are the current mainstays of nonsurgical treatment in advanced melanoma, and their indications and efficacy continue to broaden as combination therapies, and sequencing of these therapies are further investigated. Novel targets in either discipline are being identified; however, the greater promise relies on new mechanisms of therapy. Intratumoral therapy, adoptive cell therapy, and vaccines have produced promising early results, and some have even achieved FDA approval in the management of advanced melanoma. Cytokine therapy, meanwhile, is experiencing a resurgence as scientists are able to strengthen efficacy and mitigate adverse effects through modification of previously known molecules.

The next few years will also see the completion of large trials that might broaden the applications of current tools and establish the efficacy of new tools. Specifically, we can expect a clearer understanding of the neoadjuvant landscape, and the potential resultant shift toward neoadjuvant management, while anticipating the addition of several adjunct therapies in the adjuvant setting.

CLINICS CARE POINTS

- Surgical resection remains the mainstay of treatment for resectable advanced melanoma.
- Immunotherapy and targeted therapy have been established as effective adjuncts in the adjuvant setting.
- They have also demonstrated agency as primary treatment in cases of unresectable or metastatic melanoma.
- Checkpoint inhibition with a PD-1 inhibitor, specifically, is first-line therapy for unresectable or metastatic melanoma.
- Several trials are underway to determine the ideal combination of immunotherapy and targeted therapy, and its sequence or dosing schedule.
- Early results demonstrate that immunotherapy, targeted therapy, and certain novel

therapies are effective in the neoadjuvant setting

- Trials are underway to determine if earlier-stage melanoma will benefit from a neoadjuvant approach as well, potentially expanding the patient population that benefits from these therapies.
- Advances in intratumoral oncolytic therapy and vaccine therapy show great promise as an adjunctive treatment.
- Intratumoral oncolytic therapy may carry the benefit of a local and systemic response in the way of an abscopal effect.
- Cytokines are being revisited and modified to harness their efficacy while limiting their adverse effect profiles.
- Adoptive cell therapy, primarily in the form of tumor-infiltrating lymphocytes, may play a significant role in future treatment regimens because of its ability to induce a tumor-specific, targeted immune response.

DISCLOSURE

The authors have nothing to disclose.

REFERENCES

1. Hodi FS, O'Day SJ, McDermott DF, et al. Improved survival with ipilimumab in patients with metastatic melanoma. N Engl J Med 2010;363(8):711–23.
2. Hamid O, Robert C, Daud A, et al. Five-year survival outcomes for patients with advanced melanoma treated with pembrolizumab in KEYNOTE-001. Ann Oncol 2019;30(4):582–8.
3. Ribas A, Puzanov I, Dummer R, et al. Pembrolizumab versus investigator-choice chemotherapy for ipilimumab-refractory melanoma (KEYNOTE-002): a randomised, controlled, phase 2 trial. Lancet Oncol 2015;16(8):908–18.
4. Robert C, Ribas A, Schachter J, et al. Pembrolizumab versus ipilimumab in advanced melanoma (KEYNOTE-006): post-hoc 5-year results from an open-label, multicentre, randomised, controlled, phase 3 study. Lancet Oncol 2019;20(9):1239–51.
5. Larkin J, Chiarion-Sileni V, Gonzalez R, et al. Combined nivolumab and ipilimumab or monotherapy in untreated melanoma. N Engl J Med 2015;373(1): 23–34.
6. Eggermont AMM, Blank CU, Mandala M, et al. Adjuvant pembrolizumab versus placebo in resected stage III melanoma. N Engl J Med 2018;378(19): 1789–801.
7. Weber J, Mandala M, Del Vecchio M, et al. Adjuvant nivolumab versus ipilimumab in resected stage III or IV melanoma. N Engl J Med 2017;377(19):1824–35.
8. Eggermont AMM, Blank CU, Mandala M, et al. Longer follow-up confirms recurrence-free survival benefit of adjuvant pembrolizumab in high-risk stage III melanoma: updated results from the EORTC 1325-MG/KEYNOTE-054 trial. J Clin Oncol 2020; 38(33):3925–36.
9. Ascierto PA, Del Vecchio M, Mandalá M, et al. Adjuvant nivolumab versus ipilimumab in resected stage IIIB-C and stage IV melanoma (CheckMate 238): 4-year results from a multicentre, double-blind, randomised, controlled, phase 3 trial. Lancet Oncol 2020; 21(11):1465–77.
10. Rosa K. Adjuvant nivolumab/ipilimumab fails to significantly improve RFS in high-risk melanoma. Available at: https://www.onclive.com/view/adjuvant-nivolumab-ipilimumab-fails-to-significantly-improve-rfs-in-high-risk-melanoma. Accessed February 20, 2021
11. Yushak M, Mehnert J, Luke J, et al. Approaches to high-risk resected stage II and III melanoma. Am Soc Clin Oncol Educ Book 2019;39:e207–11.
12. Geoerger B, Kang HJ, Yalon-Oren M, et al. Pembrolizumab in paediatric patients with advanced melanoma or a PD-L1-positive, advanced, relapsed, or refractory solid tumour or lymphoma (KEYNOTE-051): interim analysis of an open-label, single-arm, phase 1-2 trial. Lancet Oncol 2020;21(1):121–33.
13. Wang Y, Zhou S, Yang F, et al. Treatment-related adverse events of PD-1 and PD-L1 inhibitors in clinical trials: a systematic review and meta-analysis. JAMA Oncol 2019;5(7):1008–19.
14. Gutzmer R, Stroyakovskiy D, Gogas H, et al. Atezolizumab, vemurafenib, and cobimetinib as first-line treatment for unresectable advanced BRAF. Lancet 2020;395(10240):1835–44.
15. Blank CU, Rozeman EA, Fanchi LF, et al. Neoadjuvant versus adjuvant ipilimumab plus nivolumab in macroscopic stage III melanoma. Nat Med 2018; 24(11):1655–61.
16. Rozeman EA, Menzies AM, van Akkooi ACJ, et al. Identification of the optimal combination dosing schedule of neoadjuvant ipilimumab plus nivolumab in macroscopic stage III melanoma (OpACIN-neo): a multicentre, phase 2, randomised, controlled trial. Lancet Oncol 2019;20(7):948–60.
17. Atkinson V, Khattak A, Haydon A, et al. Eftilagimod alpha, a soluble lymphocyte activation gene-3 (LAG-3) protein plus pembrolizumab in patients with metastatic melanoma. J Immunother Cancer 2020;8(2):e001681.
18. Long GV, Dummer R, Hamid O, et al. Epacadostat plus pembrolizumab versus placebo plus pembrolizumab in patients with unresectable or metastatic melanoma (ECHO-301/KEYNOTE-252): a phase 3, randomised, double-blind study. Lancet Oncol 2019;20(8):1083–97.

19. Arnace-Fernandez AM, O'Day SJ, de la Cruz Merino L, et al. LBA44 Lenvatinib (len) plus pembrolizumab (pembro) for advanced melanoma (MEL) that progressed on a PD-1 or PD-L1 inhibitor: initial results of LEAP-004. Presented at: European Society for Medical Oncology; 2020. Virtual, 19-21 September, 2020.

20. Wolf Y, Anderson AC, Kuchroo VK. TIM3 comes of age as an inhibitory receptor. Nat Rev Immunol 2020;20(3):173–85.

21. Bagheri H, Pourhanifeh MH, Derakhshan M, et al. CXCL-10: a new candidate for melanoma therapy? Cell Oncol (Dordr) 2020;43(3):353–65.

22. Chauvin JM, Zarour HM. TIGIT in cancer immunotherapy. J Immunother Cancer 2020;8(2):e000957.

23. Savoia P, Fava P, Casoni F, et al. Targeting the ERK signaling pathway in melanoma. Int J Mol Sci 2019; 20(6):1483.

24. Chapman PB, Hauschild A, Robert C, et al. Improved survival with vemurafenib in melanoma with BRAF V600E mutation. N Engl J Med 2011; 364(26):2507–16.

25. Hauschild A, Grob JJ, Demidov LV, et al. Dabrafenib in BRAF-mutated metastatic melanoma: a multicentre, open-label, phase 3 randomised controlled trial. Lancet 2012;380(9839):358–65.

26. Long GV, Stroyakovskiy D, Gogas H, et al. Combined BRAF and MEK inhibition versus BRAF inhibition alone in melanoma. N Engl J Med 2014;371(20): 1877–88.

27. Grob JJ, Amonkar MM, Karaszewska B, et al. Comparison of dabrafenib and trametinib combination therapy with vemurafenib monotherapy on health-related quality of life in patients with unresectable or metastatic cutaneous BRAF Val600-mutation-positive melanoma (COMBI-v): results of a phase 3, open-label, randomised trial. Lancet Oncol 2015;16(13):1389–98.

28. Amaria RN, Prieto PA, Tetzlaff MT, et al. Neoadjuvant plus adjuvant dabrafenib and trametinib versus standard of care in patients with high-risk, surgically resectable melanoma: a single-centre, open-label, randomised, phase 2 trial. Lancet Oncol 2018; 19(2):181–93.

29. Heidorn SJ, Milagre C, Whittaker S, et al. Kinase-dead BRAF and oncogenic RAS cooperate to drive tumor progression through CRAF. Cell 2010;140(2):209–21.

30. Martinez-Garcia M, Banerji U, Albanell J, et al. First-in-human, phase I dose-escalation study of the safety, pharmacokinetics, and pharmacodynamics of RO5126766, a first-in-class dual MEK/RAF inhibitor in patients with solid tumors. Clin Cancer Res 2012;18(17):4806–19.

31. Moschos SJ, Sullivan RJ, Hwu WJ, et al. Development of MK-8353, an orally administered ERK1/2 inhibitor, in patients with advanced solid tumors. JCI Insight 2018;3(4):e92352.

32. Janku F, Elana E, Tyer G, et al. Phase I dose-finding study of oral ERK1/2 inhibitor LTT462 in patients (pts) with advanced solid tumors harboring MAPK pathway alterations. J Clin Oncol 2020;38(15_suppl):3640.

33. Hoeflich KP, Merchant M, Orr C, et al. Intermittent administration of MEK inhibitor GDC-0973 plus PI3K inhibitor GDC-0941 triggers robust apoptosis and tumor growth inhibition. Cancer Res 2012; 72(1):210–9.

34. Bardia A, Gounder M, Rodon J, et al. Phase Ib study of combination therapy with MEK inhibitor binimetinib and phosphatidylinositol 3-kinase inhibitor Buparlisib in patients with advanced solid tumors with RAS/RAF alterations. Oncologist 2020;25(1): e160–9.

35. Ascierto PA, Flaherty K, Goff S. Emerging strategies in systemic therapy for the treatment of melanoma. Am Soc Clin Oncol Educ Book 2018;38:751–8.

36. Ferrucci PF, Di Giacomo AM, Del Vecchio M, et al. KEYNOTE-022 part 3: a randomized, double-blind, phase 2 study of pembrolizumab, dabrafenib, and trametinib in. J Immunother Cancer 2020;8(2): e001806.

37. Ascierto P. LBA45 - first report of efficacy and safety from the phase II study SECOMBIT (SEquential COMBo Immuno and Targeted therapy study). Presented at: European Society for Medical Oncology; 2020; Virtual. Session Proffered Paper - Melanoma and other skin tumours.

38. Rosenberg SA, Restifo NP. Adoptive cell transfer as personalized immunotherapy for human cancer. Science 2015;348(6230):62–8.

39. Andtbacka RH, Kaufman HL, Collichio F, et al. Talimogene Laherparepvec improves durable response rate in patients with advanced melanoma. J Clin Oncol 2015;33(25):2780–8.

40. Dummer R, Gyorki DE, Berger AC, et al. 3-year results of the phase 2 randomized trial for talimogene laherparepvec (T-VEC) neoadjuvant treatment plus surgery vs surgery in patients with resectable stage IIIB-IVM1a melanoma. Poster presented at: Society of Immunotherapy for Cancer (SITC) Annual Meeting; November 11-14, 2020. Poster 432.

41. Danielli R, Patuzzo R, Di Giacomo AM, et al. Intralesional administration of L19-IL2/L19-TNF in stage III or stage IVM1a melanoma patients: results of a phase II study. Cancer Immunol Immunother 2015; 64(8):999–1009.

42. Haymaker C, Andtbacka D, Johnson M, et al. 1083MO - Final results from ILLUMINATE-204, a phase I/II trial of intratumoral tilsotolimod in combination with ipilimumab in PD-1 inhibitor refractory advanced melanoma. Presented at: European society for medical oncology virtual congress; 2020; Session Mini Oral - Melanoma and other skin tumors.

43. Viralytics presents new CAVATAK ® data at the 11th international oncolytic virus conference. Oxford: Viralytics; 2018.

44. Andtbacka R, Ross M, Agarwala S, et al. Final results of a phase II multicenter trial of HF10, a replication-competent HSV-1 oncolytic virus, and ipilimumab combination treatment in patients with stage IIIB-IV unresectable or metastatic melanoma. Presented at: annual meeting of the american society of clinical oncology, ASCO; 2017; United States.

45. Yokota K, Isei T, Uhara H, et al. 1625 - final results from phase II of combination with canerpaturev (formerly HF10), an oncolytic viral immunotherapy, and ipilimumab in unresectable or metastatic melanoma in 2nd-or later line treatment. Presented at: European society for medical oncology 2019 congress; 2019; Session Poster Display session 3.

46. Thompson JF, Agarwala SS, Smithers BM, et al. Phase 2 study of intralesional PV-10 in refractory metastatic melanoma. Ann Surg Oncol 2015;22(7): 2135–42.

47. Diab A, Tykodi S, Daniels G. Progression-free survival and biomarker correlates of response with BEMPEG plus NIVO in previously untreated patients with metastatic melanoma: results from the PIVOT-02 study. Presented at: society for immunotherapy of cancer 35th anniversary annual meeting & preconference programs 2020; virtual.

48. Weide B, Eigentler T, Catania C, et al. A phase II study of the L19IL2 immunocytokine in combination with dacarbazine in advanced metastatic melanoma patients. Cancer Immunol Immunother 2019;68(9): 1547–59.

49. Glitza IC, Goff SL, Ross M, et al. And now for something completely different: immunotherapy beyond checkpoints in melanoma. Am Soc Clin Oncol Educ Book 2020;40:1–12.

50. Saranik A, Khushalani N, Chesney JA, et al. Long-term follow up of lifileucel (LN-144) cryopreserved autologous tumor infiltrating lymphocyte therapy in patients with advanced melanoma progressed on multiple prior therapies. J Clin Oncol 2020;38(15 suppl):1006.

51. Simon B, Uslu U. CAR-T cell therapy in melanoma: a future success story? Exp Dermatol 2018;27(12): 1315–21.

52. Schwartzentruber DJ, Lawson DH, Richards JM, et al. gp100 peptide vaccine and interleukin-2 in patients with advanced melanoma. N Engl J Med 2011; 364(22):2119–27.

53. Hu Y, Kim H, Blackwell CM, et al. Long-term outcomes of helper peptide vaccination for metastatic melanoma. Ann Surg 2015;262(3):456–64 [discussion 462-4].

54. Dreno B, Thompson JF, Smithers BM, et al. MAGE-A3 immunotherapeutic as adjuvant therapy for patients with resected, MAGE-A3-positive, stage III melanoma (DERMA): a double-blind, randomised, placebo-controlled, phase 3 trial. Lancet Oncol 2018;19(7):916–29.

55. Loquai C, Hassel J, Oehm P, et al. A shared tumor-antigen RNA-lipoplex vaccine with/without anti-PD1 in patients with checkpoint-inhibition experienced melanoma. J Clin Oncol 2020;38(15 suppl):3136.

56. Dillman RO, Cornforth AN, Nistor GI, et al. Randomized phase II trial of autologous dendritic cell vaccines versus autologous tumor cell vaccines in metastatic melanoma: 5-year follow up and additional analyses. J Immunother Cancer 2018;6(1):19.

57. Slingluff CL, Petroni GR, Yamshchikov GV, et al. Clinical and immunologic results of a randomized phase II trial of vaccination using four melanoma peptides either administered in granulocyte-macrophage colony-stimulating factor in adjuvant or pulsed on dendritic cells. J Clin Oncol 2003;21(21):4016–26.

58. Squibb B-M. An investigational immuno-therapy study of nivolumab combined with ipilimumab compared to nivolumab by itself after complete surgical Removal of stage IIIb/c/d or stage IV melanoma 2017. Available at: https://ClinicalTrials.gov/show/NCT03068455. Accessed March 01, 2021.

59. Sharp M, Corp D. A study of pembrolizumab (MK-3475) in pediatric participants with an advanced solid tumor or lymphoma (MK-3475-051/KEYNOTE-051). 2015. Available at: https://ClinicalTrials.gov/show/NCT02332668.

60. Kirkwood J, Squibb B-M. Nivolumab, BMS-936558 in combination with relatlimab, BMS-986016 in patients with metastatic melanoma naïve to prior immunotherapy in the metastatic setting. 2019. Available at: https://ClinicalTrials.gov/show/NCT03743766.

61. Merck Sharp & Dohme Corp, Eisai Inc. Efficacy and safety of lenvatinib (E7080/MK-7902) plus pembrolizumab (MK-3475) for advanced melanoma in anti-programmed death-1/programmed death-ligand 1 (PD-1/L1)-Exposed participants (MK-7902-004/E7080-G000-225/LEAP-004). 2019. Available at: https://ClinicalTrials.gov/show/NCT03776136.

62. Melanoma Institute Australia. Neoadjuvant dabrafenib + trametinib for AJCC stage IIIB-C BRAF V600 mutation positive melanoma 2014. Available at: https://ClinicalTrials.gov/show/NCT01972347.

63. Sunnybrook Health Sciences Centre. Study of neoadjuvant use of vemurafenib plus cobimetinib for BRAF mutant melanoma with palpable lymph node metastases 2015. Available at: https://ClinicalTrials.gov/show/NCT02036086.

64. Eli Lilly and Company. A study of LY3214996 administered alone or in combination with other agents in participants with advanced/metastatic cancer. 2016. Available at: https://ClinicalTrials.gov/show/NCT02857270.

65. Merck Sharp & Dohme Corp, Pharmaceuticals N. A study of the safety and efficacy of pembrolizumab

(MK-3475) in combination with trametinib and dabrafenib in participants with advanced melanoma (MK-3475-022/KEYNOTE-022). 2014. Available at: https://ClinicalTrials.gov/show/NCT02130466.

66. Hoffmann-La Roche. A study of atezolizumab plus cobimetinib and vemurafenib versus placebo plus cobimetinib and vemurafenib in previously untreated BRAFv600 mutation-positive patients with metastatic or unresectable locally advanced melanoma 2017. Available at: https://ClinicalTrials.gov/show/NCT02908672.

67. Mayo Clinic, National Cancer Institute (NCI), Genentech, Inc. Neoadjuvant combination targeted and immunotherapy for patients with high-risk stage III melanoma 2018. Available at: https://ClinicalTrials.gov/show/NCT03554083.

68. Melanoma Institute Australia, Merck Sharp & Dohme Corp, Novartis. Neoadjuvant dabrafenib, trametinib and/or pembrolizumab in BRAF mutant resectable stage III melanoma. 2017. Available at: https://ClinicalTrials.gov/show/NCT02858921.

69. National Cancer Institute (NCI). Dabrafenib and trametinib followed by ipilimumab and nivolumab or ipilimumab and nivolumab followed by dabrafenib and trametinib in treating patients with stage III-IV BRAFV600 melanoma 2015. Available at: https://ClinicalTrials.gov/show/NCT02224781.

70. Fondazione Melanoma Onlus, Clinical Research Technology S.r.l.. Sequential combo immuno and target therapy (SECOMBIT) study 2016. Available at: https://ClinicalTrials.gov/show/NCT02631447.

71. European Organisation for Research and Treatment of Cancer - EORTC. Immunotherapy with ipilimumab and nivolumab preceded or not by a targeted therapy with encorafenib and binimetinib 2018. Available at: https://ClinicalTrials.gov/show/NCT03235245.

72. University Hospital Essen. Evaluating the efficacy and safety of a sequencing schedule of cobimetinib plus vemurafenib followed by immunotherapy with an anti- PD-L1 antibody in patients with unresectable or metastatic BRAF V600 mutant melanoma. 2016. Available at: https://ClinicalTrials.gov/show/NCT02902029.

73. Amgen. Efficacy and safety of talimogene laherparepvec neoadjuvant treatment plus surgery versus surgery alone for melanoma 2015. Available at: https://ClinicalTrials.gov/show/NCT02211131.

74. University of California D, Amgen. Neoadjuvant T-VEC in High risk early melanoma. 2020. Available at: https://ClinicalTrials.gov/show/NCT04427306.

75. Amgen, Sharp M, Corp D. Pembrolizumab with or without talimogene Laherparepvec or talimogene Laherparepvec placebo in unresected melanoma (KEYNOTE-034). 2014. Available at: https://ClinicalTrials.gov/show/NCT02263508.

76. Philogen S.p.A. Efficacy of daromun neoadjuvant intratumoral treatment in clinical stage IIIB/C melanoma patients 2018. Available at: https://ClinicalTrials.gov/show/NCT03567889.

77. Idera Pharmaceuticals Inc, Bristol-Myers Squibb. A study of IMO-2125 in combination with ipilimumab versus ipilimumab alone in subjects with anti-PD-1 refractory melanoma (ILLUMINATE-301). 2018. Available at: https://ClinicalTrials.gov/show/NCT03445533.

78. Provectus Biopharmaceuticals Inc, Provectus Pharmaceuticals. PV-10 in combination with pembrolizumab for treatment of metastatic melanoma 2015. Available at: https://ClinicalTrials.gov/show/NCT02557321.

79. Nektar Therapeutics, Bristol-Myers Squibb. A dose escalation and cohort expansion study of NKTR-214 in combination with nivolumab and other anti-cancer therapies in patients with select advanced solid tumors (PIVOT-02) 2016. Available at: https://ClinicalTrials.gov/show/NCT02983045.

80. Bristol-Myers Squibb, Nektar Therapeutics. A study of NKTR-214 combined with nivolumab vs nivolumab alone in participants with previously untreated inoperable or metastatic melanoma 2018. Available at: https://ClinicalTrials.gov/show/NCT03635983.

81. Iovance Biotherapeutics, Inc. Study of Lifileucel (LN-144), autologous tumor infiltrating lymphocytes, in The treatment of patients with metastatic melanoma 2015. Available at: https://ClinicalTrials.gov/show/NCT02360579.

82. BioNTech RNA Pharmaceuticals Gmb, BioNTech SE (BioNTech RNA Pharmaceuticals GmbH). Evaluation of the safety and tolerability of i.v. Administration of a cancer vaccine in patients with advanced melanoma 2015. Available at: https://ClinicalTrials.gov/show/NCT02410733.

83. Dummer R, Ascierto PA, Gogas HJ, et al. Encorafenib plus binimetinib versus vemurafenib or encorafenib in patients with BRAF-mutant melanoma (COLUMBUS): a multicentre, open-label, randomised phase 3 trial. Lancet Oncol 2018;19(5):603–15.

UNITED STATES POSTAL SERVICE®
Statement of Ownership, Management, and Circulation
(All Periodicals Publications Except Requester Publications)

1. Publication Title: CLINICS IN PLASTIC SURGERY

2. Publication Number: 006 – 530

3. Filing Date: 9/18/2021

4. Issue Frequency: JAN, APR, JUL, OCT

5. Number of Issues Published Annually: 4

6. Annual Subscription Price: $543.00

7. Complete Mailing Address of Known Office of Publication (Not printer) (Street, city, county, state, and ZIP+4®)
ELSEVIER INC.
230 Park Avenue, Suite 800
New York, NY 10169

Contact Person: Malathi Samayan
Telephone (Include area code): 91-44-4299-4507

8. Complete Mailing Address of Headquarters or General Business Office of Publisher (Not printer)
ELSEVIER INC.
230 Park Avenue, Suite 800
New York, NY 10169

9. Full Names and Complete Mailing Addresses of Publisher, Editor, and Managing Editor (Do not leave blank)

Publisher (Name and complete mailing address)
Dolores Meloni, ELSEVIER INC.
1600 JOHN F KENNEDY BLVD. SUITE 1800
PHILADELPHIA, PA 19103-2899

Editor (Name and complete mailing address)
STACY EASTMAN, ELSEVIER INC.
1600 JOHN F KENNEDY BLVD. SUITE 1800
PHILADELPHIA, PA 19103-2899

Managing Editor (Name and complete mailing address)
PATRICK MANLEY, ELSEVIER INC.
1600 JOHN F KENNEDY BLVD. SUITE 1800
PHILADELPHIA, PA 19103-2899

10. Owner (Do not leave blank. If the publication is owned by a corporation, give the name and address of the corporation immediately followed by the names and addresses of all stockholders owning or holding 1 percent or more of the total amount of stock. If not owned by a corporation, give the names and addresses of the individual owners. If owned by a partnership or other unincorporated firm, give its name and address as well as those of each individual owner. If the publication is published by a nonprofit organization, give its name and address.)

Full Name	Complete Mailing Address
WHOLLY OWNED SUBSIDIARY OF REED/ELSEVIER, US HOLDINGS	1600 JOHN F KENNEDY BLVD. SUITE 1800 PHILADELPHIA, PA 19103-2899

11. Known Bondholders, Mortgagees, and Other Security Holders Owning or Holding 1 Percent or More of Total Amount of Bonds, Mortgages, or Other Securities. If none, check box ☑ None

Full Name	Complete Mailing Address
N/A	

12. Tax Status (For completion by nonprofit organizations authorized to mail at nonprofit rates) (Check one)
The purpose, function, and nonprofit status of this organization and the exempt status for federal income tax purposes:
☑ Has Not Changed During Preceding 12 Months
☐ Has Changed During Preceding 12 Months (Publisher must submit explanation of change with this statement)

13. Publication Title: CLINICS IN PLASTIC SURGERY

14. Issue Date for Circulation Data Below: JULY 2021

15. Extent and Nature of Circulation

		Average No. Copies Each Issue During Preceding 12 Months	No. Copies of Single Issue Published Nearest to Filing Date
a. Total Number of Copies (Net press run)		268	235
b. Paid Circulation (By Mail and Outside the Mail)	(1) Mailed Outside-County Paid Subscriptions Stated on PS Form 3541 (Include paid distribution above nominal rate, advertiser's proof copies, and exchange copies)	131	116
	(2) Mailed In-County Paid Subscriptions Stated on PS Form 3541 (Include paid distribution above nominal rate, advertiser's proof copies, and exchange copies)	0	0
	(3) Paid Distribution Outside the Mails Including Sales Through Dealers and Carriers, Street Vendors, Counter Sales, and Other Paid Distribution Outside USPS®	83	73
	(4) Paid Distribution by Other Classes of Mail Through the USPS (e.g. First-Class Mail®)	0	0
c. Total Paid Distribution (Sum of 15b (1), (2), (3), and (4))		214	189
d. Free or Nominal Rate Distribution (By Mail and Outside the Mail)	(1) Free or Nominal Rate Outside-County Copies included on PS Form 3541	33	25
	(2) Free or Nominal Rate In-County Copies Included on PS Form 3541	0	0
	(3) Free or Nominal Rate Copies Mailed at Other Classes Through the USPS (e.g. First-Class Mail)	0	0
	(4) Free or Nominal Rate Distribution Outside the Mail (Carriers or other means)	0	0
e. Total Free or Nominal Rate Distribution (Sum of 15d (1), (2), (3) and (4))		33	25
f. Total Distribution (Sum of 15c and 15e)		247	214
g. Copies not Distributed (See Instructions to Publishers #4 (page #3))		21	21
h. Total (Sum of 15f and g)		268	235
i. Percent Paid (15c divided by 15f times 100)		86.63%	88.31%

* If you are claiming electronic copies, go to line 16 on page 3. If you are not claiming electronic copies, skip to line 17 on page 3.

16. Electronic Copy Circulation

	Average No. Copies Each Issue During Preceding 12 Months	No. Copies of Single Issue Published Nearest to Filing Date
a. Paid Electronic Copies	►	
b. Total Paid Print Copies (Line 15c) + Paid Electronic Copies (Line 16a)	►	
c. Total Print Distribution (Line 15f) + Paid Electronic Copies (Line 16a)	►	
d. Percent Paid (Both Print & Electronic Copies) (16b divided by 16c × 100)	►	

☒ I certify that 50% of all my distributed copies (electronic and print) are paid above a nominal price.

17. Publication of Statement of Ownership
☒ If the publication is a general publication, publication of this statement is required. Will be printed in the OCTOBER 2021 issue of this publication.
☐ Publication not required.

18. Signature and Title of Editor, Publisher, Business Manager, or Owner
Malathi Samayan
Malathi Samayan - Distribution Controller

Date: 9/18/2021

I certify that all information furnished on this form is true and complete. I understand that anyone who furnishes false or misleading information on this form or who omits material or information requested on the form may be subject to criminal sanctions (including fines and imprisonment) and/or civil sanctions (including civil penalties).

PS Form **3526**, July 2014 [Page 1 of 4 (see instructions page 4)] PSN: 7530-01-000-9931 PRIVACY NOTICE: See our privacy policy on www.usps.com.

PS Form **3526**, July 2014 (Page 3 of 4)

PRIVACY NOTICE: See our privacy policy on www.usps.com

Printed and bound by CPI Group (UK) Ltd, Croydon, CR0 4YY

08/05/2025

01864700-0020